Respiratory Medicine

Series Editors

Sharon I. S. Rounds
Alpert Medical School of Brown University
Providence, RI, USA

Anne Dixon
University of Vermont, College of Medicine
Burlington, VT, USA

Lynn M. Schnapp
Medical University of South Carolina
Charleston, SC, USA

More information about this series at http://www.springer.com/series/7665

David A. Kaminsky • Charles G. Irvin
Editors

Pulmonary Function Testing

Principles and Practice

Humana Press

ATS
We help the world breathe®
PULMONARY • CRITICAL CARE • SLEEP

Editors
David A. Kaminsky
University of Vermont
Burlington, VT
USA

Charles G. Irvin
University of Vermont
Burlington, VT
USA

ISSN 2197-7372 ISSN 2197-7380 (electronic)
Respiratory Medicine
ISBN 978-3-030-06806-6 ISBN 978-3-319-94159-2 (eBook)
https://doi.org/10.1007/978-3-319-94159-2

This Humana press imprint is published by the registered company Springer Nature Switzerland AG
The registered company address is: Gewerbestrasse 11, 6330 Cham, Switzerland

Preface

Welcome to *Pulmonary Function Testing: Principles and Practice*. You might ask why do we need another book on pulmonary function tests (PFTs)? We have been involved in teaching PFTs to students, residents, and fellows for many years and have realized that there appear to be two main types of educational resources available. On the one hand, there are many classic books about pulmonary physiology, such as West's *Respiratory Physiology: The Essentials* and the American Physiological Society's *Handbook of Physiology*. And there are also many excellent references about how to perform and interpret pulmonary function tests, such as Ruppel's *Manual of Pulmonary Function Testing* and Wanger's *Pulmonary Function Testing: A Practical Approach*. What we felt was needed was a resource that combined the best of both worlds, including not only details about how each PFT is performed and interpreted but also the physiological basis of each test. In addition, this level of content would best be geared toward the postgraduate trainee or fellow in pulmonary medicine and should include a section on the practical "how to" run a PFT lab. This book is the result of our vision and goals. We have purposely included authors that are both pulmonary physicians and scientists, each with expertise in their field. We hope you find *Pulmonary Function Testing: Principles and Practice* ideally suited to your education and training in pulmonary physiology and how to perform and interpret PFTs.

Burlington, VT, USA

David A. Kaminsky
Charles G. Irvin

Acknowledgment

We dedicate this book to the memory of Reuben Cherniack, MD. Reuben was not only a world-class pulmonary physiologist but also a friend and mentor to both of us when we worked with him at National Jewish Health and the University of Colorado Health Sciences Center in Denver. Reuben inspired in us a love for pulmonary physiology and a desire to apply that knowledge for the benefit of patients with the most severe of lung disease. He continually challenged us to understand, teach, and perform PFTs at the highest level of excellence.

David A. Kaminsky
Charles G. Irvin

Contents

Contributors

Tony G. Babb, PhD Division of Pulmonary and Critical Care Medicine, Department of Internal Medicine, University of Texas Southwestern Medical Center and Institute for Exercise and Environmental Medicine, Texas Health Presbyterian Hospital, Dallas, TX, USA

Jason H. T. Bates, PhD University of Vermont Larner College of Medicine, Burlington, VT, USA

Susan Blonshine, RRT, RPFT, AE-C, FAARC TechEd Consultants, Inc., Mason, MI, USA

Louis-Philippe Boulet, MD, FRCPC Institut universitaire de cardiologie et de pneumologie de Québec, Québec, Canada

John D. Brannan, PhD Department of Respiratory and Sleep Medicine, John Hunter Hospital, Newcastle, NSW, Australia

Robert H. Brown, MD, MPH Departments of Anesthesiology, Medicine, Division of Pulmonary and Critical Care Medicine, Environmental Health and Engineering and Radiology, Johns Hopkins Medical Institutions, Baltimore, MD, USA

Brendan G. Cooper, BSc, MSc, PhD Lung Function and Sleep Department, Queen Elizabeth Hospital Birmingham, Birmingham, UK

Bruce H. Culver, MD Pulmonary, Critical Care and Sleep Medicine, University of Washington School of Medicine, Seattle, WA, USA

Matthew J. Fogarty, PhD Department of Physiology and Biomedical Engineering, Mayo Clinic, Rochester, MN, USA

School of Biomedical Sciences, The University of Queensland, Brisbane, Australia

Krystelle Godbout, MD, FRCPC Institut universitaire de cardiologie et de pneumologie de Québec, Québec, Canada

Brian L. Graham, PhD Division of Respirology, Critical Care and Sleep Medicine, University of Saskatchewan, Saskatoon, SK, Canada

Graham L. Hall, BASc, PhD, CRFS Children's Lung Health, Telethon Kids Institute, Subiaco, WA, Australia

School of Physiotherapy and Exercise Science, Faculty of Health Science, Curtin University, Bentley, Perth, WA, Australia

Teal S. Hallstrand, MD, MPH Department of Medicine, Division of Pulmonary, Critical Care and Sleep Medicine, University of Washington, Seattle, WA, USA

Center for Lung Biology, University of Washington, Seattle, WA, USA

Theresa Harvey-Dunstan, BSc (Physiotherapy), MSc Centre for Exercise and Rehabilitation Science, NIHR Leicester Biomedical Research Centre – Respiratory, Glenfield Hospital, Leicester, UK

Faculty of the College of Medicine, Biological Sciences and Psychology, University of Leicester, Leicester, UK

Jeffrey Haynes, RRT, RPFT, FAARC Pulmonary Function Laboratory, St. Joseph Hospital, Nashua, NH, USA

Anne E. Holland, BAppSc(Physiotherapy), PhD Alfred Health, Melbourne, VIC, Australia

Department of Rehabilitation, Nutrition and Sport, La Trobe University, Bundoora, VIC, Australia

Institute for Breathing and Sleep, Austin Health, Heidelberg, VIC, Australia

Yuh Chin Huang, MD Division of Pulmonary and Critical Care Medicine, Department of Medicine, Duke University, Durham, NC, USA

Katrina Hynes, MHA, RRT, RPFT Pulmonary Function Laboratory, Mayo Clinic, Rochester, MN, USA

Charles G. Irvin, PhD Department of Medicine, Vermont Lung Center, University of Vermont Larner College of Medicine, Burlington, VT, USA

David A. Kaminsky, MD Pulmonary Disease and Critical Care Medicine, University of Vermont Larner College of Medicine, Burlington, VT, USA

Gregory King, MD Woolcock Institute of Medical Research, The University of Sydney, Sydney, NSW, Australia

Annemarie L. Lee, BPhysio, MPhysio, PhD Rehabilitation, Nutrition and Sport, La Trobe University, Bundoora, VIC, Australia

Institute for Breathing and Sleep, Austin Health, Heidelberg, VIC, Australia

Faculty of Medicine, Nursing and Health Sciences, Monash University, Frankston, VIC, Australia

Neil MacIntyre, MD Division of Pulmonary and Critical Care Medicine, Department of Medicine, Duke University, Durham, NC, USA

Meredith C. McCormack, MD, MHS Pulmonary Function Laboratory, Pulmonary and Critical Care Medicine, Johns Hopkins University, Baltimore, MD, USA

Wayne Mitzner, PhD Environmental Health and Engineering, Johns Hopkins Bloomberg School of Public Health, Baltimore, MD, USA

J. Alberto Neder, MD, PhD Respiratory Investigation Unit and Laboratory of Clinical Exercise Physiology, Division of Respirology and Sleep Medicine, Department of Medicine, Queen's University and Kingston General Hospital, Kingston, ON, Canada

Denis E. O'Donnell, MD, FRCPI, FRCPC, FERS Respiratory Investigation Unit and Laboratory of Clinical Exercise Physiology, Division of Respirology and Sleep Medicine, Department of Medicine, Queen's University and Kingston General Hospital, Kingston, ON, Canada

Jeremy Richards, MD, MA Division of Pulmonary, Critical Care, and Sleep Medicine, Beth Israel Deaconess Medical Center, Harvard Medical School, Boston, MA, USA

Richard M. Schwartzstein, MD Division of Pulmonary, Critical Care, and Sleep Medicine, Beth Israel Deaconess Medical Center, Harvard Medical School, Boston, MA, USA

Gary C. Sieck, PhD Department of Physiology and Biomedical Engineering, Mayo Clinic, Rochester, MN, USA

Sally Singh, BSc, PhD Centre for Exercise and Rehabilitation Science, NIHR Leicester Biomedical Research Centre – Respiratory, Glenfield Hospital, Leicester, UK

Faculty of the College of Medicine, Biological Sciences and Psychology, University of Leicester, Leicester, UK

Sanja Stanojevic, MSc, PhD Translational Medicine, The Hospital for Sick Children, Toronto, ON, Canada

James A. Stockley, BSc, PhD Lung Function and Sleep Department, Queen Elizabeth Hospital Birmingham, Birmingham, UK

Jeff Thiboutot, MD Department of Medicine, Division of Pulmonary and Critical Care Medicine, Johns Hopkins Medical Institutions, Baltimore, MD, USA

Bruce R. Thompson, MD, MPH Head Physiology Service, Department of Respiratory Medicine, Central Clinical School, The Alfred Hospital and Monash University, Melbourne, VIC, Australia

Andrew R. Tomlinson, MD Division of Pulmonary and Critical Care Medicine, Department of Internal Medicine, University of Texas Southwestern Medical Center and Institute for Exercise and Environmental Medicine, Texas Health Presbyterian Hospital, Dallas, TX, USA

Sylvia Verbanck, PhD Respiratory Division, University Hospital, UZ Brussel, Brussels, Belgium

Jack Wanger, MSc, RPFT, RRT, FAARC Pulmonary Function Testing and Clinical Trials Consultant, Rochester, MN, USA

Daniel J. Weiner, MD, FCCP, ATSF University of Pittsburgh School of Medicine, Pulmonary Function Laboratory, Antonio J. and Janet Palumbo Cystic Fibrosis Center, Children's Hospital of Pittsburgh of UPMC, Pittsburgh, PA, USA

Tianshi David Wu, MD Division of Pulmonary and Critical Care Medicine, Johns Hopkins University School of Medicine, Baltimore, MD, USA

Chapter 1
Introduction to the Structure and Function of the Lung

Jeff Thiboutot, Bruce R. Thompson, and Robert H. Brown

1.1 Pulmonary Structure

The primary function of the lungs is gas exchange. Knowledge of the anatomy and airflow pathways is important to understand how gas moves to the blood from the atmosphere. Human airway anatomy starts at the oro- and nasopharynx and terminates at the alveoli. The airways along this path can be divided into two zones: (1) conducting zone, consisting of large and medium airways that are responsible for mass transport of air from the atmosphere to the alveoli without gas exchange occurring, and (2) respiratory zone, consisting of small airways with alveolar sacs in their walls (airways <2 mm) and alveoli that participate in gas exchange with the blood.

J. Thiboutot
Department of Medicine, Division of Pulmonary and Critical Care Medicine,
Johns Hopkins Medical Institutions, Baltimore, MD, USA
e-mail: jthibou1@jhmi.edu

B. R. Thompson
Head Physiology Service, Department of Respiratory Medicine, Central Clinical School,
The Alfred Hospital and Monash University, Melbourne, VIC, Australia
e-mail: B.Thompson@alfred.org.au

R. H. Brown (✉)
Departments of Anesthesiology, Medicine, Division of Pulmonary and Critical Care
Medicine, Environmental Health and Engineering and Radiology, Johns Hopkins Medical
Institutions, Baltimore, MD, USA
e-mail: rbrown@jhmi.edu

D. A. Kaminsky, C. G. Irvin (eds.), *Pulmonary Function Testing*,
Respiratory Medicine, https://doi.org/10.1007/978-3-319-94159-2_1

1.1.1 Conducting Zone

Air moves through the mouth and nares to the oro- and nasopharynx. The oro- and nasopharynx combine to form the hypopharynx which houses the epiglottis, larynx, and upper esophageal sphincter. The larynx is a complex structure that contains the vocal cords and forms a passage for movement of air from the hypopharynx to the trachea. The trachea is a flexible single tubular airway passage which is kept patent by a series of c-shaped collagenous rings. Between the rings are smooth muscle and fibroelastic tissue. The posterior wall of the trachea contains no cartilaginous support and is comprised of a longitudinally oriented membrane that contains smooth muscle (Fig. 1.1). The trachea is 10–12 cm in length and is divided into an upper extrathoracic portion and a lower intrathoracic portion, separated at the level of superior aspect of the manubrium. At the angle of Louis (manubriosternal junction), the trachea divides into the left and right main stem (primary) bronchi at the main carina. The main stem bronchi then rapidly branch into shorter, smaller (secondary) lobar bronchi, then (tertiary) segmental bronchi, and then subsegemental bronchi until terminating into bronchioles. Like the trachea, bronchi are flexible and contain less collagenous support than the trachea, and the folded mucosa is encircled by a layer of smooth muscle (Fig. 1.2). Tertiary bronchi give rise to the terminal component of the conducting system, bronchioles, which are generally less than 1 mm in diameter. Bronchioles do not contain collagenous support but contain folded mucosa with a ring of smooth muscle (Fig. 1.3). The most distal bronchioles are named terminal bronchioles and also contain a thin layer of smooth muscle (Fig. 1.4). Since no gas exchange occurs in the conducting zone, this entire region is considered anatomical dead space (see Chap. 5), the total volume of which is ~150 mL.

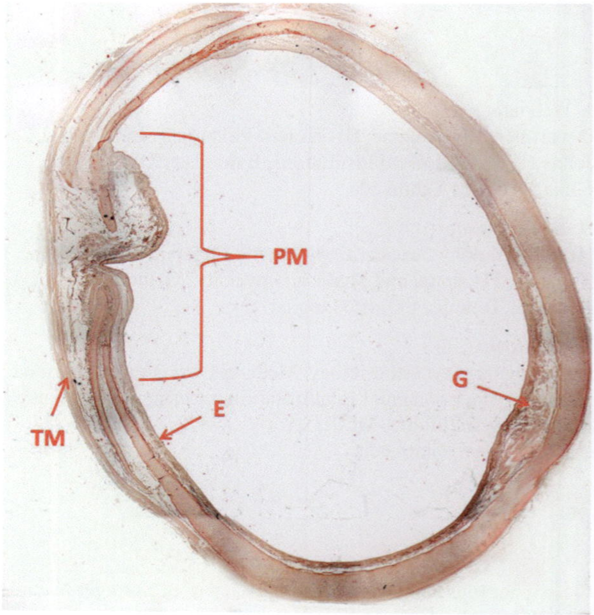

Fig. 1.1 Trachea histology. PM posterior membrane, TM trachealis muscle, G glands, E epithelium

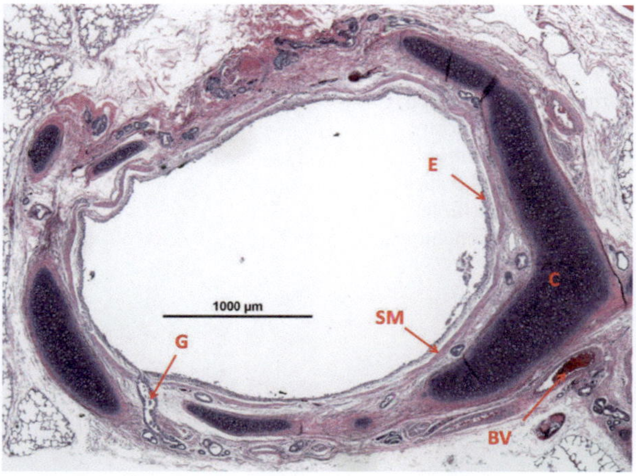

Fig. 1.2 Bronchus histology. Cross section of bronchus depicting microstructure of the airway wall. SM smooth muscle, C cartilage, G gland, BV blood vessel (bronchial circulation), E epithelium

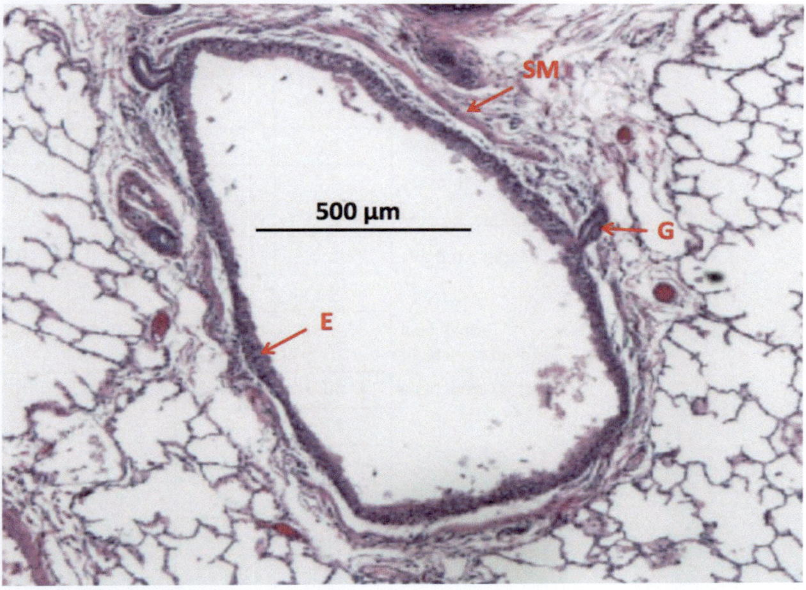

Fig. 1.3 Bronchiole histology. SM smooth muscle, G gland, E epithelium

1.1.2 Respiratory Zone

The respiratory zone begins as terminal bronchioles and subsequently divides into respiratory bronchioles forming anatomical units called acini. While respiratory bronchioles are still conducting airways, they contain alveolar sacs that can participate in gas exchange. The respiratory bronchioles divide into alveolar ducts that are completely lined with alveolar sacs. The alveolar ducts terminate with thin walled

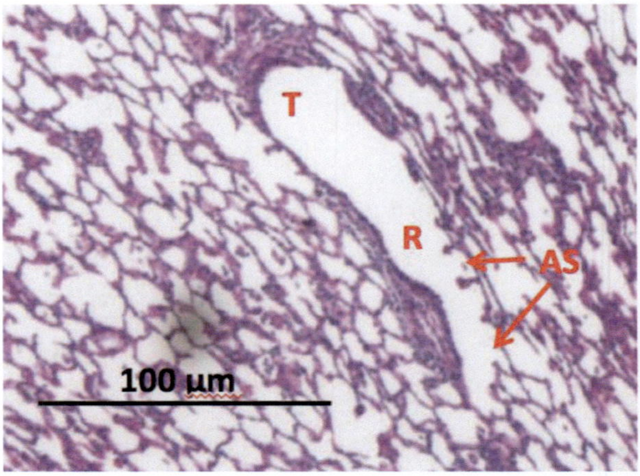

Fig. 1.4 Terminal bronchiole and respiratory bronchiole histology. Terminal bronchiole on end branching to form respiratory bronchiole lined with alveolar sacs. T terminal bronchiole, R respiratory bronchiole, AS alveolar sacs

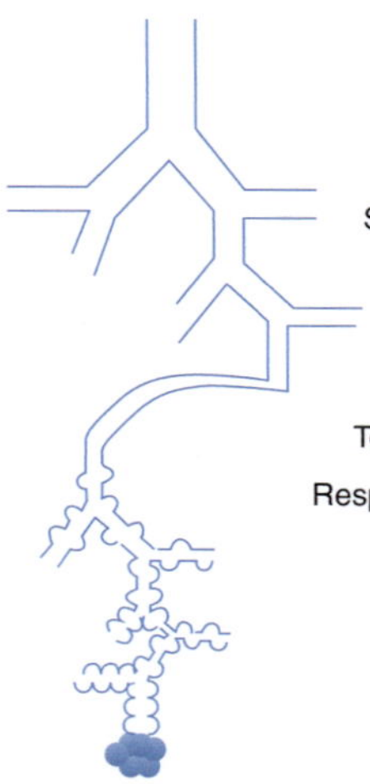

	Generation	Number of airways	Diameter, cm	Total Cross-sectional Area, cm^2
Trachea	0	1	2.0	2.5
Main bronchi	1	2	1.3	2.3
Secondary bronchi	2	4	0.8	2.1
Tertiary bronchi	3	8	0.5	2.0
	4	16	0.4	2.5
Bronchioles Terminal bronchiole	5–15	$32–3\times10^4$	0.3–0.06	3.1–180
Respiratory bronchiole	16	$6x10^4$	0.05	10^4
	17	10^5		
	18	3×10^5		
Alveolar ducts	19	10^5	0.04	10^5
Alveolar sacs	20	10^6		
	21	2×10^6		

Fig. 1.5 Bronchial tree, size, and number of airways

alveolar sacs and are the primary location for gas exchange. Due to this rapid branching, the cross-sectional area for gas exchange exponentially increases with each division. It is estimated that the total cross-sectional area of the lungs is approximately 50–75 m^2 (Fig. 1.5). The volume of the respiratory zone is the majority of a subject's total lung capacity. Figure 1.6 depicts the rapidly branching nature of the airway tree.

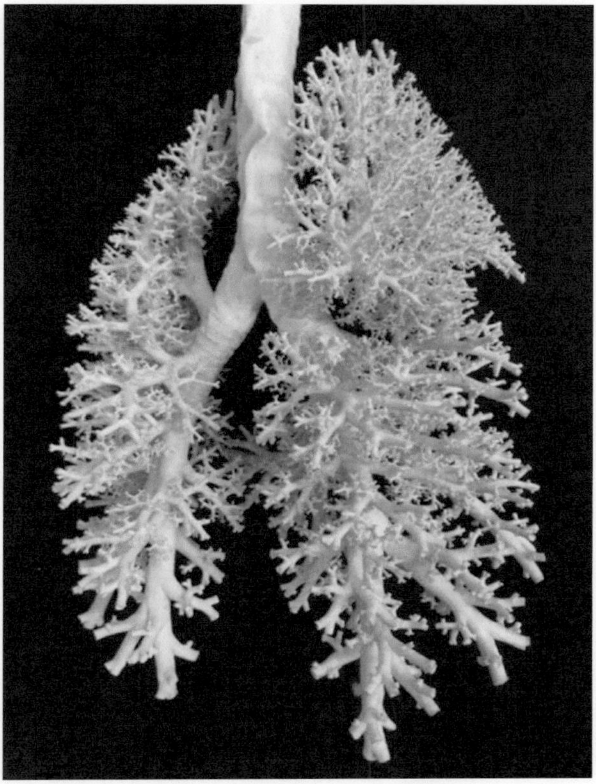

Fig. 1.6 Silicone cast of the airway tree

1.1.3 Pulmonary Vasculature

With the primary function of the lungs being gas exchange, the lungs are dependent on adequate perfusion. The right heart pumps deoxygenated blood from the systemic circulation through the pulmonary circulation via the pulmonary artery. The main pulmonary artery bifurcates to a left and right side each supplying the ipsilateral lung. The pulmonary arteries then sequentially divide, following alongside the airway tree. Like the respiratory tree, the pulmonary arteries rapidly divide until forming a series of capillaries, about the diameter of a single red blood cell, that form networks around the alveoli, providing interfaces for gas exchange. Oxygenated blood is returned to the left heart via pulmonary veins and then out to the systemic circulation. As the entire cardiac output is circulated through the lungs, one of the unique features of the pulmonary circulation is its low resistance to flow, being about one tenth the resistance of the systemic circulation. This gives the lungs the ability to handle a large cardiac output at relatively low pulmonary pressures.

Because of the anatomic arrangement of the pulmonary vasculature along the airways, and the influence of gravity on blood flow and pulmonary compliance, the lung is uniquely situated to bring more blood flow to dependent regions that are better ventilated and less blood flow to nondependent regions that are less well ventilated. This matching of ventilation and perfusion is a key physiologic aspect of how the lung optimizes the efficiency of gas exchange.

The lungs have a dual blood supply, primarily from the pulmonary circulation but supported by bronchial arteries. The bronchial arteries arise from the aorta and intercostal arteries providing oxygenated blood to the airways and lung supporting tissues and ending at the level of the terminal bronchioles. As the bronchial arteries arise from peripheral arterial circulation, they deliver oxygenated blood to the lung tissues. They also supply blood to the lower third of the esophagus, the vagus nerve, the visceral pleura, the pericardium, the hilar lymph nodes and the vasa vasorum of the thoracic aorta and pulmonary arteries and veins. Venous drainage from the lower trachea and lobar bronchi is via the bronchial veins to the right atrium. However, venous drainage from the more distal lung is via anastomoses between the bronchial veins and pulmonary veins to the left atrium is to the right atrium via the azygous system from the airways down to the lower trachea and lobar bronchi.

1.1.4 Muscles of Respiration

During inhalation, negative pressure at the pleura draws air in through the oro- and nasopharynx to the respiratory zone for gas exchange. The negative pleural pressure is primarily generated by contraction and flattening of the diaphragm. Inhalation can also be aided by accessory muscles, largely being the external intercostals, sternocleidomastoid, and scalenes which stabilize, lift, and expand the rib cage.

Expiration is a passive process during quiet breathing, moving air out of the thorax by relaxation and elastic recoil of the lungs and diaphragm. However, during active breathing, exhalation can be supported by contraction of the internal intercostals (pulling the ribs down) and abdominal muscles (contracting the abdominal compartment to elevate the diaphragm).

1.2 How Lung Function Is Based on Structure

1.2.1 Conditioning and Host Defense

Before gas can be exchanged with the blood, air from the atmosphere must be conditioned for hospitable delivery to the sensitive alveoli. The epithelium of the conducting airways plays a critical role in preconditioning air for exchange. The relatively dry air of the atmosphere must be humidified before delivery to the alveoli. The respiratory epithelium of the trachea and bronchi contain goblet cells that produce epithelial lining fluid, containing mucus and watery secretions that act to warm and humidify the air. Large air pollutants are filtered at the nares. The epithelial lining fluid of the trachea and bronchi acts to trap particles, and the trachea's ciliated epithelium transports it up toward the pharynx, where it is then swallowed or expectorated. This is a key defense mechanism to protect the lung from pollutants and infection.

1.2.2 Gas Delivery to the Alveoli

During quiet breathing, about 500 mL of air is inhaled. However, because of the anatomical dead space of about 150 ml in the conducting zone, not all of this volume is delivered to the alveoli. For this reason, it is important to understand the different static lung volumes (see Chap. 3). With normal quiet breathing, the volume of each breath is termed tidal volume. The vital capacity (VC) is the amount of air moved after maximal inhalation and exhalation. Functional residual capacity (FRC) is the amount of air left in the lungs after quiet exhalation. However, because complete collapse of the alveoli and conducting zone does not occur even after maximal expiration, there is a residual volume (RV) that still remains in the lungs (Fig. 1.7). Residual volume (and FRC) cannot be assessed by simply measuring airflow at the mouth (i.e., spirometry); therefore more advanced pulmonary function testing techniques are needed to derive these volumes (see Lung Volume Measurement). Total lung capacity (TLC) is a total volume of air in the lungs, the sum of vital capacity and residual volume.

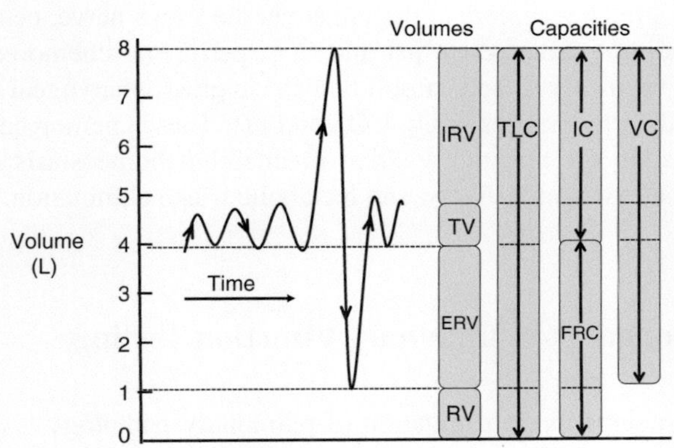

Fig. 1.7 Lung volumes and capacities. A spirogram (volume vs. time) of an individual who is first breathing quietly (reading from left to right), then takes a maximal inhalation to total lung capacity (TLC), then exhales slowly to residual volume (RV), and then returns to quiet breathing. On the right are the four lung volumes: inspiratory reserve volume (IRV), tidal volume (TV), expiratory reserve volume (ERV), and RV. Lung capacities are the combination of lung volumes and are as follows: TLC shown here as RV + ERV + TV + IRV, inspiratory capacity (IC) shown here as TV + IRV, functional residual capacity (FRC) shown here as ERV + RV, and vital capacity shown here as IRV + TV + ERV

1.2.3 Gas Exchange at the Alveoli

The alveolar/capillary interface is the site of gas exchange. The alveolar epithelium contains two cell types: (1) type 1 pneumocytes (95% of alveolar area) (these are very thin flat cells through which gas exchange occurs) and (2) type 2 pneumocytes (5% of alveolar area) (these secrete surfactant to maintain alveolar stability and contribute to host defense in the lung). The type 1 pneumocytes are in extremely close proximity to the vascular endothelium of the capillary (~0.25 μm) through which gases can easily cross. The rapid branching of the respiratory tree leads to an exponential increase in the total cross-sectional surface area for exchange to occur. This in turn decreases the velocity of air moving across the alveoli and permits sufficient time for gas exchange within the capillary bed. Equilibrium between the alveolar gas and blood in the capillary happens extremely quickly, so efficient that each red blood cell fully takes up oxygen in only about 0.25 s of the approximately 0.75 s it spends in the capillary bed.

1.2.4 Drivers of Respiration

The control center for respiration is located in the respiratory center in the medulla in the brainstem (See Chap. 9). Neurons in the medulla contain pacemaker cells that are self-excitatory and stimulate the diaphragm and external intercostals via the phrenic nerve. Higher cortical centers aid in the control of respiration to permit airflow through the vocal cords to allow speech. Respiratory drive is modulated by feedback from stretch receptors in the lungs via the vagus nerve, central chemoreceptors responding to changes in pH and CO_2, peripheral chemoreceptors in the aortic arch via vagus nerve, and carotid bodies via glossopharyngeal nerve, the latter two responding to changes in O_2, CO_2, and pH. These chemoreceptors are ultimately responsible for respiratory drive maintaining homeostasis of the blood, ensuring adequate oxygen delivery, and metabolic waste elimination.

1.3 Components of Pulmonary Function Testing

One of the first steps in the evaluation of pulmonary pathology is assessment of pulmonary function. While static imaging can give us clues to structural morphology, they offer little information of the dynamic function of the lungs. Pulmonary function testing (PFT) is a series of tests, most often performed in a PFT lab, which evaluates the global function of the lungs. There are three primary goals of pulmonary function testing: (1) assessment of airflow obstruction, (2) measurement of lung volumes, and (3) assessment of diffusion of gases across the alveoli/capillary interface. Additionally, 6-min walk testing (6MWT), incremental and endurance shuttle walk testing (ISWT, ESWT), and cardiopulmonary exercise testing (CPET) can offer a broader assessment of the cardiac, pulmonary, and peripheral circulatory interactions, helpful in the evaluation of dyspnea. Finally, tests of respiratory muscle strength and drive may additionally be helpful in the evaluation of disease state.

1.3.1 Spirometry

Spirometry is performed by breathing through a sealed mouthpiece (with closed nares) to measure how much and how quickly airflow is generated by the lungs. Most often, airflow is measured using a pneumotachometer, based on the measured pressure drop across a fine metal screen. This generates data on flow and calculated volume. Three of the most critical outputs from spirometry are (1) the volume of forced air exhaled in the first one second (FEV_1); (2) the total volume of air that can be forcefully exhaled voluntarily, the forced vital capacity (FVC); and (3) the ratio of FEV_1/FVC. These offer a global assessment of how much and how fast air can be exhaled from the lungs, which is essential in the evaluation of airflow obstruction (e.g., asthma, COPD).

Using spirometry, flow-volume loops are also generated (Fig. 1.8). These graphical depictions describe the normal pattern of airflow during an entire forced respiratory cycle (inhalation and exhalation), plotting flow on the y-axis and volume on the x-axis. The flow-volume loop pattern can take on characteristic shapes based on certain pathologies. Slowly emptying airways, intra- and extrathoracic airway obstruction, and vocal cord dysfunction are a few of the helpful characteristic patterns that can be evaluated on flow-volume loops (see Chap. 7).

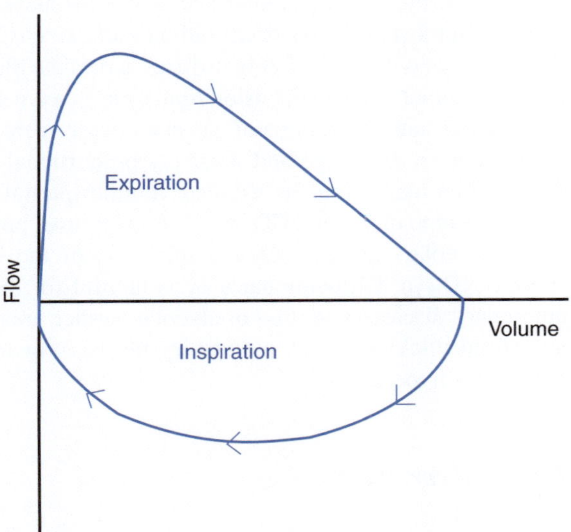

Fig. 1.8 Flow-volume loop. Example of normal flow-volume loop

1.3.2 Lung Volume Measurement

As spirometry can only measure the amount of air forcibly exhaled, assessment of the residual air (RV and FRC) or total lung volume (TLC) is not possible with this method. As changes in lung volumes are a common finding in obstructive lung disease (e.g., hyperinflation, increased TLC; air trapping, increased RV), interstitial lung disease (decreased TLC), and obesity (decreased ERV), additional techniques are needed to measure the various lung volumes for accurate diagnostics.

Lung volumes are most commonly measured by two techniques, (1) body plethysmography and (2) closed-circuit inert gas dilution. Body plethysmography is based on Boyle's law ($P_1V_1 = P_2V_2$) by placing the patient in an airtight box and having them breathe against a closed shutter after quiet exhalation. Change in the box pressure between inhalation and exhalation permits calculation in the change in volume in the box. This change in volume is the FRC. By doing other breathing maneuvers such as inspiratory capacity and vital capacity, calculations of RV and TLC can be performed. Lung volumes can also be measured using the inert gas washout technique. This method capitalizes on the conservation of mass principle ($C_1V_1 = C_2V_2$) to determine lung volumes. A known volume and concentration of gas (usually helium) is quietly inhaled over a series of breaths. After equilibrium has been reached, the concentration of gas at end exhalation is measured, permitting calculation of FRC, RV, and TLC (see Chap. 3).

1.3.3 Diffusing Capacity

Measurement of diffusion capacity enables a combined assessment of the area and thickness of the blood-gas interface as well as assessment of pulmonary capillary volume. In most circumstances, carbon monoxide (CO) is used as it is a diffusion-limited gas and therefore freely diffuses across the blood-gas interface and does not have a potential to reach diffusion limitation as oxygen does (see Chap. 6). The laws of diffusion state the volume of gas that diffuses across a membrane is proportional to the area for exchange and inversely proportional to the thickness of the membrane. Thus measuring the exhaled volume (partial pressure) of CO following a known volume of inhaled CO, over a known time, provides a combined assessment of the alveolar surface area and thickness of the interstitium, termed diffusing capacity (D_{LCO}). Diffusing capacity is helpful for the diagnosis and evaluation of pulmonary diseases with loss of alveolar surface area (e.g., emphysema), increased interstitial thickness (e.g., pulmonary fibrosis), or loss of capillary volume (e.g., pulmonary hypertension).

1.3.4 Exercise Testing

A relatively simple, yet standardized and robust, assessment of one's pulmonary reserve can be achieved by performing a 6-min walk test (6MWT). It does not require any specific instruments and can easily be performed in almost any location. Patients walk on flat ground at a self-paced rate for 6 min, and the distances traveled are measured. It provides a combined global functional assessment of the integrated pulmonary, cardiac, and peripheral circulatory systems. Another important field exercise test is the shuttle walk test, which is classically considered as two different tests, the incremental shuttle walk test (ISWT) and the endurance shuttle walk test (ESWT). Both tests are commonly used outside the United States, where the ISWT is a good measure of maximal exercise capacity and the ESWT provides information on exercise endurance. While the 6MWT, ISWT, and ESWT do not provide specific assessment of the individual physiological systems, more complex testing via cardiopulmonary exercise testing (CPET) can provide useful information on the individual limitations of each of these systems (cardiac, pulmonary, circulatory), helpful for the advanced evaluation of dyspnea (see Chap. 12).

1.3.5 Tests of Respiratory Drive and Muscle Strength

Pulmonary function tests are also available to assess various aspects of the neuromuscular contribution to breathing. Specifically, the drive to breathe in response to hypoxia and hypercapnia is assessed by measuring the change in minute ventilation in response to progressive hypoxemia or hypercapnia, respectively. An overall measure of drive to breathe is also assessed by measuring the inspiratory pressure that occurs within the first 100 ms of inhalation, termed the "P100" or "P0.1." The function of the respiratory muscles themselves is usually assessed by measuring the maximal inspiratory and maximal expiratory pressures (MIP, MEP).

1.3.6 What Is on the Horizon?

New technologies are being developed and tested to advance and supplement the current landscape of pulmonary function testing. As spirometry is effort dependent and requires cooperation, a newer technology is the forced oscillation technique (FOT) which uses small amplitude pressure waves superimposed on normal breathing to assess airflow obstruction and small airway disease. FOT can be helpful in diagnoses in the pediatric population, as it requires little cooperation (see Chap. 8). Multiple-breath nitrogen washout (MBNW) is another emerging technique that can be used to calculate the lung clearance index (LCI) that measures global ventilation inhomogeneity but also is able to compartmentalize the ventilation heterogeneity into conducting airways (Scond) and more peripheral acinar airways (Sacin). This has potential to serve as a highly sensitive marker for assessing changes in airway status in diseases such as asthma, cystic fibrosis, and lung transplantation.

1.3.7 What Are We Trying to Achieve with the Report?

While no single diagnosis can be made with PFTs alone, they are designed to aid in the diagnosis as well as follow the response to therapy and the progression of disease. The raw data from PFTs are compiled to generate a report. The report provides physiologic analysis and interpretation of the findings, often with a differential diagnosis of disease processes that may cause the physiologic alterations. In interpreting these findings, the limitations of PFTs must be considered. PFTs are a critical tool utilized in the management of pulmonary disease. However, they should be interpreted with consideration of the patient's presentation, history, physical exam, radiologic, and other findings.

1.4 Conclusion

To properly understand and interpret pulmonary function testing, knowledge of structural and functional interactions of the pulmonary system is needed. Respiration is modulated by central and peripheral chemoreceptors that provide feedback to the muscle of respiration to augment respiratory depth and rate. These muscles generate negative pleural pressure that draws air through the conducting zones of the lung to alveoli where gas exchange occurs. Pulmonary circulation supports delivery of deoxygenated blood and metabolites to the lung. Pulmonary disease can occur along any portion of this complex physiologic process, and pulmonary function tests play a vital role in management of pulmonary disease. The most common pulmonary tests are (1) spirometry, providing information primarily on airflow obstruction and lung volumes; (2) plethysmography or He dilution, measuring total lung volumes; and (3) diffusing capacity, measured using CO to assess overall gas exchange property of the lung. Pulmonary function testing is critical in the diagnosis, and evaluation of progression, and response to therapy in pulmonary disease.

Selected References

Berry CE, Wise RA. Interpretation of pulmonary function test: issues and controversies. Clin Rev Aller Immunol. 2009;37:173–80.

Blakemore WS, Forster RE, Morton JW. Ogilvie CM. A standardized breath holding technique for the clinical measurement of the diffusing capacity of the lung for carbon monoxide. J Clin Invest. 1957;36:1–17.

Bokov P, Delclaux C. Interpretation and use of routine pulmonary function tests: spirometry, static lung volumes, lung diffusion, arterial blood gas, methacholine challenge test and 6-minute walk test. La Revue de medecine interne. 2016;37:100–10.

Coates AL, Peslin R, Rodenstein D, Stocks J. Measurement of lung volumes by plethysmography. Eur Respir J. 1997;10:1415–27.

Flesch JD, Dine CJ. Lung volumes: measurement, clinical use, and coding. Chest. 2012;142:506–10.

Hyatt RE, Black LF. The flow-volume curve. A current perspective. Am Rev Respir Dis. 1973;107:191–9.

Permutt S, Martin HB. Static pressure-volume characteristics of lungs in normal males. J Appl Physiol. 1960;15:819–25.

Suarez CJ, Dintzis SM, Frevert CW. 9 - Respiratory. Comparative anatomy and histology. San Diego: Academic Press; 2012. p. 121–34.

Sylvester JT, Goldberg HS, Permutt S. The role of the vasculature in the regulation of cardiac output. Clin Chest Med. 1983;4:111–26.

Vaz Fragoso CA, Cain HC, Casaburi R, et al. Spirometry, static lung volumes, and diffusing capacity. Respir Care. 2017;62:1137–47.

Woodson BT. A method to describe the pharyngeal airway. Laryngoscope. 2015;125:1233–8.

Zeballos RJ, Weisman IM. Behind the scenes of cardiopulmonary exercise testing. Clin Chest Med. 1994;15:193–213.

Chapter 2
The History of Pulmonary Function Testing

Tianshi David Wu, Meredith C. McCormack, and Wayne Mitzner

2.1 Spirometry

2.1.1 1846: Hutchinson and the Spirometer

Although experimentalists have measured lung volumes as early as the seventeenth century, modern spirometry can trace its roots to John Hutchinson. Hutchinson, who obtained a medical degree after initially working as a life insurance salesman, became interested in spirometry through his observations of an association between lung volumes and pulmonary disease and by tangential measurements of lung volumes by fellow physician Charles Thackrah in 1831. The major illness at the time was phthisis, or pulmonary tuberculosis, and because of his combined interest in life insurance and medicine, Hutchinson sought to develop a measurement tool to aid in its diagnosis.

In his seminal paper, published in Transactions of the Medical and Chirurgical Society of London, in 1846, Hutchinson reviewed five measures that form the basis of modern spirometry today: first, the residual air, conceptualized as the amount of

T. D. Wu
Division of Pulmonary and Critical Care Medicine, Johns Hopkins University School of Medicine, Baltimore, MD, USA
e-mail: twu38@jhmi.edu

M. C. McCormack (✉)
Pulmonary Function Laboratory, Pulmonary and Critical Care Medicine, Johns Hopkins University, Baltimore, MD, USA
e-mail: mmccor16@jhmi.edu

W. Mitzner
Environmental Health and Engineering, Johns Hopkins Bloomberg School of Public Health, Baltimore, MD, USA
e-mail: wmitzner@jhu.edu

D. A. Kaminsky, C. G. Irvin (eds.), *Pulmonary Function Testing*, Respiratory Medicine, https://doi.org/10.1007/978-3-319-94159-2_2

air remaining at the lungs at the end of maximal expiration, now known as the residual volume (though not measurable with a spirometer); second, the reserve air, the maximal volume of air that can be expired from the nadir of natural breathing, now known as the expiratory reserve volume; third, the breathing air, the volume of air inspired or expired in a breath during natural breathing, now known as the tidal volume; fourth, the complemental air, the volume of air that can still be inspired at the apex of natural breathing, now known as the inspiratory reserve volume; and fifth, perhaps the most famous among these, the vital capacity, the volume of air "given by a full expiration following the deepest inspiration," which is equal to the sum of reserve air, complementary air, and breathing air. Hutchinson was specifically interested in the vital capacity, believing that its measure carried diagnostic and prognostic value, and he introduced a device that he called the "spirometer" to measure it (named from *spiro*, which is Latin for breathe out or exhale) (Fig. 2.1).

Hutchinson was the first to suggest that vital capacity was heavily influenced by subject height and age. Most critically, he found that the vital capacity was altered by disease and suggested that this "difference is sufficiently strong to

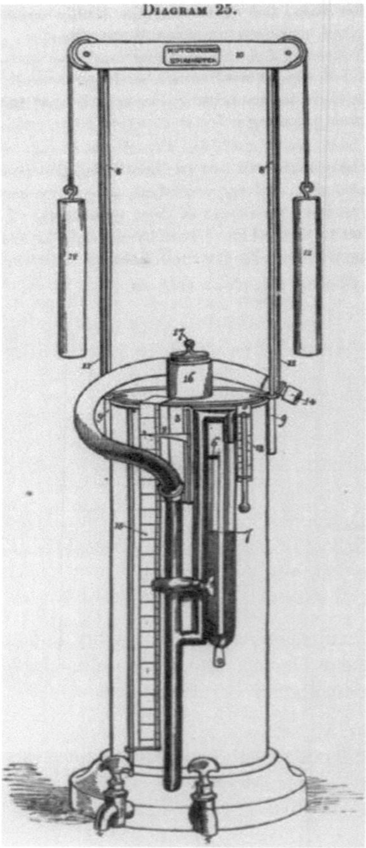

Fig. 2.1 The original Hutchinson spirometer

merit consideration," resulting in the early hypothesis that spirometry has diagnostic and prognostic potential. And likely because of his early background selling life insurance, he advocated the use of the spirometer in actuarial estimations.

The original Hutchinson spirometer was a water seal spirometer. It consisted of an inverted, counterweighted cylinder in a large water chamber. The patient would breathe into a pneumatic tube, and the increased volume in the system translated into vertical motion of the bell. Numerous variations followed in the century after—portable, able to record volume tracings over time—but the basic design was so robust and elegant in its simplicity that one can still buy water seal spirometers that look very similar to the Hutchinson original.

Despite Hutchinson's promotions, his spirometer was mainly adopted in research settings, including an ambitious project by the US Sanitary Commission to document the vital capacity of Union soldiers during the American Civil War, as larger vital capacity was believed to be directly correlated with body vitality and vigor (and hence better fighters). Although the relevance and applicability of Hutchinson's work are readily apparent today, it would not be until more than 50 years later, with discoveries of other important measures in lung disease, that contemporary clinicians began to appreciate the importance of the vital capacity.

At age 40, Hutchinson sailed to Australia, likely to join the Australian gold rush, and died from uncertain causes in 1861 at the age of 50. His early work on lung physiology laid the foundations for future innovations in pulmonary function testing.

2.1.2 *1925: Fleisch, the Pneumotach, and Early Dynamic Measurements of Breathing*

Beyond incremental innovations in the spirometer, such as the ability to graphically record measurements, the field remained largely stagnant until the early twentieth century. A golden age in pulmonary function testing began in the 1920s, driven by the increasing interest in thoracic surgery that required assessment of preoperative respiratory fitness, by the increasing prevalence of occupational lung disease, and by the respiratory distress often experienced by pilots during the First World War. Asthma and emphysema were also becoming recognized as clinical problems, and physicians became interested in objectively quantifying disability and the severity of disease.

Although significant advances had been made to spirometers, airflow was not measured directly, and dynamic breathing was difficult to measure, in large part due to mechanical challenges. Early efforts in the 1920s to measure flow rates were hampered by inadequate equipment and measurement error.

Alfred Fleisch, a Swiss physiologist, developed a simple device to measure flow rates and volumes in 1925. He employed multiple (90) small (2 mm) tubes in parallel calculated to ensure laminar flow so that the flow would be proportional to the pressure difference at two points along the tubes. He quantified the small

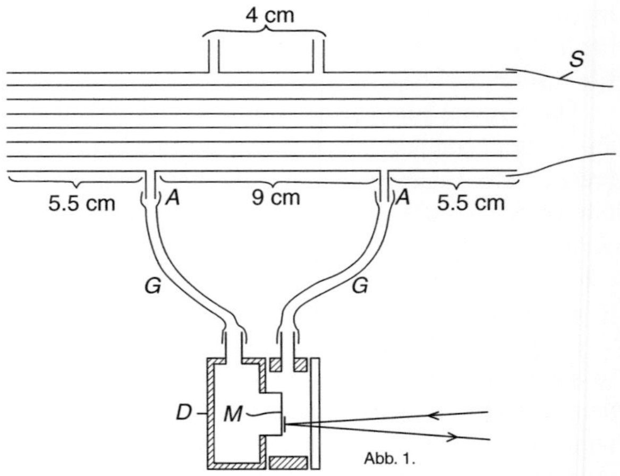

Fig. 2.2 Fleisch pneumotachograph

pressure changes using a novel optical device. In human volunteers he demonstrated the device's utility showing dynamic inspiratory and expiratory flows with simultaneous integration to obtain dynamic volumes. Figure 2.2 shows his drawing of this first pneumotachograph. Pneumotachs along with further innovations to the spirometer from the 1920s and onward allowed for rapid advances in spirometry.

2.1.3 1933: Hermannsen and the Maximum Voluntary Ventilation

Johannes Hermannsen, a German physiologist, proposed measurement of the maximum breathing capacity (MBC) in 1933. This measurement was the total volume of air that a subject inhaled and exhaled over a minute when instructed to breathe as quickly and as deeply as possible. Investigators realized that individuals with lower MBC were also more dyspneic and, perhaps more importantly, that the ratio of MBC to vital capacity, termed *capacity ratio* by some, was decreased when artificial resistance to ventilation was added to the system (e.g., breathing through a narrowed straw). This was the first indication that the rate of ventilation was affected by obstruction and would foreshadow the fundamental dichotomization of ventilatory disease into obstructive and restrictive patterns.

At the time, the MBC was criticized for being too strenuous on participants, especially those who were ill. Others noted that the MBC was affected by a variety of non-pulmonary conditions, especially neuromuscular disease, and was therefore not a very specific measure for lung disease. Although the MBC became popular as a means for preoperative evaluation, these valid criticisms encouraged others to develop alternative methods of assessing pulmonary function.

Hermannsen is remembered as the first physiologist to define a durable and reproducible measure of dynamic ventilatory capacity. Today, the maximum breathing capacity is known as the maximum voluntary ventilation (MVV), a measurement that is rarely done outside of research and specific clinical settings.

2.1.4 1938: Barach, Cournand, and the Classification of Breathing Abnormalities

Alvan Barach, an American physician, made the first observation that asthma and emphysema were associated with decreased rates of exhalation. In his 1938 paper, entitled "Physiological methods in the diagnosis and treatment of asthma and emphysema," Barach noted diminished expiratory flow rates in adults with asthma or emphysema and noted complete or partial reversal of these abnormalities with inhalation of nebulized epinephrine. This was perhaps the first report quantifying the effective use of a bronchodilator.

These and other studies began yielding rich information on the scope and variety of breathing abnormalities. André Cournand and Dickinson Richards, working at Columbia University's Bellevue Hospital, built on these findings with a series of landmark experiments relating abnormalities in pulmonary physiology with derangements in dynamic measurements of breathing. They noted that ventilatory insufficiencies can be partitioned into those attributable to narrowing of the airways, termed obstruction, or attributable to structural stiffening of the lungs, termed restriction, and further remarked that abnormalities in breathing may also be caused by deficiencies in respiratory gas exchange between the lung and capillaries. These fundamental proposals were foundational for subsequent classification of respiratory disease.

2.1.5 1947: Tiffeneau, Gaensler, and the FEV_1

Meanwhile, Robert Tiffeneau and André Pinelli, French physicians, sought a simpler and less taxing measure of pulmonary health than the MBC. They noted that individuals performing the maneuver would increase their respiratory rate to approximately 30 breaths per second and that a major determinant of the MBC was the volume of air moved during forceful exhalation. They formally proposed this measurement as the volume of air that can be exhaled during one cycle of forceful expiration from maximal inspiration. Noting the average respiratory rate augmentation during rapid breathing, they also defined that this volume should be measured over 1 s. Tiffeneau and Pinelli introduced this measurement, the *capacité pulmonaire utilisable à l'effort (CPUE)*, or the pulmonary capacity utilizable with exertion, in 1947. This was the first definition of what would become the FEV_1.

Tiffeneau and colleagues noted that the CPUE was influenced by the vital capacity, and they were also the first to introduce the ratio of CPUE to vital capacity and define its normal bounds. They noted that worse ventilatory disease was associated with lower values of CPUE. Also strikingly, they related changes in the CPUE to changes in airway disease as well as acute changes induced with bronchodilator and bronchoconstriction challenges (to be discussed later).

Despite these important seminal contributions, the work of Tiffeneau was not well-appreciated outside of France at the time. It wouldn't be until 1951, with the parallel work by Edward Gaensler at Boston University in the United States, that the modern-day FEV_1 became more prominent.

Gaensler, who was formally trained as a thoracic surgeon, also appreciated the need for standardized measurements of lung function and like Tiffeneau was interested in measuring the initial volume of a forced expiratory maneuver. He proposed that these volume measurements be made across a constant time and termed this the "timed vital capacity," generally equivalent to Tiffeneau and Pinelli's CPUE. He demonstrated that the timed vital capacity correlated closely with the MBC and was also more reproducible. After some years of controversy over optimal timing, measuring the exhaled air from a maximal inspiration over the first second of exhalation became the standard. Gaensler, who remained at Boston University through his academic career, was also notable for introducing a method to dynamically measure vital capacity and for proposing the briefly popular air velocity index, the ratio of percentage predicted MBC over percentage predicted vital capacity, as a method of differentiating obstructive from restrictive lung disease.

Importantly, along with Tiffeneau, Gaensler also advocated measuring the ratio of timed vital capacity to the total vital capacity, the predecessor to the FEV_1/FVC ratio, and observed that this measure decreased in states of obstruction. Investigators began to relate decreases in the ratio to illness, especially in emphysema, and the timed vital capacity began to gain prominence over the MBC as the primary marker of pulmonary disease.

2.1.6 1955–1959: Fowler, Wright, and Expiratory Flow Rates

Interest increased, predominantly in the United States, with alternative methods of measuring ventilatory function. These were driven mainly by observations that measurements of expiratory volume or maximum voluntary ventilation involved "cumbersome" machinery and that the initial phase of expiration was often difficult to accurately capture.

In 1955, Ward Fowler and colleagues noted significant variation in the initial expiratory flow rates of individuals performing forced maximal exhalation. Instead, he advocated measuring mean flow over the mid-part of the expiratory curve, essentially what is now called FEF_{25-75}.

Wright, citing these same limitations, suggested that published variability in the forced exhalations was mainly a result of equipment error rather than physiologic

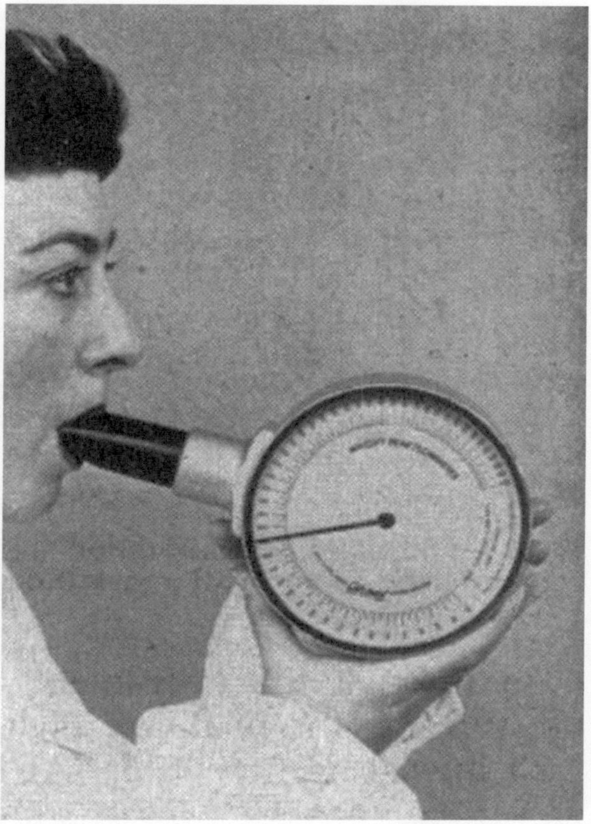

Fig. 2.3 Wright peak flow meter

differences. He introduced the peak flowmeter in 1959 (Fig. 2.3), a portable hand-held device, and advocated for its use by citing high correlation between changes in the peak expiratory flow rate and the FEV_1. The Wright peak flowmeter, which he later miniaturized, remains in use today.

2.1.7 1956: Standardization of Terminology

Compared to 1846, the toolbox of pulmonary function testing had grown substantially more crowded a century later. Different nomenclatures had been used by various investigators to relate to equivalent concepts, creating difficulty in disseminating knowledge across the field.

In 1956, the British Medical Society, recognizing a need to standardize terminology in the field, convened a meeting to establish a consensus in definitions. They defined the volume of air forcibly expired as FEV_x, where x is the time span of measurement, the forced vital capacity as FVC, the maximum volume of air a person can breathe over 1 min as MBC (maximum breathing capacity), and the volume of air someone can breathe on maximum hyperventilation for a given time as the MVV (maximum voluntary ventilation). Although there was no critical determination of how long the forced expiratory volume should be measured, in the meeting, participants had "general agreement" that measuring over 1 s was the most appropriate. The committee further defined that the FEV and FVC should be obtained during forced, maximal exhalation starting from total lung capacity (TLC), recognizing that these values are altered depending on participant effort and what phase of respiration they are measured in. When the vital capacity is not measured with forcible exhalation, the committee recommended representing this as the VC instead of the FVC.

This terminology remains in use today with minimal changes. MBC and MVV are now often used interchangeably, with the latter being measured over 12 s and used as a surrogate to represent the maximum breathing capacity.

Of note, a year prior in 1955, a group of French investigators recommended that the volume expired in the first second be referred to as the "volume expiratoire maximum seconde" (VEMS) and that the ratio of this measurement to vital capacity be referred to as the VEMS/CV ("capacité vitale"). Although having slightly different interpretations than the English equivalents, these terms remain in use in France.

2.1.8 1954–1958: Hyatt, Fry, Miller, Permutt, Mead, and the Flow–Volume Loop

Robert Hyatt is considered the "father of the flow-volume loop" and was the first to describe its measurement and interpretation (Fig. 2.4). Hyatt, an American physician, made a series of critical discoveries on lung mechanics during his time as an investigator at the National Heart Institute, the predecessor to the National Heart, Lung, and Blood Institute. In 1954, Don Fry presented the first quantitative analysis to explain the underlying mechanics of forced expiration, including the counterintuitive concept of the isovolume pressure-flow curve. While examining such curves in human subjects, Hyatt made the observation that maximum expiratory flow was determined primarily by lung volume and not transpulmonary pressure. Recognizing that expiratory flow limitation caused flattening of these curves, he realized that a plot of volume against flow would allow visual identification of this pathology. He introduced this intuitive plot of ventilatory function in 1958 (Fig. 2.5).

Hyatt transitioned to the Mayo Clinic in 1962, where he would later identify with his mentee R. Drew Miller the value of the flow-volume loop's inspiratory limb in the detection of upper airway abnormalities. He remained at Mayo until his retirement in 1987, passing away in 2016 at the age of 91.

Although this early work from Fry and Hyatt laid the experimental and analytical foundation for analyzing forced exhalation as a pulmonary function test, what was not yet understood was how the flow limitation actually occurred. Such analysis was first described in the same year in two different ways by two different independent research groups led by Sol Permutt and Jere Mead, respectively. Both groups utilized intuitive and heuristic arguments still being taught to pulmonary

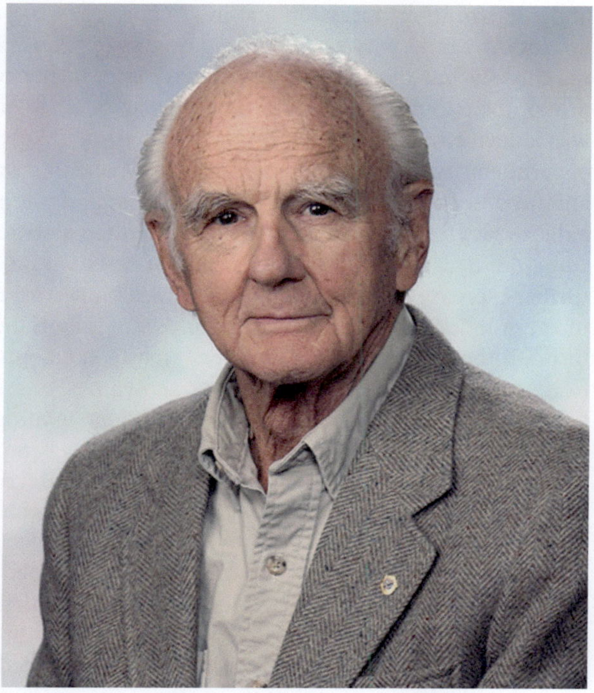

Fig. 2.4 Robert Hyatt (picture courtesy of Mayo Clinic)

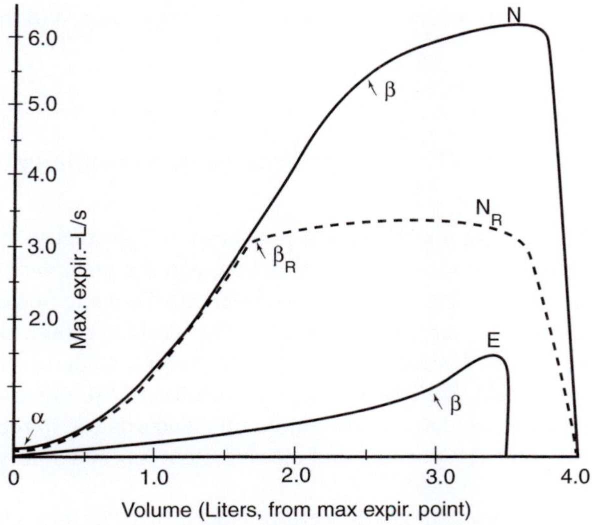

Fig. 2.5 Flow-volume loops shown in the original paper. The curve *N* is a normal subject, while the curve *E* is a subject with emphysema

physiologists and clinicians. Mead's group developed the simple concept of the equal pressure point (EPP), which defined a point in the airway where the pressure in the airway lumen equaled the pleural pressure. Thus during a forced expiration, airways downstream to this EPP (downstream is toward the alveoli) would be under dynamic compression tending to collapse. Any further increases in expiratory effort would only serve to increase this dynamic compression, thereby resisting any further increases in expiratory flow. In the other analysis by Permutt's group, the expiratory flow limitation was modeled using a Starling resistor. This was a device originally used by Ernest Starling to keep a constant afterload in his experiments with an isolated perfused heart, and this vascular application was later analyzed in detail by Permutt and Riley. The Permutt group then adapted this vascular model to the airways, where they defined a critical airway transmural pressure (defined as Ptm') at which a bronchus would collapse, thereby limiting further increases in flow and is sometimes known as the "waterfall" model. Each of these independent models highlights the importance of the resistance to flow through the upstream (i.e., smaller) airway segments, since the anatomic location of these collapsing airways was shown by Peter Macklem and associates to lie in larger airways. This mechanical understanding added important support for the use of forced exhalation as a relatively simple noninvasive pulmonary function test to detect pathologic changes in smaller airways. The maximal expiratory flow then becomes a function of the lung elastic recoil pressure and the resistance of the smaller airways. The importance of collapsible airways in determining maximal flow was also further refined by Dawson and Elliot in 1977, who applied the wave speed principle to airflow limitation, which they adapted from observations of fluid flowing through a collapsible tube. In this model, flow limitation was determined by the speed at which a local pressure wave could propagate within the walls of the conduit. In the case of the airway, the mechanical determinants of airflow limitation included the cross-sectional area of the airway, the airway wall compliance, and the density of the gas within the airway.

2.1.9 1977: Standardization of Spirometry

Recognizing the increasing popularity of spirometry, the wide array of spirometers available to measure lung function, and the great variation with which these measurements were obtained, the American Thoracic Society convened a workshop to discuss standards for spirometry. The working group, numbering 22 scientists from around the United States, met in Snowbird, Utah, in 1977. The resultant statement "Snowbird Workshop on Standardization of Spirometry" was the first document to establish guidelines and minimum standards for spirometry. These included standards for test conduct and measurement reproducibility and were updated in 1987 and again in 1995.

European standards were produced in 1983 through the European Community for Steel and Coal and then updated in 1993 under the European Respiratory Society. The American Thoracic Society and the European Respiratory Society ultimately harmonized recommendations in a joint update published in 2005.

2.2 Lung Volumes

The history of quantifying lung volumes predates spirometry and was grounded in the study of gases and diffusion. The earliest lung volumes were measured from cadaveric specimens, but physiologic measurements in living individuals did not gain prominence until the early twentieth century. There was early interest in the curious observation that air remained in the lungs at the end of forced expiration—the residual volume—before evolving into our contemporary understanding of the complementary information provided between lung volumes and spirometry.

2.2.1 1800: Davy and Active Dilution

The first individual to physiologically measure lung volumes was Sir Humphry Davy. Sir Davy, born in 1778 in Cornwall, was trained as a surgeon-apothecary but was interested in chemistry and physics. Perhaps more known for his discovery and promotion of the euphoric effects of nitrous oxide, he is recognized in the field of pulmonary function testing as the first to describe a closed-circuit gas dilution system to measure lung volumes.

Sir Davy, in his descriptive studies on nitrous oxide, became interested in measuring the residual volume. He produced a reservoir of pure hydrogen and deeply inhaled and exhaled several times from this reservoir, starting from complete expiration. He subsequently measured the volume of hydrogen remaining in the reservoir and reasoned, because the air in his lungs was admixed with the air in the reservoir, that the magnitude of the decrease in hydrogen volume in the reservoir would be proportional to the residual volume. By changing the phase of respiration from which he started his experiment, he was able to calculate his residual volume and total lung capacity. Unsurprisingly, Sir Davy also described numerous adverse effects of breathing pure hydrogen, and thus this specific method was not adopted for any more general application. Similar to the limited application of the Hutchinson spirometer, it would be more than a century before closed-circuit methods began to be applied for routine measurement of lung volumes..

2.2.2 1882: Pflüger and Early Plethysmography

Eduard Pflüger, a German physiologist, proposed an alternative method of measuring lung volumes in 1882. His device, which he called the "pneumometer," was an early plethysmograph that sought to take advantage of the Boyle-Mariotte law, which held that the pressure and volume exerted by a gas were inversely proportional. He described a subject who would be seated inside an airtight cabinet. The subject would breathe forcefully through a mouthpiece, connected to a tube open to the outside, which would then be suddenly occluded. Subsequent pressure changes at the tube would be compared against volume changes detected by a spirometer attached to the cabinet. Pflüger reasoned that the volume of air decreased in the cabinet would be equivalent to the volume of air breathed into the lungs, and further, knowing the volume and pressure changes in the lungs with breathing and the pressure in the lungs at rest would allow calculation of the volume in the lungs at rest, that is, the functional residual capacity.

This technique to derive lung volumes from plethysmography, while fundamentally no different today, was highly prone to technical error when it was initially introduced. Although ultimately prophetic, Pflüger's pneumometer would not be successfully adapted until 70 years later, through the seminal work of Arthur Dubois, to be discussed.

2.2.3 1907: Bohr and Initial Measurements of Lung Volumes

Christian Bohr, a Danish physician born in 1855, was a notable contributor to the field of respiratory physiology. Among his many accomplishments, he was the discoverer of the Bohr effect, describing altered affinity for hemoglobin's binding ability for oxygen in the presence of hydrogen and carbon dioxide, and he would mentor Marie and August Krogh, pioneers in the diffusing capacity, to be discussed later.

Bohr's contribution to the measurement of lung volumes came in 1907, when he published an article describing volumes of the lungs in normal and diseased states. Using a combination of gas dilution methods and spirometry, he painstakingly described how body position, size and shape, and the presence of emphysema altered these values. He was the first to advocate for the measurement of all lung volumes from one subject, and he emphasized the importance of the relationship to residual volume and total lung capacity.

2.2.4 1923–1932: Van Slyke, Binger, Christie, and Passive Dilution

The closed-circuit gas dilution systems described by Davy and other investigators relied on the participant forcibly breathing from a reservoir of gas, such that complete equilibrium between the lung and the reservoir occurred as quickly as possible. If mixing did not occur quickly enough, tissue respiration—the production of carbon dioxide and consumption of oxygen—would violate the assumptions of the closed system and cause inaccurate measurements of lung volume. This shortcoming was particularly relevant for ill participants who could not generate sufficiently vigorous ventilatory forces.

Van Slyke and Binger, researchers from the Rockefeller Institute in New York, proposed a solution in 1923. Instead of relying on the amount of dilution of a principal gas within the reservoir, their procedure utilized the ratio of two relatively insoluble gases—hydrogen and nitrogen—to relate to the lung volume. Participants were connected to a system to which a known volume of hydrogen was introduced, approximating the estimated volume of nitrogen in the lung. After a period of passive breathing, the ratio of nitrogen to hydrogen in the reservoir was measured. Because this ratio is constant in a closed system, and because the amount of hydrogen introduced to the system is known, the amount of nitrogen originally in the lung can be derived; because nitrogen constitutes 79% of ambient air, the total volume of the lung can be calculated.

In comparison to active dilution methods, van Slyke's passive method allowed accurate measurement of lung volumes over longer time periods and produced accurate results in less than 6 min. However, two nontrivial considerations prevented significant adoption of their methods: first, the procedure required pure hydrogen, and there was concern over its explosive potential; and second, the hydrogen was occasionally contaminated with arsine, resulting in production of arsenic gas.

Noting these shortcomings, Ronald Christie, a Scottish physician and physiologist, described an alternative passive dilution method in 1932. While at McGill University in Montreal, he published a series of seminal papers in the *Journal of Clinical Investigation* on pulmonary and pleural mechanics. The first of these described a dilution method utilizing oxygen as the principal gas.

Christie's method involved the introduction of a known volume of pure oxygen to subjects breathing in a closed system, with the resultant lung volume calculated based on the proportional reduction in nitrogen. Unlike hydrogen, however, oxygen is actively removed from the system by the lungs, and Christie's method therefore required the subject's oxygen consumption at rest be measured.

To give insight to how active the field was at the time, Christie noted in his article the crowded and confusing terminologies for lung volumes in use at the time. He observed that "perhaps no realm of physiology is there a more confusing medley of terms than in that which deals with the lung volume and its various subdivisions" and complained that many terms were synonymous, were difficult to measure accurately, or were of no clinical or physiological significance.

2.2.5 1940: Darling and Nitrogen Washout

There were some serious downsides to Christie's passive closed-circuit method: the calculation of how much oxygen consumed by the subject was difficult, the magnitude of nitrogen dilution was often low (resulting in high likelihood of measurement error), and adequate mixing of gases could not be guaranteed.

Robert Darling, in the final section of a 1940 three-part treatise on nitrogen handling in the body, introduced the multi-breath nitrogen washout method for estimating lung volumes. In contrast to previous methods, the nitrogen washout method was an open system requiring breathing pure oxygen.

In the Darling method, the subject breathes pure oxygen, and the total expired volume from numerous breaths over 7 min is collected. The exhaled concentration of nitrogen at the beginning and end of the experiment is then measured, representing the alveolar concentration of nitrogen at both time points. The amount of nitrogen in the expired volume is calculated from the volume of "washout" and its concentration of nitrogen, and knowing this amount and the change in nitrogen concentration that it causes, the volume that this nitrogen originally occupied can be derived. If the subject starts breathing oxygen from the end of expiration, this volume then represents the functional residual capacity.

Decades later, with the advent of plethysmography, investigators would note that the nitrogen washout method comparatively underestimated lung volumes in individuals with emphysema. This was initially attributed wholly to "trapped gas," such as that in bullae, and is not fully detected by washout methods. George Emmanauel, from Columbia in New York, would later prove in 1961 that this difference was instead due to underestimation of alveolar nitrogen after 7 min of washout, and he would introduce a modified procedure that more accurately measured lung volumes in these patients.

The multi-breath nitrogen washout test remains in use and relies on these same principles. Technological advances, such as real-time gas analyzers, have vastly improved the accuracy of the test today.

2.2.6 1941: Meneely and Helium Dilution

George Meneely, an American physician and scientist, also noted difficulties with the Christie oxygen dilution method. He was especially aware of the potential for error due to mismeasurement of basal oxygen consumption, and he remained interested in using a nonabsorbed principal gas. Instead of hydrogen, as was originally employed by van Slyke, he proposed helium, which had the same desirable properties without the potential for explosion.

The Meneely helium dilution method was similar in principle to van Slyke's and was a closed system. The subject would rebreathe from a reservoir with a known volume and initial concentration of helium, and the subsequent equilibrated concentration would be measured to derive the lung volume. Unlike van Slyke's method, the subject could breathe passively, as the concentration of other gases was clamped with a carbon dioxide scrubber and periodic instillation of oxygen.

This helium dilution method, with some later modification, remains in use. Meneely would go on to become instrumental in the field of nuclear medicine, and he would later found the Louisiana State University Medical Center.

2.2.7 *1949–1972: Fowler, Buist, Closing Volume, and Single–Breath Nitrogen Washout*

Ward S. Fowler, the same individual who later advocated for mid-expiratory flow rates, was interested in quantifying the volume of dead space in the 1940s. While a junior scientist at the University of Pennsylvania, under the tutelage of Julius Comroe, he conducted a series of fundamental respiratory experiments. In one of the most well-known, he plotted the concentration of exhaled nitrogen against exhaled volume after a participant inhaled from a reservoir of pure oxygen. He noted that the concentration of exhaled nitrogen by volume slowly increased to a plateau from zero, as the exhaled air transitioned from dead space air to alveolar air. He reasoned that the integral of the concentration-volume relationship divided by the total exhaled volume represented the mixed expired nitrogen concentration, and knowing this and the alveolar nitrogen concentration, one could estimate the anatomic dead space of the subject. Fowler would go on to note that the plateau of nitrogen concentration would not actually be a plateau in patients with pulmonary disease, and he would relate that change to nonhomogeneous mixing of air in these subjects, constituting a fundamental observation in pulmonary pathophysiology. The slope of this region of the curve (called phase III) remains a contemporary index of lung pathology.

A modification to this technique was proposed by Sonia Buist and colleagues in 1973 (Fig. 2.6). A subject would breathe down to his or her residual volume and would inhale to total lung capacity from a reservoir of 100% oxygen. The same Fowler nitrogen-volume plot would be produced. The plateau of nitrogen concentration described by Fowler would be seen, but as the person breathed down to residual volume, there would be an inflection point where the nitrogen concentra-

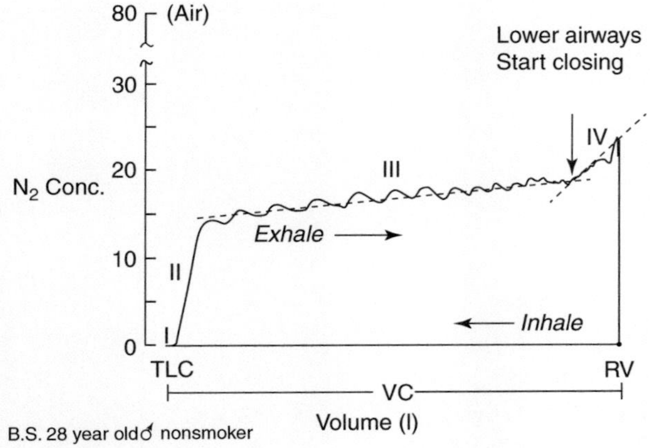

Fig. 2.6 Nitrogen-volume curve for determination of closing volume (marked as IV in this original drawing from Buist)

tion would increase again. The transition volume at this inflection point near residual volume was termed the "closing volume," and Buist and others proposed that elevations in closing volume (from its ratio to total lung capacity or vital capacity) would detect peripheral airways disease. From this procedure, a straightforward application of the alveolar dilution equation could also estimate the total lung capacity, and the whole approach used in this curve is now known as the single-breath nitrogen washout method.

Closing volume and the single-breath washout method did not gain significant adoption, in large part because they proved nonspecific and not very reproducible in persons with significant pulmonary disease. However, these procedures are still occasionally performed, and they remain important historical milestones in the field.

2.2.8 1956: Dubois, Comroe, and Modern Plethysmography

A short time after Fowler's experiments on dead space, Arthur Dubois, also at the University of Pennsylvania and mentored by Julius Comroe, described the first functional whole-body plethysmograph in 1956.

Recognizing the principle of the Boyle-Mariotte law and its potential application to lung volumes suggested by Pflüger in 1882, Dubois made the critical observation that only small respiratory efforts needed to be made after occlusion of the mouthpiece to derive an accurate representation of the pressures and volumes within the lung. Recognition of this fundamental "panting" procedure, in combination with other technological advancements made since the nineteenth century, allowed Dubois to construct a viable plethysmograph (Fig. 2.7).

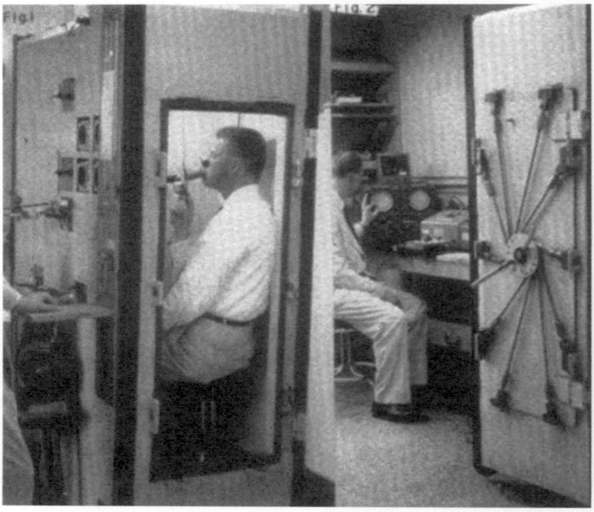

Fig. 2.7 The original plethysmograph, opened (*left*) and closed (*right*); Dubois is shown in right panel

Perhaps the most significant advancement made by Dubois was that of the measurement of airway resistance (R_{aw}). The major impediment to an accurate measurement of R_{aw} is the fact that pressure in alveoli cannot be measured directly. By comparing the plethysmograph pressure and volume changes with and without a closed shutter, he showed how alveolar pressure could be accurately estimated, and this allowed him to measure airway resistance. The articles written by Dubois describing this technique and the whole-body plethysmograph remain two highly cited articles in the *Journal of Clinical Investigation*.

2.3 Diffusing Capacity

2.3.1 1915: Marie Krogh and the Single-Breath Technique

It may be argued that the central figure in the measurement of pulmonary diffusing capacity was Marie Krogh (Fig. 2.8). Born in 1874 as Marie Jorgensen, she trained in medicine at the University of Copenhagen and as a student worked in the lab of

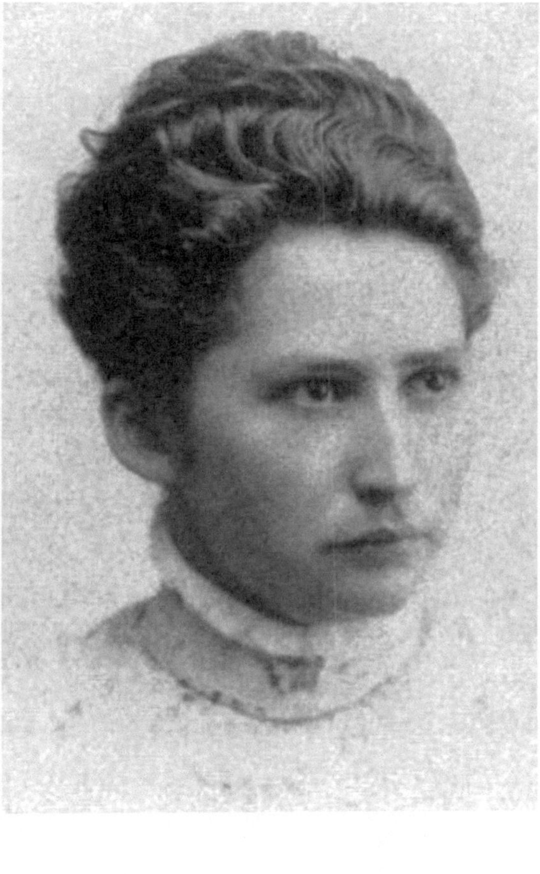

Fig. 2.8 Marie Krogh

Christian Bohr, studying respiratory physiology and the mechanism of oxygen transport into the body. There, she met her husband and future Nobel Laureate, August Krogh, and the two formed a close personal and scientific collaboration. Her life was marked by competing external interests—as a child, she was discouraged from entering university to care for her family, and shortly after completing medical school, she gave birth to four children between 1908 and 1918. She pursued her research interests diligently through these events and, in a series of publications in 1915, related the fundamental methods of assessing pulmonary diffusing capacity using carbon monoxide.

A controversy existed in the early 1900s on whether the lung passively diffused oxygen or was responsible for actively secreting it, an idea driven by experiments from Bohr and John Haldane showing lower oxygen tension in alveoli than in blood. August, through a series of publications in1909, refuted a series of these experiments—including that of his mentor—and suggested that the lung merely functioned to absorb oxygen passively from the external environment. In this work, Marie and August, using themselves as subjects, calculated the diffusing capacity for oxygen in the lung using carbon monoxide, a gas with similar diffusion properties although much higher affinity for hemoglobin.

Marie reasoned that carbon monoxide, an "indifferent gas," would pass freely by diffusion through the pulmonary epithelium and would be immediately bound by circulating hemoglobin. This binding would keep the partial pressure of CO in the blood near zero, and thus the rate of CO diffusion would be constant and could be calculated from the difference in exhaled concentrations of carbon monoxide over a set time period. This rate constant, when subsequently multiplied by the total alveolar volume, would produce a measurement of the diffusing capacity for CO. A simple ratio, related to the solubilities and molecular weights of oxygen and carbon monoxide, would then give a calculated diffusing capacity for oxygen.

Despite the work of Marie and August, continued controversy over the role of the oxygen handling in the lung spurred Marie to perform more thorough experiments. She recruited a cohort of 38 human subjects, 8 of whom had pulmonary disease, and measured diffusing capacity for carbon monoxide during states of work and rest. Calculating the expected diffusion constant for oxygen, she concluded that passive diffusion would be sufficient to satisfy oxygen demands in all cases and also made the important observation that diffusing capacity is increased by exercise, presumably due to increases in pulmonary blood flow. The summary of this work, published in 1915, is the foundational document for measuring the diffusing capacity of carbon monoxide.

In practice, the Krogh method required two measurements of expired air in order to calculate a differential concentration of carbon monoxide. The subject would exhale to residual volume and would inspire a mixture of 1% CO, exhale partially for the first sample, hold their breath for 10 s, and exhale fully for the second sample. The alveolar volume was calculated by summing the inspiratory vital capacity, measured during the CO maneuver, with the residual volume, measured by a hydrogen dilution method.

2.3.2 1954–1957: Forster, Ogilvie, and Standardization of the Single-Breath Technique

Robert Forster, and later joined by Colin Ogilvie, both from the University of Pennsylvania, standardized and improved Krogh's method in 1954. By inserting a helium tracer in the reservoir of carbon monoxide, the initial alveolar concentration of CO could be estimated, obviating the need to collect two expired samples and also allowing residual volume to be simultaneously calculated. Ogilvie and colleagues generated predictive equations, showed decrements in diffusing capacity with pathologic states, and discussed situations in which the test may give erroneous results. Notably, although it was known that exercise and increased pulmonary blood-flow altered results, the influence of hemoglobin concentration was not stated.

Despite many factors that altered its value, the diffusing capacity for carbon monoxide was rapidly adopted into clinical practice as an easy-to-perform test that was sensitive to pulmonary pathology not detectable by other noninvasive methods at the time. In a retrospective penned in 1992, Ogilvie would write that when he originally presented his results to Julius Comroe (the chair of the physiology department at the time), Comroe said that he "didn't know what we were measuring, but we seemed to be measuring it extremely well." Indeed, in European settings the diffusing capacity is referred to as the "transfer factor," reflecting recognition of other components that influence its value.

2.3.3 1955: Filley, Bates, and the Steady–State Technique

A potential limitation of the single-breath technique was its reliance on a patient who could actively breathe deeply and breath hold. Recognizing this, Giles Filley and colleagues of the Trudeau-Saranac Institute in New York introduced in 1955 a passive method for determining the diffusing capacity of carbon monoxide. In this method, the subject breathed 0.1% carbon monoxide for several minutes. Under this condition, the rate of CO absorption by the lung reaches a steady state, and the ratio of this rate to the alveolar concentration of CO would equal the diffusing capacity. Filley utilized an arterial blood gas measure of CO_2, collected at the end of the experiment, in order to calculate the alveolar CO concentration.

David Bates, a British physician who in the course of his training was also mentored by Julius Comroe, introduced a small modification to the Filley technique by measuring alveolar CO concentration with an end-tidal CO monitor, removing the need for an arterial blood gas. Later, investigators would note only a modest correlation between end-tidal CO and alveolar CO, limiting the applicability of this technique.

Because the steady-state technique took comparatively longer than the single-breath method, and because it generally didn't produce meaningfully different results, it is not used today.

2.3.4 1957: Roughton and the Partitioning of the Diffusion Coefficient

Meanwhile, Forster turned his attention to the kinetics of carbon monoxide uptake by hemoglobin. Krogh, 40 years prior, assumed that hemoglobin would instantaneously bind to carbon monoxide, but contemporary experiments suggested that this assumption was inaccurate. Forster was joined by FJW Roughton and in 1957 jointly advanced what became known as the Roughton-Forster equation.

$$\frac{1}{D_L} = \frac{1}{D_M} + \frac{1}{\theta V_c}$$

where D_L is the measured diffusing capacity, D_M is the true membrane diffusing capacity, θ is the rate of gas absorption by 1 mL of blood per minute per 1 mm of Hg pressure gradient, and V_c is the total volume of blood in the pulmonary capillaries.

This equation partitioned the diffusing capacity of carbon monoxide into two components: the first, the resistance provided by the alveolar capillary membrane and, the second, resistance provided by carbon monoxide binding to hemoglobin. Although important in the conceptual understanding of the underlying determinants of the diffusing capacity, in practice, these two components are often coupled, limiting its clinical utility. Nevertheless, in pathologies where there is damage to the membrane available for diffusion, there is often also a loss of capillary blood volume, so both changes often work in concert.

2.3.5 1983: Borland, Guénard, and the Diffusing Capacity of Nitric Oxide

Initial interest in nitric oxide was in its potential role in the development of cigarette-related emphysema. Colin Borland and colleagues of Cambridge University in the United Kingdom were the first to measure the diffusing capacity of nitric oxide in 1983. Borland developed a method of simultaneously measuring DL_{CO} and DL_{NO}, noting that the latter was almost fivefold higher, a difference that could not be explained by the greater diffusivity of nitric oxide. These findings were replicated around the same time by Hervé Guénard in Paris.

There was initial enthusiasm that nitric oxide's strong affinity for hemoglobin would allow its θ as represented in the Roughton-Forster equation to be essentially infinite, such that DL_{NO} would be a true representation of alveolar membrane conductance. Subsequent studies by Borland showed this to be false. Currently, perhaps owing to the entrenched use of the DL_{CO}, the DL_{NO} is not routinely measured in clinical practice. Professional society recommendations, however, advocate for its use, especially when considered in conjunction with $DL_{CO.}$ The ratio of DL_{NO}/DL_{CO} has been studied in a variety of disease states and shows excellent potential as a diagnostic tool to determine the source of abnormalities in gas transfer.

2.4 Bronchoprovocation Testing

The history of bronchoprovocation testing traces its origins to the study of allergic diseases, particularly asthma, and it is in many ways nestled within the history of spirometry. Physician Alvin Barach, in 1938, made the initial observation that nebulized epinephrine reversed the reduction in expiratory flow rates seen in asthmatics, giving way to the role of bronchodilators as a treatment for asthma. The reverse—the use of bronchoprovocation—arose thereafter as a means to diagnose it.

2.4.1 1873: Blackley and the Antigen Challenge

The first documented use of bronchoprovocation was performed by Charles Blackley in 1873. A medical physician from the United Kingdom, Blackley was interested in the mechanisms behind allergic rhinitis and asthma. In his treatise, "Experimental Researches on the Causes and Nature of Catarrhus Aestivus," Blackley introduced experimental evidence that hay fever and asthma were predominantly caused by exposure to various forms of pollen. He isolated pollen and dust from various sources and tested them on a small group of experimental subjects—himself being the most predominant one, reproducing symptoms of asthma by inhaling the candidate substances. Blackley did not have access to pulmonary testing at the time, and understanding of respiratory physiology in asthma was still nascent, but his early use of bronchoprovocation testing predicted its utility as a tool in the diagnosis of asthma.

2.4.2 1921–1932: Alexander, Paddock, Weiss, and Parenteral Bronchoprovocation

Harry Alexander and Royce Paddock, both from Cornell University in New York, published the first systematic report of bronchoprovocation with parenteral agents in 1921. They sought to investigate the effects of sympathetic and parasympathetic tone on asthma symptoms, and they recruited 20 patients with asthma and gave them intravenous quantities of epinephrine and pilocarpine. They noted that participants would have "asthmatic breathing" when exposed to either agent. Eleven years later, Soma Weiss, at Harvard Medical School, published results of his experiments with parenteral histamine in normal and ill subjects, noting that those with pulmonary disease often responded to histamine with symptoms of bronchial constriction. These early experiments were fundamental in understanding the biological mechanism through which asthma induced bronchoconstriction.

2.4.3 1933: Samter and the Histamine Challenge

Max Samter, born in 1908 in Berlin, was a notable German physician and scientist who made significant contributions to allergy and immunology. Samter, perhaps most well-known for the clinical triad (asthma, nasal polyposis, aspirin sensitivity) that bears his name, made many of his discoveries while still a medical intern in Germany. In 1933, he reported on the use of an aerosolized method for challenging patients with asthma with histamine, precipitating clinically significant exacerbations in nearly half of them. This method, the forerunner to modern bronchoprovocation testing, would set the stage for its clinical use.

2.4.4 1941: Tiffeneau, Inhaled Acetylcholine, and the Methacholine Challenge

Robert Tiffeneau, in creating his method for measuring expiratory flow and FEV_1, also performed a series of experiments showing changes in these values after exposure to a variety of aerosolized medications. He and his colleagues demonstrated in a group of subjects with asthma that exposure to acetylcholine led to reductions in FEV_1 and that these reductions were rescued with inhaled isoproterenol. Tiffeneau suggested that bronchoprovocation may have value in the diagnosis of airway hyperresponsiveness and in particular asthma.

However, due to the lack of understanding of airway hyperresponsiveness in normal individuals and standardization of the procedure, the use of acetylcholine and later the synthetic agent methacholine did not become standard clinical practice until the 1960s.

2.4.5 1951: Herxheimer and an Early Bronchoprovocation Test

Herbert Herxheimer, a German physician who emigrated to the United Kingdom in 1938, was also a pioneer in allergy and immunology, being credited with the discovery of the slow reacting substance of anaphylaxis and bradykinin. As a clinician, he was concerned about the difficulty of identifying effective treatments for asthma, complaining that "a high proportion of psychological successes is

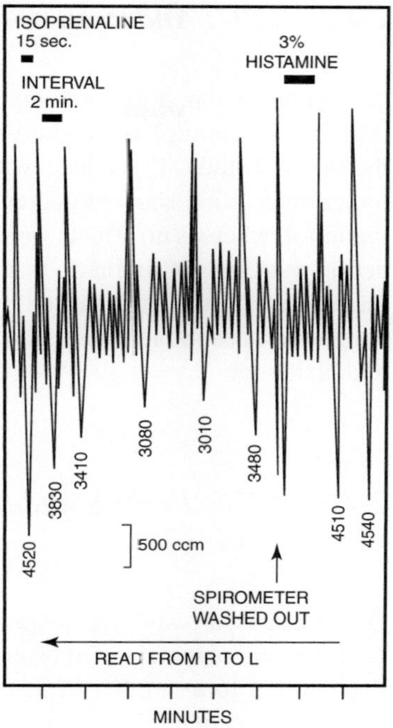

Fig. 2.9 Changes in vital capacity on exposure to histamine and isoprenaline documented by Herxheimer

assured whatever treatment is adopted, so that objective successes are swamped…" To remedy this, he proposed the first bronchoprovocation testing system, a device that allowed a variety of substances to be aerosolized and inhaled by a subject while simultaneously measuring spirometry. He proposed that "psychological" asthma can be differentiated in this way from true asthma through the use of control substances. It was known at the time, through work of Samter and Herxheimer, that individuals with asthma were susceptible to aerosols of histamine and acetylcholine, and he demonstrated reduction and subsequent recovery of vital capacity on exposure to these substances and isoprenaline (Fig. 2.9).

2.4.6 1970–1980s: Exercise Testing

Noting the presence of exercise-induced bronchoconstriction and exercise-induced asthma in some patients, interest arose in the early 1970s in the use of exercise testing as an indirect method of bronchoprovocation. In contrast to histamine, acetylcholine, and methacholine, which directly acted on airway smooth muscle to cause bronchoconstriction, indirect methods cause stress on cells and mediators in the airway, precipitating bronchoconstriction through standard inflammatory pathways. Standards were initially published for exercise testing in 1979 and were further updated by national professional societies, to be discussed.

2.4.7 1997: Anderson and the Mannitol Indirect Challenge

Sandra Anderson, a pulmonologist and researcher from the University of Sydney, introduced mannitol as an additional indirect bronchoprovocation agent in 1997. In the original study, 43 subjects with asthma and proven bronchial hyperreactivity to hypertonic saline showed decrements in FEV_1 when challenged with dry-powder mannitol, whereas no effects were seen in seven control subjects. The mechanism of action was thought similar to that occurring during exercise testing—dehydration of the airways, in this case caused by transient increases in osmolarity. Further studies suggested acceptable safety and comparable performance with hypertonic saline and histamine.

2.4.8 1975–1999: Standardization of Bronchoprovocation Testing

By the 1970s, airway hyperresponsiveness by direct and indirect methods was being assessed with a variety of substances and maneuvers. Variation in interpretation and conduct led to a number of attempts at standardization. In the United States, the American Academy of Allergy convened a workshop in 1975. The resultant document, "Standardization of bronchial inhalation challenge procedures," established procedures and standards for antigen, methacholine, and histamine.

The European Respiratory Society convened a series of task forces in the 1990s to establish European standards for direct and indirect bronchoprovocation testing, and the American Thoracic Society outlined criteria for methacholine and exercise challenge testing in 2000. Some harmonization between the European Respiratory Society and the American Thoracic Society occurred with methacholine challenge procedures in 2017.

2.5 Conclusion

Spirometry, which traces its modern origins to Hutchinson, is now the first-line tool in the diagnosis of functional lung disease. Through the benefit of computer technology, standardization, and advancements in miniaturization, rigorous and reproducible spirometry can be reliably performed in the primary care physician's office. Perhaps satisfying Hutchinson's original intent, spirometers have become widely disseminated, and professional societies recommend their use by generalists as a standard of care.

Lung volumes and measurement of diffusing capacity, from the pioneering works of Davy and Krogh, are now routinely performed in the pulmonary function laboratory. They are instrumental in the advanced diagnosis of lung disease and firmly remain in the toolbox of the pulmonologist. Bronchoprovocation testing, by comparison, has declined in popularity, concurrent to our greater appreciation that the presence of airway hyperreactivity is possible even in otherwise normal and asymptomatic individuals.

We hope the reader has gained an appreciation for the diverse history behind the modern-day pulmonary function test and for the people who were instrumental in the process. From its beginnings in the physiology laboratory, pulmonary function testing is now a fundamental tool in medicine today.

Acknowledgments The authors wish to thank Dr. Jimmie Sylvester for his insight and very helpful comments critiquing an earlier version of this document.

Selected References

Alexander HL, Paddock R. Bronchial asthma: response to pilocarpine and epinephrine. Arch Int Med. 1921;27(2):184–91.

American Physiological Society. Robert E. Hyatt. 2016; Obituary for Robert E. Hyatt. Available at: http://www.the-aps.org/mm/Membership/Obituaries/Robert-E-Hyatt.html. 2017.

American Thoracic Society. Snowbird workshop on standardization of spirometry. Amer Rev Respir Dis. 1979;119:831.

American Thoracic Society. Standardization of spirometry-1987 update. Am Rev Respir Dis. 1987;136:1285–98.

American Thoracic Society Standardization of Spirometry, 1994 Update. 2012.

Anderson SD, Brannan J, Spring J, et al. A new method for bronchial-provocation testing in asthmatic subjects using a dry powder of mannitol. Am J Respir Crit Care Med. 1997;156(3 Pt 1):758–65.

Barach AL. Physiological methods in the diagnosis and treatment of asthma and emphysema. Ann Intern Med. 1938;12(4):454–81.

Bates DV, Boucot NG, Dormer AE. The pulmonary diffusing capacity in normal subjects. J Physiol. 1955;129(2):237–52.

Blackley CH. Experimental researches on the causes and nature of catarrhus aestivus (hay-fever or hay-asthma). London: Baillière, Tindall & Cox; 1873.

Borland CD, Dunningham H, Bottrill F, et al. Significant blood resistance to nitric oxide transfer in the lung. J Appl Physiol. 2010;108(5):1052–60.

Braun L. Spirometry, measurement, and race in the nineteenth century. J Hist Med Allied Sci. 2005;60(2):135–69.

Buist AS, Ross BB. Closing volume as a simple, sensitive test for the detection of peripheral airway disease. Chest J. 1973a;63(4_Supplement):29S–30S.

Buist AS, Ross BB. Predicted values for closing volumes using a modified single breath nitrogen test. Am Rev Respir Dis. 1973b;107(5):744–52.

Chai H, Farr RS, Froehlich LA, et al. Standardization of bronchial inhalation challenge procedures. J Allergy Clin Immunol. 1975;56(4):323–7.

Christie RV. The lung volume and its subdivisions: i. Methods of measurement. J Clin Invest. 1932;11(6):1099–118.

Coates AL, Wanger J, Cockcroft DW, et al. ERS technical standard on bronchial challenge testing: general considerations and performance of methacholine challenge tests. Eur Respir J. 2017;49(5):1601526.

Cohen SG. In lasting tribute: max Samter, MD. J Aller Clin Immunol. 1999;104(2):274–5.

Comroe JH Jr, Botelho SY, Dubois AB. Design of a body plethysmograph for studying cardiopulmonary physiology. J Appl Physiol. 1959;14(3):439–44.

Cournand A, Richards D Jr, Darling R. Graphic tracings of respiration in study of pulmonary disease. Am Rev Tuberc. 1939;40(487):79.

Crapo R, Casaburi R, Coates A, et al. Guidelines for methacholine and exercise challenge testing-1999. This official statement of the American Thoracic Society was adopted by the ATS Board of Directors, July 1999. Am J Respir Crit Care Med. 2000;161(1):309.

Cropp GJ. The exercise bronchoprovocation test: standardization of procedures and evaluation of response. J Allergy Clin Immunol. 1979;64(6):627–33.

Darling RC, Cournand A, Richards DW. Studies on the intrapulmonary mixture of gases. Iii. An open circuit method for measuring residual air. J Clin Investig. 1940;19(4):609–18.

Davy H. Researches, chemical and philosophical, chiefly concerning nitrous oxide, or dephlogisticated nitrous air, and its respiration. London: J. Johnson; 1800.

Dawson SV, Elliott EA. Wave-speed limitation on expiratory flow – a unifying concept. J Appl Physiol Respirat Environ Exercise Physiol. 1977;43:498–515.

D'Silva JL, Mendel D. The maximum breathing capacity test. Thorax. 1950;5(4):325.

Dubois AB, Botelho SY, Bedell GN, Marshall R, Comroe JH Jr. A rapid plethysmographic method for measuring thoracic gas volume: a comparison with a nitrogen washout method for measuring functional residual capacity in normal subjects. J Clin Invest. 1956a;35(3):322–6.

Dubois AB, Botelho SY, Comroe JH Jr. A new method for measuring airway resistance in man using a body plethysmograph: values in normal subjects and in patients with respiratory disease. J Clin Invest. 1956b;35(3):327–35.

Emmanuel G, Briscoe W, Cournand A. A method for the determination of the volume of air in the lungs: measurements in chronic pulmonary emphysema. J Clin Investig. 1961;40(2):329.

Filley GF, MacIntosh DJ, Wright GW. Carbon monoxide uptake and pulmonary diffusing capacity in normal subjects at rest and during exercise. J Clin Investig. 1954;33(4):530–9.

Forster R, Fowler W, Bates D, Van Lingen B. The absorption of carbon monoxide by the lungs during breathholding. J Clin Investig. 1954;33(8):1135.

Fowler WS. Lung function studies. III. Uneven pulmonary ventilation in normal subjects and in patients with pulmonary disease. J Appl Physiol. 1949;2(6):283–99.

Fry DL, Ebert RV, Stead WW, Brown CC. The mechanics of pulmonary ventilation in normal subjects and in patients with emphysema. Am J Med. 1954;16(1):80–97.

Gaensler EA. Air velocity index; a numerical expression of the functionally effective portion of ventilation. Am Rev Tuberc. 1950;62(1-A):17–28.

Gaensler EA. An instrument for dynamic vital capacity measurements. Science. 1951a;114(2965):444–6.

Gaensler EA. Analysis of ventilatory defect by timed capacity measurement. Am Rev Tuberc. 1951b;64:256–78.

Gandevia B, Hugh-Jones P. Terminology for measurements of Ventilatory capacity: a report to the thoracic society. Thorax. 1957;12(4):290–3.

Gibson G. Spirometry: then and now. Breathe. 2005;1(3):206–16.

Guenard H, Varene N, Vaida P. Determination of lung capillary blood volume and membrane diffusing capacity in man by the measurements of NO and CO transfer. Respir Physiol. 1987;70(1):113–20.

Herxheimer H. Induced asthma in man. Lancet. 1951;257(6669):1337–41.

Hirdes J, Van Veen G. Spirometric lungfunction investigations. II. The form of the expiration curve under normal and pathological conditions. Acta Tuberc Scand. 1952;26(3):264.

Hughes J, Bates D. Historical review: the carbon monoxide diffusing capacity (Dl CO) and its membrane (Dm) and red cell (Θ· Vc) components. Respir Physiol Neurobiol. 2003;138(2):115–42.

Hughes JMB, van der Lee I. The TL, NO/TL, CO ratio in pulmonary function test interpretation. Eur Respir J. 2013;41(2):453–61.

Hutchinson J. On the capacity of the lungs, and on the respiratory functions, with a view of establishing a precise and easy method of detecting disease by the spirometer. Medico-chirurgical transactions. 1846;29:137.

Hyatt RE, Schilder DP, Fry DL. Relationship between maximum expiratory flow and degree of lung inflation. J Appl Physiol. 1958;13(3):331–6.

Klocke RA. Dead space: simplicity to complexity. J Appl Physiol (Bethesda, MD) 1985. 2006;100(1):1–2.

Knowlton F, Starling E. The influence of variations in temperature and blood-pressure on the performance of the isolated mammalian heart. J Physiol. 1912;44(3):206–19.

Krogh M. The diffusion of gases through the lungs of man. J Physiol. 1915;49(4):271–300.

Leuallen EC, Fowler WS. Maximal midexpiratory flow. Am Rev Tuberc. 1955;72(6):783–800.

Macklem PT, Mead J. Factors determining maximum expiratory flow in dogs. J Appl Physiol. 1968;25(2):159–69.

Macklem PT, Wilson N. Measurement of intrabronchial pressure in man. J Appl Physiol. 1965;20(4):653–63.

Matheson HW, Spies SN, Gray JS, Barnum DR. Ventilatory function tests. Ii. Factors affecting the voluntary ventilation capacity. J Clin Investig. 1950;29(6):682–7.

Mead J. Mechanics of the lung and chest wall. In: West JB, editor. Respiratory physiology: people and ideas. New York: Oxford University Press; 1996.

Mead J, Turner J, Macklem P, Little J. Significance of the relationship between lung recoil and maximum expiratory flow. J Appl Physiol. 1967;22(1):95–108.

Meneely GR, Kaltreider NL. The volume of the lung determined by helium dilution. Description of the method and comparison with other procedures. J Clin Investig. 1949;28(1):129–39.

Miller RD, Hyatt RE. Obstructing lesions of the larynx and trachea: clinical and physiologic characteristics. Mayo Clin Proc. 1969 Mar; 44(3): 145–61.

Miller RD, Hyatt RE. Evaluation of obstructing lesions of the trachea and larynx by flow-volume loops. Am Rev Respir Dis. 1973;108(3):475–81.

Miller MR, Hankinson J, Brusasco V, et al. Standardisation of spirometry. Eur Respir J. 2005;26(2):319–38.

Mitzner W. Mechanics of the lung in the 20th century. Compr Physiol. 2011;1:2009–27.

Morrell MJ. One hundred years of pulmonary function testing: a perspective on 'the diffusion of gases through the lungs of man' by Marie Krogh. J Physiol. 2015;593(2):351–2.

Needham CD, Rogan MC, McDonald I. Normal standards for lung volumes, intrapulmonary gas-mixing, and maximum breathing capacity. Thorax. 1954;9(4):313–25.

Ogilvie C. Measurement of gas transfer in the lung-a citation-classic commentary on a standardized breath holding technique for the clinical measurement of the diffusing-capacity of the lung for carbon-monoxide by Ogilvie, Cm, Forster, Re, Blakemore, Ws And Morton, Jw. Curr Contents/Clin Med. 1992;14:10.

Ogilvie C, Forster R, Blakemore WS, Morton J. A standardized breath holding technique for the clinical measurement of the diffusing capacity of the lung for carbon monoxide. J Clin Investig. 1957;36(1 Pt 1):1.

Otis A. A history of respiratory mechanics. In: Fishman A, editor. Handbook of physiology; section 3: the respiratory system. Bethesda: American Physiological Society; 1986.

Peabody FW, Wentworth JA. Clinical studies of the respiration: IV. The vital capacity of the lungs and its relation to dyspnea. Arch Intern Med. 1917;20(3):443–67.

Perkins J. Historical development of respiratory physiology. In: Fenn W, Rahn H, editors. Handbook of physiology; Section 3: Respiration. Washington, DC: American Physiological Society; 1964.

Permutt S, Riley R. Hemodynamics of collapsible vessels with tone: the vascular waterfall. J Appl Physiol. 1963;18(5):924–32.

Pride N, Permutt S, Riley R, Bromberger-Barnea B. Determinants of maximal expiratory flow from the lungs. J Appl Physiol. 1967;23(5):646–62.

Quanjer PH. Standardized lung function testing. Report working Party'Standardization of lung function Tests', European Community for coal and steel. Bull Eur Physiopathol Respir. 1983;19:1–95.

Proctor DF, ed. A History of Breathing Physiology. Lung Biology in Health and Disease, vol. 83. New York: Marcel Dekker, 1995

Quanjer P, Tammeling G, Cotes J, Pedersen O, Perlin R, Yernault J. Lung volumes and forced ventilatory flows. Report working party. Standardization of lung function test European Community for steel and oral official statement of the European Respiratory Society. Eur Respir J. 1993;6(5):40.

Rodarte JR, Hyatt RE, Westbrook PR. Determination of lung volume by single- and multiple-breath nitrogen washout. Am Rev Respir Dis. 1976;114(1):131–6.

Roughton FJ, Forster RE. Relative importance of diffusion and chemical reaction rates in determining rate of exchange of gases in the human lung, with special reference to true diffusing capacity of pulmonary membrane and volume of blood in the lung capillaries. J Appl Physiol. 1957;11(2):290–302.

Samter M. Herbert Herxheimer, 90 years of age, died after a brief illness in October 1985. J Allergy Clin Immunol. 1987;79(1):121.

Schmidt-Nielsen B. August and Marie Krogh and respiratory physiology. J Appl Physiol. 1984;57(2):293–303.

Spriggs EA. John Hutchinson, the inventor of the spirometer – his north country background, life in London, and scientific achievements. Med Hist. 1977;21(4):357–64.

Spriggs E. The history of spirometry. Br J Dis Chest. 1978;72:165–80.

Sterk P, Fabbri L, Quanjer PH, et al. Standardized challenge testing with pharmacological, physical and sensitizing stimuli in adults. Eur Respir J. 1993;6(Suppl 16):53–83.

Taylor G, Walker J. Charles Harrison Blackley, 1820–1900. Clin Exp Allergy. 1973;3(2):103–8.

Tiffeneau R, Pinelli A. Air circulant et air captif dans l'exploration de la fonction ventilatrice pulmonaire. Paris Med. 1947;37(52):624–8.

Tiffeneau R, Beauvallet M. Epreuve de bronchoconstriction et de bronchodilation par aerosols. Bull Acad Med. 1945;129:165–8.

Van Slyke DD, Binger CA. The determination of lung volume without forced breathing. J Exp Med. 1923;37(4):457–70.

Weiss S, Robb GP, Ellis LB. The systemic effects of histamine in man: with special reference to the responses of the cardiovascular system. Arch Intern Med. 1932;49(3):360–96.

West JB. Translations in respiratory physiology. Stroudsburg: Dowden, Hutchinson & Ross; 1975.

West JB. The birth of clinical body plethysmography: it was a good week. J Clin Investig. 2004;114(8):1043–5.

West JB. History of respiratory mechanics prior to world war II. Compr Physiol. 2012;2:609–19.

West JB. Humphry Davy, nitrous oxide, the pneumatic institution, and the royal institution. Am J Phys Lung Cell Mol Phys. 2014;307(9):L661–7.

Westcott FH, Gillson RE. The treatment of bronchial asthma by inhalation therapy with vital capacity studies. J Allergy. 1943;14(5):420–7.

Wright BM. A miniature Wright peak-flow meter. Br Med J. 1978;2(6152):1627–8.

Wright BM, McKerrow CB. Maximum forced expiratory flow rate as a measure of ventilatory capacity. Br Med J. 1959;2(5159):1041–7.

Yernault J. The birth and development of the forced expiratory manoeuvre: a tribute to Robert Tiffeneau (1910-1961). Eur Respir J. 1997;10(12):2704–10.

Yernault JC, Pride N, Laszlo G. How the measurement of residual volume developed after Davy (1800). Eur Respir J. 2000;16(3):561–4.

Zavorsky GS, Hsia CC, Hughes JMB, et al. Standardisation and application of the single-breath determination of nitric oxide uptake in the lung. Eur Respir J. 2017;49(2):1600962.

Chapter 3
Breathing In: The Determinants of Lung Volume

Charles G. Irvin and Jack Wanger

3.1 Introduction

The size of the lung is critical to the optimal function of the respiratory system and provides a protection from lung disease. Humans have about 20–30% more lung volume than is necessary for maximal exercise; it is speculated that the additional lung volume serves as a reserve so that the loss of lung volume that would most commonly occur during a bout of pneumonia would be mitigated. One measure of lung volume, the forced vital capacity (FVC), has been shown repeatedly to be the best predicator of poor health or mortality and therefore should be the mainstay of the investigation of disease or lung function. One of the goals for this chapter is to provide the reader with the fundamental knowledge to better utilize the measurement of lung volume in their clinical practice.

An important use of lung volume measurement clinically is to distinguish between a process that resides in the airways and a process that resides in the parenchyma, that is, obstructive disease versus restrictive disease. In patients with an obstructive presentation, there is evidence of increased lung volume, whereas patients with a restrictive process will have decreased lung volume. The measurement of the subdivisions of the total lung volume is often critical in establishing prognosis and diagnosis of patients presenting with vague respiratory complaints such as dyspnea, wheeze, or cough. Considering FVC in isolation of the forced expiratory volume in 1 s (FEV_1) or sending the patients for lung volume measurements can often be extremely illuminating. Indeed, it has been shown that lung volume measurements significantly add to the assessment and diagnosis of

C. G. Irvin (✉)
Department of Medicine, Vermont Lung Center,
University of Vermont Larner College of Medicine, Burlington, VT, USA
e-mail: charles.irvin@med.uvm.edu

J. Wanger
Pulmonary Function Testing and Clinical Trials Consultant, Rochester, MN, USA

D. A. Kaminsky, C. G. Irvin (eds.), *Pulmonary Function Testing*,
Respiratory Medicine, https://doi.org/10.1007/978-3-319-94159-2_3

patients presenting with nonspecific respiratory symptoms. It is surprising that these additional tests are not more frequently utilized in investigating patients attending a specialty clinic as illustrated by the cases at the end of this chapter. Hopefully by the end of this chapter, the reader will be also inclined to use lung volume assessments more often in investigating pulmonary or suspected pulmonary disease.

3.2 Definitions: Volumes and Capacities

The total lung volume can be divided into subdivisions, which can be grouped into volumes and capacities. The lung volumes and capacities are useful for detecting, characterizing, and quantifying most lung diseases (Table 3.1). Sometimes these are referred to as static lung volumes and capacities, as they are usually determined in absence of airflow or at points of zero flow.

There are four lung volumes: residual volume (RV), expiratory reserve volume (ERV), tidal volume (TV or V_T), and lastly the inspiratory reserve (IRV). There are also four lung capacities: inspiratory capacity (IC), functional residual capacity (FRC), vital capacity (VC), and total lung capacity (TLC). The capacities are the sum of two or more volumes; see Fig. 3.1. Spirometry can only be used to measure VC, TV, IC, and ERV but lung volumes are rarely used beyond the measurement of FVC, whereas TLC, FRC, and RV must be measured with another technique. These other lung volume techniques measure RV or TLC as there is the volume of gas that can not be expire (RV) or does not communicate with the atmosphere. As we will see, some of these measurements of lung volumes/capacities are more useful than others.

3.3 The Lung Volumes

Residual volume (RV) This is the volume of gas left in the lung after a full and complete expiration. The term residual comes from the fact that no matter how hard one tries there is always air left in the lung because the thorax can only be distorted so much. An increase in RV is characteristic of airway disease and gas trapping. When expressed as a ratio to the TLC, the RV/TLC in a healthy individual is approximately 20–25%, but this ratio rises with aging. It is often the first abnormality in

Table 3.1 Indications for measurement of lung volumes

Detection of lung disease
Assessment of disease severity
Distinguish between obstruction and restriction
Detection of trapped gas
Determination of airway closure or collapse

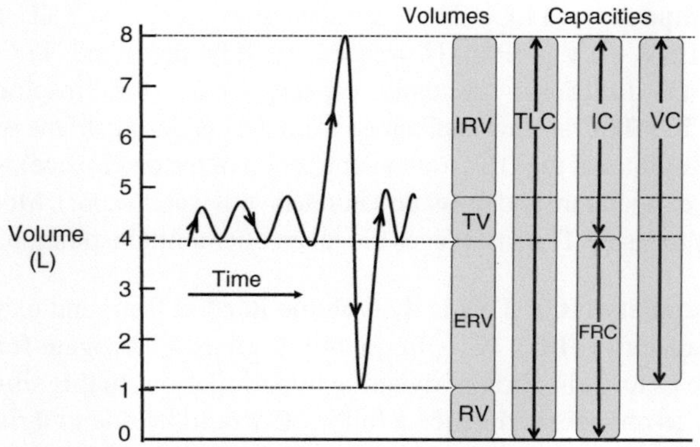

Fig. 3.1 Lung volumes and capacities. A spirogram (volume vs. time) of an individual who is first breathing quietly (reading from left to right), then takes a maximal inhalation to total lung capacity (TLC), then exhales slowly to residual volume (RV), and then returns to quiet breathing. On the right are the four lung volumes: inspiratory reserve volume (IRV), tidal volume (TV), expiratory reserve volume (ERV), and RV. Lung capacities are the combination of lung volumes and are as follows: TLC shown here as RV + ERV + TV + IRV, inspiratory capacity (IC) shown here as TV + IRV, functional residual capacity (FRC) shown here as ERV + RV, and vital capacity shown here as IRV + TV + ERV

peripheral lung disease and with treatment the last index of airway disease or gas trapping to resolve. If a patient makes a maximal expiratory effort, the elevations of RV are pathognomonic for airway disease, whereas a low RV is unusual and would almost always indicate a restrictive disorder.

Tidal volume (TV or VT) This is the volume that a person moves in and out during quiet, normal breathing. Since so many things affect the size of the TV, it has little, if any, diagnostic utility.

Expiratory reserve volume (ERV) This is the volume that is expired from the end of a normal breath. In obese patients, it is the first volume to fall, and in an obese patient who has lung disease, it can be quite small.

Inspiratory reserve volume (IRV) This is the largest volume that can be inhaled after a normal breath at the end of inspiration. As the V_T is so variable, the IRV too has little clinical utility except during exercise where the fall in IRV is associated with hyperinflation and dyspnea, especially as it approaches the TLC.

3.4 Lung Capacities

Lung capacities are simply defined as various combinations of each of the four lung volumes (e.g., FRC = ERV+ RV). Starting from the top:

Total lung capacity (TLC) This is the sum total of all four volumes (TLC = RV + ERV + TV + IRV). However, as will be described, TLC is usually the measurement of functional residual capacity plus the inspiratory capacity (TLC = FRC + IC). TLC is what is obtained from the single-breath measurement of VA during the measuremnt of the DL_{CO} (after subtraction of the dead space) when expressed as BTPS (body temperature and pressure saturated with water vapor). Most radiographic techniques also measure TLC as images are taken after a full inspiration.

Inspiratory capacity (IC) This is the volume inhaled from end expiration (FRC) to total lung capacity (TLC). IC is frequently used as a surrogate for FRC such as during exercise as an indication of dynamic hyperinflation. In this situation the TLC is assumed not to change, and hence a fall in IC would be due to a rise in FRC.

Vital capacity (VC) This is the total volume that can be moved in and out of the lung or the volume between TLC and RV. This can be done slowly (SVC) or with a maximal inspiration to the TLC followed by a forced (FVC) exhalation from TLC all the way to RV. This is the most common measurement of lung volume and in many ways the most significant. Keep in mind the VC is determined by the factors that affect TLC and RV.

Functional residual capacity (FRC) This is the volume that remains in the lung at the end of a normal tidal volume excursion or end inspiration. FRC is equal to ERV + RV. When measured, the FRC is the only lung volume measure that does not require effort. During quiet breathing, it is the equilibrium point of the respiratory system (see below).

3.5 Physiological Underpinnings of Lung Volumes

The volume of gas within the lung at any one moment is determined by (1) the overall size of the thorax which is estimated by considering the demographic measures of age, sex, race, and height, (2) the elastic forces to which the lung is subjected, and (3) the intrinsic elastic properties of the lung and thorax.

The elastic forces are those generated by the distortion of either the chest wall by the respiratory muscles or the intrinsic recoil of the lung and chest wall. The equilibrium point for the chest wall usually occurs at a volume above FRC. The normal chest wall, when there is little or no respiratory muscle activity, has an equilibrium point at approximately 66% of TLC, but above that volume, the chest wall resists further inflation. Below that point, the chest wall assists inflation because of the outward recoil. The lung on the other hand is quite different.

The elastic forces of the lung are deflationary and always generate an elastic force that resists inflation and assists deflation. Indeed, as one may recall from gross anatomy, when the lung is removed from the thorax or when the chest wall integrity is compromised by a penetrating wound, the lung will completely collapse. Hence, the elastic force of the normal lung is always an inward deflating force. The elastic recoil of the lung is largely linear up to about 80% of TLC, and then the recoil markedly increases as the inhaled volume nears TLC. The elastic recoil of the lung also varies by the previous changes in volume, which is called the lung volume history. Lung recoil is higher on inspiration and falls after the lung is inflated to TLC; this lung volume history dependence is called hysteresis. As a result elastic recoil can be highly variable and dependent on what lung volume the patient is breathing at and whether one is considering inflation or deflation.

The combination of the chest wall and lung that is referred to as the respiratory system leads to a pressure volume (PV) relationship for the combined system that has a slope (compliance or its inverse elastance) that is lower than that of the individual parts (Fig. 3.2). To better understand this increase in elasticity of the combination of two less elastic components, consider a toy balloon (lung) that is inserted inside of a second balloon (chest wall). This combined system is more difficult to inflate, i.e., it is stiffer. The point at which the PV relationship of the respiratory system crosses zero occurs at only one lung volume, and at this point, the outward (inflation) forces are equal and opposite to the inward (deflating) forces – this equilibrium point sets the FRC during quiet breathing. At lung volumes above this point, the net forces cause the lung to deflate and aid in normal expiration. At volumes below this point, the net forces favor inflation. A good example of this is the change in FRC that occurs during exercise where the FRC falls and the inflationary forces assist inspiration. Thus at any given lung volume, the static forces which cause inflation and deflation are determined by a balance between the lung and chest wall and thus set the FRC of the normal person.

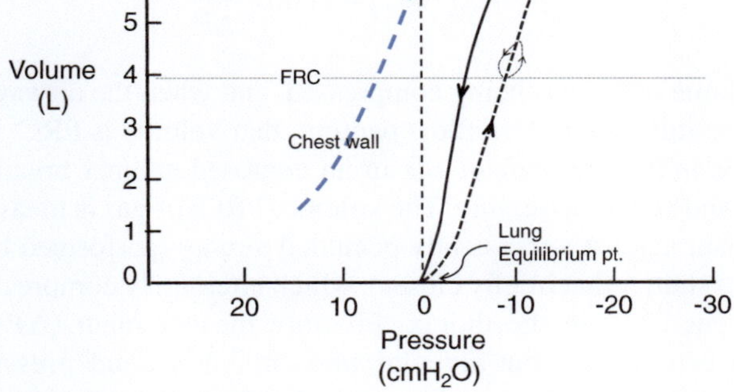

Fig. 3.2 The pressure-volume (PV) relationship. Depicted are the pressure-volume relationships of the chest wall (blue dashed line) and lung (black lines both dashed for inspiration and solid for expiration). Pressures to the right of zero are negative and resist inflation, whereas pressures to the left are positive and support inflation. Lung: the PV relationship for quiet breathing is depicted by the small loop (highly dashed line). Notice the looping of the PV curve of the lung from RV to TL – this is called hysteresis. The expiratory limb shows the typical curvilinear PV relationship where maximal recoil occurs at TLC. Chest wall: The chest wall PV, on the other hand, has an outward recoil at lung volumes below its equilibrium point at ~60% of TLC

3.6 Measuring Lung Volume

There are numerous techniques for measuring lung volume. They range from the simple spirometer to the more complex whole-body plethysmograph or the CT scanner.

Spirometry Hutchinson described the spirometer in the mid-1800s to assist insurance companies in assessing risk as he correctly surmised that smaller lungs would put people at risk. The instrument was simple: an inverted cylinder or bell in a moat of water to provide a seal and reduced friction to movement when air was introduced and some means to measure displacement of the bell to measure the slow vital capacity. With subsequent improvements by the 1960s, the spirometer could then measure the FVC, and thus the FEV_1, with fidelity. However, the spirometer can only measure VC, IRV, ERV, and tidal volume as well as inspiratory capacity. As we will discuss later under interpretation, these lung volumes and capacities are not the complete picture and are not as useful diagnostically. The principle useful measurement that can be obtained with the spirometer is FVC and when done slowly one measures the SVC.

Body plethysmograph The whole-body plethysmograph (sometimes called body box) was developed in the 1960s to rapidly measure FRC, as the FRC and hence the RV cannot be measured with a spirometer. The principle is based on Boyle's law that states

$$\mathrm{P1V1} = \mathrm{P2V2}$$

And solved for V1(FRC) (see Appendix):

$$Vtg\left(\mathrm{FRC}\right) = \mathrm{Patm} \times \frac{\Delta V}{\Delta P}$$

V_{TG} is volume of the gas being compressed, and when the airway is occluded at end expiration during rapid, shallow panting, that volume is FRC. The essence of the technique is that the patient sits in an enclosed cabinet breathing through a mouthpiece and shutter assembly. The volume (FRC) of gas is measured by having the patient pant against a transiently occluded airway (performed by blocking the airway with a shutter that briefly closes), which alternately compresses and decompresses the gas (ΔV) in the thorax. Pressure measurement (ΔP) at the mouth provides an estimate of the alveolar pressure. A second pressure transducer measures the pressure swings within the body plethysmograph during the panting maneuver and estimates the volume (ΔV) change being applied to the system. When the shutter closes at end expiration, that volume is FRC but often is referred to as V_{tg} to indicate a body plethysmograph was used to measure FRC. The measurements made with the plethysmograph are quick and very accurate. It must be kept in mind however that this volume is measuring all the gas in the thorax whether or not it is communicating with the atmosphere. So in a patient with emphysema and a large non-communicating bullae, the V_{tg} or FRC measures that gas volume as well.

Inert gas dilution – Another common way to measure FRC and RV is inert gas dilution. A considerable number of different techniques that use inert gas dilution have been developed over the years, but the basic principle is the same. For illustration let us consider the closed-circuit breathing technique. During normal breathing the patient is switched into a breathing circuit, which contains oxygen and an inert gas such as helium or neon, precisely at end exhalation, which is FRC. As the patient breathes in the circuit, the concentration of the inert gas falls as the inert gas is diluted by the total volume to which it is now mixing with, which is FRC plus the known volume of the breathing circuit. The concentration of the gas is measured until the fall in inert gas concentration reaches a minimum. Using a simple equation:

$$C1V1 = C2V2$$

where V_1 is FRC, C_1 is the known concentration of the gas at the start of dilution maneuvers, C_2 is the measured inert gas concentration at the end of the dilution period, and V_2 is the known volume of the breathing circuit plus FRC. FRC (V1) is then calculated by

$$V1 = \frac{C2V2}{C1}$$

For example, if C1 was diluted to C2 by a total volume of 5 L, and the breathing circuit is known to have a volume of 2 L, then FRC must be 3 L.

Another common approach is to breathe oxygen and measure the nitrogen in an open-circuit configuration – the nitrogen washout technique. The washout technique has the advantage of also measuring ventilation inhomogeneity that is covered in Chap. 4. A variant of the multiple breath technique is the measurement of alveolar volume (VA) that is obtained during the measurement of DL_{CO}, as described in Chap. 5. This is a single breath, 10-s breath-hold measure of TLC. This measurement is quick (~10 s) and is measured as part of a test that is already being done. The TLC measured as VA is usually within about 200 mL of the TLC measured by other means in normal persons free of lung disease. See the cases at the end of this chapter for some examples.

There are two disadvantages of the gas dilution/washout techniques. First, rebreathing or washout measurements are slow as it takes time to dilute the inert tracer gas, especially if there is airway obstruction, as seen, for example, in a patient with severe COPD where a complete dilution really never occurs. If one measures the time to a plateau of gas concentration, this is another way to measure ventilation homogeneity. As time for complete inert gas can be quite long, this slows patient flow through the laboratory. Second, these techniques measure only gas volumes in communication with the atmosphere. So in the patient described above with COPD and large bullae, the FRC (or TLC) measured with gas dilution may be significantly underestimated.

Imaging techniques Another means of measuring lung volumes is with X-ray or CT imaging. The plain film X-ray technique requires a PA and lateral film and a means of measuring area. The CT scanner has the advantage that voxels are already a volume measurement but requires eliminating the non-air-containing areas. There are several problems with using imaging techniques that include the cost of equipment, radiation exposure, the inconstant way the volume is maintained while the image is acquired, and the volume with CT that is measured in the supine position, whereas X-ray is standing at a TLC breath-hold. Like the body plethysmograph, the CT scan measures the total gas volume in the thorax whether or not it communicates with the atmosphere. There are often issues with patient effort and coordination that can make gathering adequate images difficult.

3.7 Interpretation

The interpretation of measurements of lung volume is predicated on a strong understanding of the physiologic determinants of the volumes and capacities of the respiratory system that were covered above. Measurements of lung volume provide indirect information about the elastic resistance (recoil) to distension generated by the lung parenchyma or chest wall, which is also important when considering maximal expiratory airflow. Lung volume is also a highly significant determinate of large airway resistance and smooth muscle shortening, both of which can influence bronchodilation and constriction. The influence of lung volume on airway resistance is through the tethering effects of the alveolar walls via their attachments to the airway wall. So as lung volume increases airways resistance falls, unless disease leads to an uncoupling of those parenchymal attachments, whether transitionally or permanently. See Fig. 7.6.

From the standpoint of generating both clinical insight and an interpretation of a patient's results, it is useful to consider three boundaries of lung volume that have the most clinical utility: TLC, FRC, and RV (see Fig. 3.3). While the magnitude of these boundaries is, in part, determined by common underlying factors, including height, age, sex, and race, the proportion of FRC or RV to TLC (FRC/TLC or RV/TLC) is remarkably consistent between normal individuals. This fact makes FRC/TLC and RV/TLC, much like FEV_1/FVC and especially useful in patients where the reference or predicted equations are not robust.

TLC is the maximum possible volume of the lung and is largely determined by the ability of the respiratory muscles to distort the chest wall (ribcage and abdomen) to its maximum configuration. The three factors that determine TLC are (1) respiratory muscle coordination and strength, (2) elastic recoil of the chest wall, and (3) elastic recoil of the lung. For example, a low TLC could be the result of increased stiffness of the lung and/or chest wall or respiratory muscle weakness or less than a maximal effort by the patient. As another example, a high TLC could be due to chest wall remodeling such as the barrel chest feature of chronic severe emphysema, loss of elastic recoil, and/or excessive gas trapping.

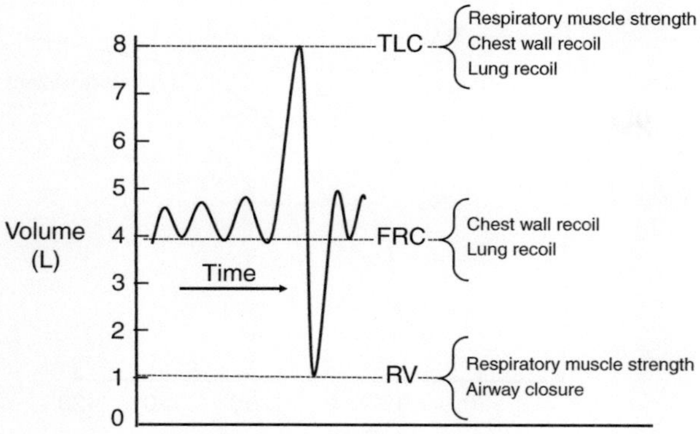

Fig. 3.3 Lung volume boundaries. There are three important lung boundaries. TLC is the maximal lung volume and is determined by the ability or strength of the respiratory muscles to distort the chest wall to its maximal configuration. Lung recoil resists that distortion. Hence, the three factors are respiratory muscle strength, chest wall recoil, and lung recoil. RV is the minimal configuration and in children is determined by the same factors as TLC. In adults however, RV is determined by respiratory muscle strength and mostly by airway closure. FRC in healthy individuals is determined by the balance of recoil between the lung and chest wall (see Fig. 3.4)

RV is the minimal possible volume of the lung. In normal adults, RV is about 20–25% of the TLC. In adults, the magnitude of the RV is largely determined by small airway closure as expiratory muscles distort the chest wall to its minimal configuration during expiration. While this is true for adults, in children the size of the RV is determined by the ability of the respiratory muscles to distort the chest wall to its minimal configuration; that is, airways do not close in normal children. Since the lung is always deflating, the lung recoil does not resist, so the major forces at play are respiratory muscle strength and chest wall elasticity. In the case of adults (>18 years), if adequate respiratory effort is exacted, RV is a measure of airway closure and by extension small airway function. Hence, an increase in RV, especially if there is a decrease in RV post-bronchodilator treatment, and providing the ERV maneuver has been done properly, is indicative of airway disease and its reversibility. On the other hand, a low RV usually occurs coincident with a low TLC or a restrictive disease.

FRC is the amount of air remaining in the lung at the end of a normal tidal breath and is the sum of the ERV and RV. In a healthy person, the FRC at end expiration is the balance between the outward recoil of the chest wall and the inward recoil of the lung (Fig. 3.4). Hence, FRC is influenced by those factors that affect the elastic properties of either the chest wall or the lung. In emphysema, for example, the FRC is increased because the loss of the inward deflationary forces allows the recoil of the chest wall to expand the thorax (up to its equilibrium point) and resets the FRC to a new equilibrium point for the chest wall and lung – the FRC is increased. In other cases, the tonic activity of the respiratory muscles can reset FRC higher due to

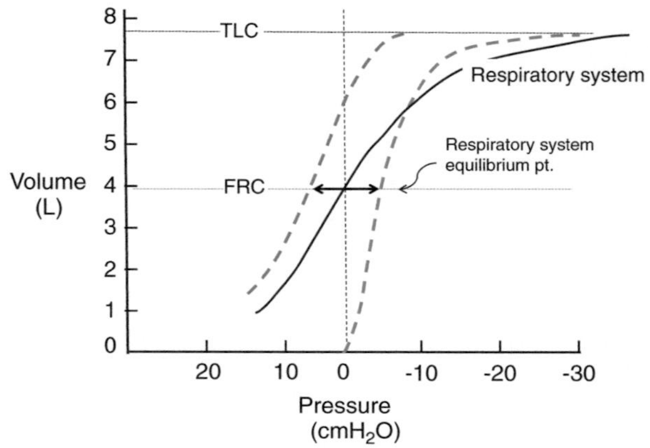

Fig. 3.4 Pressure-volume relationship of the respiratory system – determinants of FRC. The respiratory system is the sum of the elasticity of the chest wall and lung (shown as heavy, blue distal lines). Notice how the respiratory system elastance is higher and compliance is lower than either the chest wall or lung. FRC is the one point along the PV curve of the respiratory system where the inflationary force of the chest wall is equal and opposite of the lung, i.e., FRC is a balance between the chest wall and lung recoil

the increase in outward, inflationary force. To experience that, try breathing at a new, elevated FRC. You do that by maintaining tonic activity of inspiratory muscles throughout expiration, or in other words, you stiffen the chest wall and increase outward, inflationary pressures. Lastly, FRC can increase due to expiratory airflow limitation that results in an increased time constant such that not enough time is allowed for the volume of the lung to reach an equilibrium point because the drive to breathe causes the next inspiration. In the patient with severe COPD, for example, all three mechanisms (increased chest wall recoil, decreased lung recoil, and increased time constraints) can lead to profound increases in FRC.

3.8 A Generalized Approach to Interpretation of Lung Volumes

Here is provided a step-by-step series of assessments of lung volume and serves to set the stage for a written interpretation. Example interpretations are found with each of the four cases at the end of the chapter.

1. Assess the demographic information of the patient, noting age, sex, height (noting if especially tall or short), race, and weight. Age has a huge effect on lung volume, as volume increases until age 20 or so and then slowly decreases over the ensuing decades. Sex has less of an effect especially when corrected for height. Race, especially if the patient is black, needs to be taken into account. The single most important factor is height as this is a surrogate for the size of

the thorax and hence has the largest effect in determining maximal TLC. Weight has important effects. Waist size is a minor factor affecting FVC, but weight-to-height expressed as kg/cm causes FRC to fall if >0.5 and TLC to fall if >1.0. But even after taking all these factors into account, biological variability is still ±30%.

2. Assess patient effort. This may include inspiratory and expiratory maximal pressures (MEP, MIP) if determined, reproducibility of each effort and time dependence of efforts, compression artifacts on the MEFV, and perhaps – the most important – the technologist's comments. It is important to review all the effects to see how consistent the data are and to assess respiratory muscle function. If the effort is poor or if for any reason you suspect that the true TLC or RV was not reached, then the only reliable lung volume is the FRC. In this case, your ability to interpret the effects of disease can be very limited. Be sure to comment on effort and test quality in any interpretation that is written.
3. Assuming effort and the test quality are acceptable, start by assessing the TLC. If low, entertain a diagnosis of restriction. Physical examination of the chest or examination of the CT/X-ray images may prove to be adequate means to determine whether the chest wall is the source of restricted lung volumes or not. If the TLC is high, then assess RV/TLC and FRC/TLC. If either is high, then the diagnosis of airflow obstruction is supported.
4. The FRC is next on the list. If the chest wall assessment (#3 above) suggests normalcy, then FRC is an indirect assessment of lung elastic recoil. A decreased FRC is very common in the overweight and obese (BMI > 30 kg/m^2); indeed, if the FRC/TLC is not decreased, airway disease should be suspected. If the patient is not overweight/obese, then a reduced FRC is likely to indicate a restrictive process. An increase in FRC is typical of airflow obstruction with hyperinflation, although anxiety can also play a role, so assess consistency of the measurements.
5. Assessment of RV is largely an index to detect airway disease. Assuming the patient has given a good expiratory effort, elevated RV is indicative of increased airway closure, as the smaller, non-cartilaginous airways close at low lung volumes. In isolation, an increased RV is highly suggestive of small airway disease especially if the RV falls (>200 ml) with a bronchodilator treatment (and the FVC rises). An elevated RV/TLC ratio is often indicative of gas trapping, especially when associated with a low FEV_1/FVC ratio. RV is the last of the lung volumes to normalize with treatment and the first to rise in mild airway disease, e.g., the asymptomatic smoker. A low RV is highly suggestive of a restrictive process, but with extrapulmonary restriction, such as occurs in obesity or chest wall disease, the relative decrement in RV may be less than that in TLC, often yielding a mildly elevated RV/TLC ratio. Gas trapping and airway closure may also be suggested by a larger SVC compared to FVC, where the patient exerts maximal force and the airways close and more gas is trapped during the FVC maneuver.
6. Assess gas maldistribution, or poorly communicating gas, if the right measurements have been made. Poorly communicating gas is suggested when the TLC

measured by the body box (or imaging) is larger (>200 ml) than the TLC calculated by inert gas dilution measurements. For example, this is commonly seen in bullous disease, emphysema, or severe asthma. Gas maldistribution may also be seen when V_A measured during the single-breath DLCO is much lower than the TLC assessed by gas dilution or body plethysmography (VA/TLC < 0.85) (Table 3.2).

7. Mixed disease can be particularly difficult to assess depending on the relative contributions of each process. Keep in mind that most interstitial lung diseases are not totally isolated to the alveolar wall but also involve the airways, especially the small airways. Hence, in patients with ILD and a reduced TLC, one might encounter an increased RV/TLC or FRC/TLC. In patients with obesity and airway disease the FRC may not be elevated, but there is usually a rise in RV. The combination of low TLC, low FVC, normal FEV_1/FVC, and elevated RV/TLC has recently been termed "complex restriction." This pattern is commonly due to diseases involving impaired lung emptying, such as neuromuscular or chest wall disease, or subtle air trapping.
8. A final word about FVC. The FVC is determined by two boundaries, TLC and RV. A decreased FVC is due to a decrease in TLC, an increase in RV or both. A reduction in FVC and preserved FEV_1/FVC ratio does not suggest restriction until the FVC falls to 60% of predicted, and even then it is not all that helpful. Both in asthma and COPD, the FEV_1 is largely a reflection of the FVC, which in turn is determined in large part by RV. A reduced FVC, normal FEV_1/FVC, and chest size (TLC) that is not elevated may be suggestive of small airway disease. Meanwhile, a low FVC, normal FEV_1/FVC, and normal TLC has been termed "non-specific pattern," which is thought to be due to different causes, such as obstruction, restriction, chest wall disease, and neuromuscular weakness.
9. A final word about terms or words used in a written interpretation. First, there is no convention for terms to use for interpretation of lung volumes. The following are suggested terms and what they indicate (Table 3.3):
10. In cases where both lung volume and flow-volume relationships are determined, try starting with the lung volumes and then the changes in the lung volumes (>200 ml) with bronchodilator treatment. It has been shown that measurements of lung volumes add incremental information to the assessment of the patient with suggested but as of yet undiagnosed lung disease. Lung volume results also pull important insights into the pathophysiological processes at

Table 3.2 Lung volume patterns of change in common lung disease

	Obstruction	Restriction	Small airway disease
TLC	↑	↓	N
FRC	↑	↓ or ↔	N or sl↑
RV	↑	↓	↑
FRC/TLC	↑	N	N or sl↑
RV/TLC	↑	N	↑
SVC-FVC	↑ or ↔	N	N
TLC-VA	↑ or ↔	N	N or sl↑

N = normal; ↓ = reduced; ↑ = increased; ↔ = little change; sl = slightly

Table 3.3 Terms for interpretation of lung volumes

Restriction	Reduced TLC, FRC, or RV
Gas trapping	High RV/TLC
Gas trapping or	
Ventilation inhomogeneity	Low VA/TLC (<0.85)
Hyperinflation	Normal TLC with elevated FRC or FRC/TLC
Overdistension	Elevated TLC with elevated FRC/TLC and RV/TLC
Large lung volumes	Elevated TLC with normal FRC/TLC and RV/TLC

work and should be an essential part of any lung function assessment after spirometry.

3.9 Cases

Case 1

The patient is a 70-year-old white male who weighs 77 kg, is 182 cm in height, and has a BMI of 23 kg/m^2 with increasing dyspnea over the last several years. An initial spirometry showed:

Spirometry	Actual	Predicted	% predicted
FEV_1 (L)	0.99	3.51	28
FVC (L)	2.45	4.77	51
FEV_1/FVC (%)	40	74	54

The patient was referred for more complete lung function tests that included lung volume and DLCO. Lung volumes were measured with a plethysmograph as noted (V_{TG}).

	Actual	Predicted	% predicted
TLC (L)	8.96	7.43	121
FRC (V_{TG}) (L)	6.59	3.97	166
FRC/TLC	0.735	0.534	138
RV (L)	5.78	2.56	226
RV/TLC	0.656	0.345	190
SVC (L)	3.19	4.77	67
VA (L)	5.30	7.43	71

The lung volumes by plethysmograph are all very elevated, especially the RV. The SVC and VA, on the other hand, are reduced. In addition, the DLCO (not shown) is reduced (42% predicted) as well as sGaw (not shown) (19% predicted).

Interpretation: Patient effort was excellent yielding reproducible results. Lung volumes are abnormally elevated indicating overdistension, hyperinflation, and gas trapping. The marked differences between VA and TLC suggest the presence of large non-communicating air spaces consistent with emphysema and large bullae.

Note – The TLC-VA is greater than 3 l. Note also the difference between SVC and FVC suggesting dynamic airway collapse due to broken alveolar tethers typical of emphysema. The RV/TLC is greater than predicted also indicating gas trapping, and the FRC/TLC is elevated suggesting the interpretation of hyperinflation. The elevated TLC suggests overdistension and the presence of chronic COPD with remodeling of the chest wall. Subsequent CT scans showed large apical bullae. The patient has a 30 pack/year smoking history.

Case 2

The patient is a 70-year-old male with a 60 pack/year smoking history who presents with increasing dyspnea upon exertion. The patient is 175.5 cm in height, weighs 87 kg with a BMI of 28 kg/m^2. The following lung function tests were obtained. The technician noted that the patient gave a good effort and cooperation yielding reproducible results.

	Actual	Predicted	% predicted
FEV_1 (L)	1.27	2.95	43
FVC (L)	2.19	4.08	54
FEV_1/FVC (%)	58	73	79

While the spirometry is consistent with a diagnosis of COPD, further lung function tests were ordered.

	Actual	Predicted	% predicted
TLC (L)	4.02	6.86	59
FRC (V_{tg}) (L)	3.08	3.67	84
FRC/TLC	0.766	0.539	141
RV (L)	1.99	2.50	80
SVC (L)	2.03	4.08	50
VA (L)	3.32	6.86	48

The lung volumes are reduced or at the lower limits of normal. Given excellent patient effort, the low TLC is suggestive of a restrictive process especially given the low normal RV. However, there is probably some airway disease as well given the differences between SVC-FVC and TLC-VA. Consistent with that consideration is the elevated FRC that yields a high FRC/TLC. Unfortunately, the patient had taken a bronchodilator treatment an hour before testing, so post-bronchodilator results were not obtained. The DLCO was very low at 24% of predicted.

Interpretation: Excellent patient effort and cooperation. Reduced TLC and RV suggestive of a restrictive process. Airway disease is probably also present given the presence of hyperinflation and gas trapping.

Note – CT scan and biopsy revealed UIP thought to be associated with rheumatoid arthritis. Notice how if only the smoking history, low DLCO, and FEV_1 had been evaluated in this patient they would have been diagnosed with COPD. While there is some evidence of COPD, the predominant process is restrictive, so this is a good example of mixed disease.

Case 3

The patient is a 74-yery-old male with episodes of dyspnea especially with exercise. The patient is a non-smoker and has occupational exposures that suggest an occupational related process of unknown etiology. The patient is 169 cm in height and weighs 71 kg with a BMI of 25 kg/m². The patient gave good effort and cooperation as noted by the technologist's comments.

Spirometry	Actual	Predicted	% predicted
FEV_1 (L)	1.74	2.72	64
FVC (L)	2.02	3.60	56
FEV_1/FVC (%)	86	76	113

At first glance the spirometry suggests a restrictive disorder/muscle weakness. However, the peak flow was preserved within normal limits. Accordingly, more extensive tests were ordered.

Lung volumes	Actual	Predicted	% predicted
TLC (L)	3.20	6.34	50
FRC (V_{tg}) (L)	1.78	3.36	53
FRC/TLC	0.556	0.530	105
RV (L)	1.15	2.36	49
SVC (L)	2.05	56	56
VA (L)	2.88	6.34	45

All the lung volumes are moderately reduced. Note especially the reduced RV. The ratio FRC/TLC is near normal and no evidence of gas trapping (e.g., TLC-VA or SVC-FVC). In addition, the sGaw is high.

Interpretation: Patient gave good effort and the results were reproducible. A restrictive process is indicated with a reduction in all lung volumes, especially the TLC.

Note – CT scan confirmed the presence of ILD.

Case 4

The patient is a 30-year-old male who presents with vague respiratory symptoms. The patient is 71 cm in height and weighs 196 kg with a BMI of 27.5 kg/m². He is a non-smoker. The technologist reports that the results were reproducible.

Spirometry	Actual	Predicted	% predicted
FEV_1 (L)	2.22	4.56	48
FVC (L)	2.76	5.62	49
FEV_1/FVC (%)	80	81	99

The spirometry is suggestive of restrictive disease. More extensive lung function tests were ordered.

Lung volumes	Actual	Predicted	% predicted
TLC (L)	4.45	7.07	63
FRC (V_{tg}) (L)	2.75	3.48	79
RV (L)	1.66	1.68	99
SVC (L)	2.79	5.62	50
VA (L)	4.31	7.07	61

The TLC is mildly reduced with essentially normal RV and FRC that is at the lower limits of normal. The SVC and FVC are similar and the VA is similar to the TLC suggesting little in the way of gas trapping or dynamic airway collapse.

Some additional measurements are included.

	Actual	Predicted	% predicted
MEP (cmH20)	19	231	8
MIP (cmH20	−23	−125	18
MVV (L/min)	74	180	41

MEP: maximum expiratory pressure. MIP maximum inspiratory pressure. MVV: maximum voluntary ventilation.

In addition, upon reinspection the flow-volume loops (not shown) are variable and lack a well-defined peak flow. The measurements of airflow limitation assessed by the plethysmograph (not shown) showed an sGaw of 0.15 or 73% or predicted.

Interpretation. Patient's efforts were good but lack reproducibility with evidence of a restrictive process with a low TLC. Low maximal pressures and a low TLC suggest respiratory muscle weakness – consider a myopathy.

Note – The patient was referred to the neurology service and ultimately determined to have myotonic dystrophy.

Appendix

Boyle's law states that the volume of gas in a container varies inversely with the pressure within a container, assuming constant temperature. Thus, under initial conditions of pressure (P1) and volume (V1), the product equals a constant such that under new conditions P2 and V2, the following equation applies:

$$P1V1 = P2V2$$

So if P2 is a situation where a step change in P occurs (ΔP), then V2 is the new volume which is smaller, i.e., compression. During a panting maneuver against an obstruction airway (closed container), no air moves in or out, and therefore mouth pressure (Pmouth) approximates alveolar pressure (Palv); the pressure P2 and volume V2 in the lung will vary slightly by ΔP and ΔV with respect to the initial pressure P1 and volume V1 in the lung; hence,

$$\text{P1V1} = (\text{P1} + \Delta P) \times (\text{V1} + \Delta V)$$

If the obstruction is generated by a shutter closure right at end expiration or FRC (Vtg), then V1 becomes FRC and P1 is atmospheric pressure just before the shutter is closed. We therefore can solve for V1. First, the terms of the equation are rearranged:

$$\text{P1}\Delta V + \text{V1}\Delta P + \Delta V \Delta P = 0$$

Then, V1 is defined:

$$\text{V1}(\text{FRC}) = -\frac{\Delta V}{\Delta P} \times (\text{P1} + \Delta P)$$

Now we make the assumption that ΔP is very small compared to P1 + ΔP, so that P1 + ΔP is approximated by P1 alone:

$$\text{V1} = -\text{P1} \times \frac{\Delta V}{\Delta P}$$

To solve for V1, we need to know P1 (which is atmospheric pressure-Patm) and $\Delta V/\Delta P$. The latter is simply the inverse slope of the pressure tracing made during the closed-shutter panting maneuver that plots Pmouth vs. Pbox, because changes in Pmouth approximate changes in Palv (ΔP) and changes in Pbox are calibrated to measure the small volume changes in the lung (ΔV). Plugging in the inverse slope and the atmospheric pressure (P1) into the equation (and ignoring the sign) yields V1, which is FRC:

$$\text{Vtg}(\text{FRC}) = \text{Patm} \times \frac{\Delta V}{\Delta P}$$

Strictly speaking, V1 is actually thoracic gas volume (V_{tg}), since it includes all compressible gas at that moment, and the shutter may or may not have been closed precisely at FRC. Therefore, in practice one adds or subtracts the volume distance away from true FRC as determined by the position of the stable, end-expiratory lung volume recorded during the previous tidal breathing preceding the panting maneuver. This correction is sometimes called the “switch-in volume,” because it was the volume error created by switching to closed-shutter panting should that occur not precisely at FRC. When measured in a body plethysmograph, this corrected FRC is commonly reported as V_{tg} or TGV.

Selected References

Bancalari E, Clausen J. Pathophysiology of changes in absolute lung volumes. Eur Respir J. 1998;12(1):248–58.

Berry CE, Wise RA. Interpretation of pulmonary function tests: Issues and controversies. Clin Rev Aller Immunol. 2009;37:173–80.

Brown R, Leith DE, Enright PL. Multiple breath helium dilution measurement of lung volumes in adults. Eur Respir J. 1998;11(1):246–55.

Clay RD, Iyer VN, Reddy DR, Siontis B, Scanlon PD. The "complex restrictive" pulmonary function pattern: Clinical and radiologic analysis of a common but previously undescribed restrictive pattern. Chest. 2017;152:1258–65.

Coates AL, Peslin R, Rodenstein D, Stocks J. Measurement of lung volumes by plethysmography. Eur Respir J. 1997;10(6):1415–27.

Decramer M, Janssens W, Derom E, Joos G, Ninane V, Deman R, et al. Contribution of four common pulmonary function tests to diagnosis of patients with respiratory symptoms: a prospective cohort study. Lancet Respir Med. 2013;1(9):705–13.

Dykstra BJ, Scanlon PD, Kester MM, Beck KC, Enright PL. Lung volumes in 4774 patients with obstructive lung disease. Chest. 1999;115(1):68–74.

Hyatt RE, Cowl CT, Bjoraker JA, Scanlon PD. Conditions associated with an abnormal nonspecific pattern of pulmonary function tests. Chest. 2009;135(2):419–24.

Irvin CG. Lung volume: a principle determinant of airway smooth muscle function. Eur Respir J. 2003;22(1):3–5.

Irvin CG. Pulmonary physiology in asthma and COPD. In: Barnes PJ, Drazen JM, Rennard SI, Thomson NC, editors. 2nd ed. Boston: Elsevier Academic Press; 2009.

Irvin CG. Development, structure and physiology in normal lung and in asthma. In: Nguyen T, Scott J, editors. Middleton's allergy. New York: Elsevier, Inc.; 2013. Chapter 45.

Irvin CG. Lung function in asthma Up-to-Date https://www.uptodate.com/contents/pulmonary-function-testing-in-asthma 2018.

Jones RL, Nzekwu MM. The effects of body mass index on lung volumes. Chest. 2006;130(3):827–33.

Pellegrino R, Viegi G, Brusasco V, Crapo RO, Burgos F, Casaburi R, et al. Interpretative strategies for lung function tests. Eur Respir J. 2005;26(5):948–68.

Ruppel GL. What is the clinical value of lung volumes? Respir Care. 2012;57(1):26–35; discussion −8

Stocks J, Quanjer PH. Reference values for residual volume, functional residual capacity and total lung capacity. ATS Workshop on Lung Volume Measurements. Official Statement of The European Respiratory Society. Eur Respir J. 1995;8(3):492–506.

Wanger J, Clausen JL, Coates A, Pedersen OF, Brusasco V, Burgos F, et al. Standardisation of the measurement of lung volumes. Eur Respir J. 2005;26(3):511–22.

Whittaker LA, Irvin CG. Going to extremes of lung volume. J Appl Physiol. 2007;102(3):831–3.

Chapter 4
Distribution of Air: Ventilation Distribution and Heterogeneity

Gregory King and Sylvia Verbanck

4.1 Ventilatory Dead Space

4.1.1 Definition

Ventilatory dead space is the proportion of ventilation that goes to non-gas-exchanging compartments of the lung. Therefore, dead space occurs anatomically by the absence of alveolar structures in a bronchial/bronchiolar airway wall, i.e., the conducting airways. These conducting airways form the anatomical dead space, which is approximately 150 ml in healthy adults (~ 2 ml/kg). Ventilatory dead space can also be created by functional changes, when pulmonary capillary blood flow ceases to a ventilated part of the lung, i.e., when ventilation is present but no pulmonary perfusion so that the ventilation/perfusion ratio is infinite, i.e., $\dot{V}/\dot{Q} = \infty$ (because $\dot{Q} = 0$). This is thus the physiological dead space and is larger than anatomical dead space.

4.1.2 Measurement

Total ventilation (minute ventilation - $\dot{V}_E$) = alveolar ventilation ($\dot{V}_A$) + dead space ventilation ($\dot{V}_D$). Alveolar ventilation, being the part of ventilation that goes to perfused alveoli, is responsible for the exchange of CO_2. Hence $\dot{V}_D$ is measured by

G. King (✉)
Woolcock Institute of Medical Research, The University of Sydney, Sydney, NSW, Australia
e-mail: gregory.king@sydney.edu.au

S. Verbanck
Respiratory Division, University Hospital, UZ Brussel, Brussels, Belgium
e-mail: sylvia.verbanck@uzbrussel.be

D. A. Kaminsky, C. G. Irvin (eds.), *Pulmonary Function Testing*,
Respiratory Medicine, https://doi.org/10.1007/978-3-319-94159-2_4

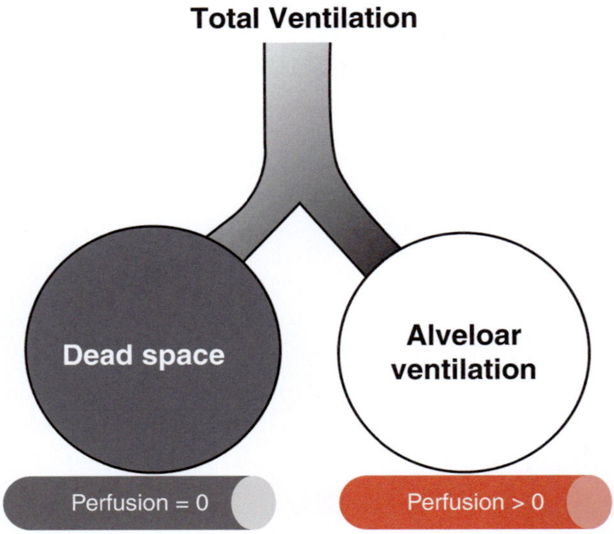

Fig. 4.1 Alveolar and dead space ventilation are represented by the two compartments. Dead space ventilation, by definition, has no pulmonary perfusion to it; therefore the CO_2 partial pressure is the same as the inspired air. Alveolar ventilation, by definition, has a measurable perfusion; therefore, its CO_2 partial pressure is the same as mixed venous. During exhalation, "dead space" gas and "alveolar ventilation" gas mix together and can be sampled at the mouth (mixed expired gas). If $\dot{V}_A$ and $\dot{V}_D$ are equal, then mixed expired CO_2 would be half that of alveolar CO_2. This proportionality thus allows calculation of $\dot{V}_D$

efficiency of CO_2 clearance from the lungs. If dead space is high, then efficiency becomes low and total ventilation ($\dot{V}_E$) will clear less CO_2 than when efficiency is high (low $\dot{V}_D$). This can be measured by looking at the difference between alveolar CO_2 and "mixed expired CO_2," the latter being a mixture of both alveolar ventilation (high CO_2 content) and dead space ventilation (negligible CO_2 content). Therefore, as dead space ventilation increases, the difference between CO_2 content in alveoli and "mixed expired CO_2" will also proportionally increase (see Fig. 4.1).

Thus $\dot{V}_D$ can be estimated by measuring the difference between alveolar CO_2 (estimated by arterial CO_2), and mixed expired CO_2 as per a simplification of the Bohr equation:

$$\text{Physiological dead space}: \frac{V_D}{V_T} = \frac{\text{PaCO}_2 - P(\text{mixed expired CO}_2)}{\text{PaCO}_2}$$

The estimation implies that ventilation perfusion mismatch will also increase dead space. That is, in lung units where ventilation is high relative to perfusion (high $\dot{V}/\dot{Q}$), alveolar CO_2 in these units will be low relative to units where $\dot{V}/\dot{Q}$ is ideal, i.e., a ratio around 1. Therefore, ventilation to those units with high $\dot{V}/\dot{Q}$ will contribute to physiological dead space.

4.1.3 Determinants in Health and Disease

Physiological dead space is increased in many common respiratory diseases, particularly obstructive airway diseases and pulmonary vascular diseases. Gas exchange studies using the multiple inert gas elimination test, also known as MIGET studies, show increased ventilatory dead space and high $\dot{V}/\dot{Q}$ in asthma and COPD. The mechanisms presumably include local vascular constriction and destruction due to inflammation and remodeling, with or without secondary pulmonary hypertension. In pulmonary vascular diseases, the decrease in pulmonary vascular blood flow may be heterogeneously distributed, and if ventilation to these units is not reduced to maintain ideal $\dot{V}/\dot{Q}$ by constricting the subtending airways, then physiological dead space will increase.

4.1.4 Clinical Relevance

In obstructive airway diseases, the concept of physiological dead space may be useful for understanding the impact of breathing pattern to gas exchange, particularly in severe disease and acute and severe exacerbations. Low tidal volumes and lung hyperinflation will have profound consequences on alveolar ventilation (hence gas exchange) when dead space is large. Dead space to tidal volume ratios (V_D/V_T) will increase with decreasing tidal volumes (given the fixed volume of the dead space). Hence the goals of treatment are to optimize tidal volumes and respiratory rate and reduce lung hyperinflation (which are all closely related to each other) by pharmacologic and ventilatory support strategies.

4.2 Ventilation Distribution

4.2.1 Definition

Ventilation distribution describes the range of ventilation that occurs within the lung. Ventilation in the lung is not homogenous, even in health. Thus ventilation being uneven throughout the lungs has been described as either "inhomogeneous" or "heterogeneous." The terms are interchangeable but heterogeneity has been the most commonly used term in research publications on ventilation distribution. The distribution of ventilation within the lungs can be characterized in terms of how much of the lung is affected by "low" or "poor" ventilation (functional) and in terms of where in the lungs those poorly ventilating units are located (topographical).

The distribution of ventilation, in a functional sense, can be measured using inert gases, i.e., gases that are not absorbed by the lung. The principle is that when ventilation is uneven or heterogeneous, taking a breath of an inert gas will result in inert gas concentrations that will differ in different parts of the lung. These can then be measured in situ (by imaging techniques) or at the mouth during the subsequent exhalation (by washout techniques).

The most fundamental way by which inert gas concentrations can differ in different lung units (see definition of lung units below) after inhalation is when there are differences in the volume of alveolar gas in lung units at the start of the breath (initial volume), as well as differences in the volume of inert gas that reaches them. This ratio, i.e., inspired volume/initial volume of lung, is named the "specific ventilation" (SV). Assuming complete dilution of inspired inert gas volume into the gas volume of the lungs, the alveolar concentration of the inert gas can be calculated by the dilution factor, which equals the ratio of inspired volume to inspired volume + initial volume. Hence, alveolar concentration of the inspired inert gas and specific ventilation are directly related (alveolar concentration equals the ratio SV/(SV + 1)). In a hypothetical lung with no ventilation heterogeneity, the specific ventilation in all parts of the lung would then correspond to the subject's pre-inspiratory volume (usually RV or FRC) and the volume of inert gas inhaled; the alveolar concentration (hence SV) would be identical everywhere in the lung. Therefore, according to this simple dilution model, the differences in alveolar concentrations of inert gases between different regions of the lung reflect differences in regional ventilation, and so the distribution of the inert gas (or "marker" gas) is a way to measure ventilation heterogeneity.

Another important concept of gas flow within the lung that is fundamental to understanding the determinants of ventilation distribution is that there is both convective gas flow (gas transport along pressure gradients) and diffusive gas flow (gas transport along concentration gradients). The specific ventilation model implicitly assumes that all lung units are supplied with inspired gas by convective flow and that dilution of inspired with the pre-inspiratory alveolar gas is instantaneous due to rapid diffusive equilibration within each lung unit. Considering that in the human lung, convective gas transport is taken over by diffusive gas transport around branching generation 15, the lung units for which gas concentrations reflect differences in specific ventilation are bigger than the fundamental gas exchanging units of the lung, i.e., the acini, which are about 0.1 cm^3 at FRC. Within these acinar units that are small in volume but large in number, a complex mechanism of interplay between convection and diffusion also generates alveolar concentration differences between intra-acinar air spaces.

Most of the present chapter will be dedicated to the inert gas concentration differences arising from specific ventilation differences between lung units larger than acini.

4.2.2 Determinants in Health

The topographical distribution of the inert gas concentrations can be measured using three-dimensional ventilation imaging techniques, which include single photon emission computed tomography (SPECT), positron emission tomography

(PET), and magnetic resonance imaging with hyperpolarized helium3 (H3 MRI) or Xenon-129. Other imaging techniques measure ventilation distribution in a given plane, such as oxygen-enhanced MRI (called specific ventilation imaging, SVI) using 100% oxygen breathing based on the rate that oxygen fills the alveoli, or electrical impedance tomography (EIT) using changes in electrical impedance at the chest wall surface to infer ventilation distribution within the lung slice circumscribed by the electrode belt. Recently, registration algorithms have been applied to high-resolution CT images obtained at two lung inflations to produce three-dimensional maps of local SV. The above imaging modalities used to quantify ventilation heterogeneity in situ differ widely in terms of spatial resolution, due to limitations imposed by the radiation exposure that is deemed acceptable and by the technology of the radiation detectors themselves.

One of the very first ways in which the distribution of ventilation was measured was by scintigraphy, using small radiation counters placed onto the chest wall to measure the distribution of Xe133, a radioactive isotope of an inert gas. This and subsequent studies in different body postures confirmed the role of gravity in determining the distribution of ventilation in healthy subjects, with ventilation being greatest in the lowest lung units in the line of gravity. In the upright posture, specific ventilation is greatest at the lung base (highest inspired volume relative to initial volume) and decreases in the cranial direction.

The underlying basis of the gravitational gradient of regional ventilation in healthy human lungs is the lungs' elastic properties. The pressure volume curve (Fig. 4.2) should be well known to many. It has a curvilinear shape which describes the increase in lung elastic recoil pressure with increasing lung volume. Above FRC, as lung inflation progresses, elastic recoil also increases, relatively linearly, until at a certain volume above which pressure then increases rapidly for very little change in volume (the "genu" or "knee-bend"). This characteristic shape and pressure-volume behavior of the lung are responsible for the distribution of regional ventilation. Below FRC, the shape of the curve changes again and becomes flatter. This is due to airways being closed near RV. As the lung inflates, the airways open,

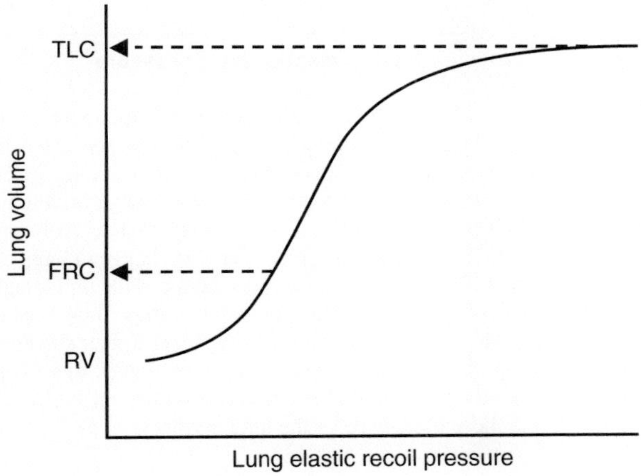

Fig. 4.2 Pressure-volume curve of the lung, measured between RV and TLC. Measurements are usually made using an esophageal balloon, placed near the lung base. However, it is assumed that the pressure-volume characteristics of the lungs are completely uniform

and the slope of the curve increases abruptly with these additional lung units now inflating.

It is assumed that the pressure-volume characteristics of the lung are uniform throughout its entirety. However, the lungs are "suspended" from the top of the chest cavity. At FRC, this then results in the lung tissue being more stretched at the top of the lungs, compared with lower down the lung. Greater distension of the lungs means that lung recoil pressure is greater at the top, i.e., the lung apex operates at a higher portion of the pressure volume curve (as arrowed in Fig. 4.3). Therefore, the top of the lungs is more distended, the alveolar walls are under greater tension, and this region of the lung is operating on the stiffer or "less-compliant" part of the pressure-volume curve. The gradient is approximately 0.2 $cmH_2O/l/s$ per cm of lung height. Therefore, in a lung of 25 cm in height, the transpulmonary pressure may vary from around 8 cmH_2O at the top of the lung to 3 cmH_2O at the bottom.

During a tidal inspiratory breath, the change in pressure across the lung (ΔP in Fig. 4.3) is uniform. The corresponding changes in regional lung volume (ΔV in Fig. 4.3) are greater at the bottom than the top; hence ventilation is greater at the bottom. The greater inert gas concentration in the bottom lung region is thus the combined result of a smaller regional volume at the beginning of inspiration (at FRC) and this region receiving a greater portion of the inhaled volume.

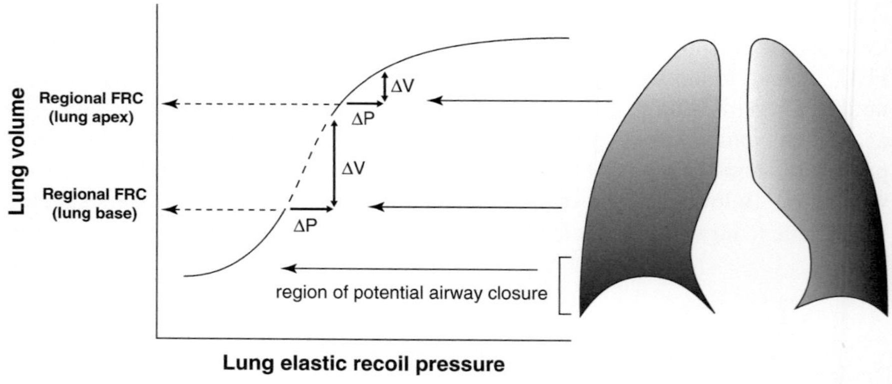

Fig. 4.3 Differences in regional inflation at FRC explain why ventilation differs on a gravitational basis in healthy lungs. The lung apex is subject to greater distending pressure, i.e., on a higher (and stiffer) part of the pressure-volume curve. Therefore, for any given change in pressure (ΔP) during a tidal breath, there is a smaller corresponding change in volume (ΔV or inspired volume) compared with lower in the lung, i.e., the change in lung volume at the base starting from FRC ("regional FRC (lung base)") is greater than the change in lung volume near the apex starting from FRC ("regional FRC (lung apex)"). The shading of the lung diagram demonstrates the gradient of ventilation along the gravitational gradient, during tidal breathing. Darker shading represents greater regional ventilation at the lung bases, and lighter shading represents less regional ventilation further up the lung. At the very base of the lungs, there is a zone where ventilation may be absent, due to airway closure. This zone is only apparent in older age where, during tidal breathing, ventilation to these basal parts of the lung is zero

Airway closure during tidal breathing can be a phenomenon of normal lungs, e.g., normal aging or in obese subjects. Airway closure occurs at the base because lung distending pressure is lowest there, and with decreasing elastic recoil pressure with increasing age, the part of the lung affected by closure increases.

4.2.3 Determinants in Disease

Most is known about changes in ventilation distribution in airway disease, and understanding and measurement of ventilation distribution are probably most relevant in airway diseases. Regional ventilation, i.e., the ventilation in a localized region of the lung, could be altered and differ from that of its neighbor, due to changes in the parenchyma or changes in the airways. In asthma and COPD, there are likely to be changes to both parenchyma and airways.

The inflammatory processes in COPD reduce the lung parenchyma's structure, leading to alveolar enlargement and loss of elastic recoil. There are similar changes in asthma but much subtler than in COPD. There are also changes in airway structure in both asthma and COPD, which alter their function. In asthma, changes in the structure of the airways affect the entire airway wall. Collectively, the changes are referred to as airway remodeling and involve changes to the airway smooth muscle, matrix including the reticular membrane underlying the mucosa which becomes characteristically thickened, mucous glands, and blood vessels. The net result is thickening of the airways and increased airway narrowing and airway closure. In COPD, airway remodeling also occurs, but this is different compared to asthma. There is obliteration of terminal and respiratory bronchioles as well as thinning of the airways walls of small airways.

The combined functional result of pathological changes to the lung parenchyma, its attachment to the airways and to the airways themselves, is airway narrowing and airway closure that is patchy and heterogeneous. Thus, the organization of regional ventilation that is seen in healthy lungs, which is predominantly gravity dependent, is now much more disorganized and "patchy" in distribution. The topographical distribution of ventilation has been well characterized by three-dimensional imaging studies in COPD and in asthma. The images from these studies indicate that there are patchy areas of non-ventilated and poorly-ventilated lung that are apparently randomly located. The pathophysiological basis of this functional abnormality is poorly understood, but functionally, it is likely to be due to the heterogeneous distribution of abnormalities of parenchyma and airways. Although the imaging studies provide a global description of the distribution of ventilation, and show that these regions can be large, subtending from large airways, the determinants of the distribution of ventilation can, in fact, also be large clusters of much smaller airways.

Ventilation in any given region of the lung is determined by the compliance of the lung tissue and resistance of its subtending airways. Multiplying resistance (R) and compliance (C) gives a term known as the time constant (τ), i.e., $\tau = R \times C$, and its unit is seconds. Those lung units that have long time constants, either from increased R or decreased C or both, ventilate poorly. Therefore, the increase in ventilation heterogeneity that is typical in asthmatic and COPD lungs can be conceptually described as having an increased range of time constants. This implies that there are some parts of the lungs that ventilate well (short time constants, high flows) and some parts that ventilate poorly (long time constants, low flows). The units might be anatomically co-located, which is what can be observed on ventilation scans, but they can also be scattered around the lungs and may be far apart. This concept that there are poorly ventilating units with long τ is important in understanding how inert gas washout tests are interpreted.

4.2.4 Measurement

Inert gas washout tests were developed 70 years ago with the description of the single-breath nitrogen washout test (SBNW). The SBNW test requires inspiration of 100% oxygen, which dilutes and washes out the nitrogen that is "resident" in the alveoli. Thus, SBNW tests have also been referred to as "resident gas" techniques, which distinguish them from inhaled inert gas tests (wash-in tests), e.g., with argon or helium. To highlight the effect of airway closure, a small bolus of argon or helium gas – instead of a full inspiration – is introduced at the start of the inhalation. The pure oxygen (or inert gases) can be inhaled from any pre-inspiratory volume and the inspired volume can also be varied. The effects of varying pre-inspiratory lung volume and inspired volume provide useful information on the nature of ventilation distribution. In the SBNW, after inhalation of pure oxygen, the subject exhales at a slow even rate, and the concentrations of the expired nitrogen gas are sampled continuously; a typical example of the expired N_2 concentration versus expired volume is in Fig. 4.4.

A useful way to understand the SNBW is by using a two-compartment concept of the lung, putting all the relatively well-ventilated lung units (high SV, short τ) into one functional compartment and the relatively poorly functioning units (low SV, long τ) into another. See Fig. 4.5. This results in two units with two averaged (and different) inert gas concentrations at the end of the inert gas inhalation. During exhalation, the concentrations from these units are then recombined to a concentration in the parent airway (or at the mouth, where the washout gas can be sampled) according to their relative contribution to the expiratory flow (or volume) from each unit. In particular, concentration at the mouth equals (conc1.ΔV1 + conc2.ΔV2)/(ΔV1 + ΔV2). This means that if both units exhale at a different but constant rate ($\dot{V}$ 1 and $\dot{V}$ 2), overall washout concentration will be a ventilation-weighted average of both unit concentrations. Importantly, in that hypothetical case, the washout concentration during the phase III will be constant, resulting in a zero phase III slope. This is because the relative contributions from both compartments at any point in the expiration are constant. However, even in healthy subjects, SBNW

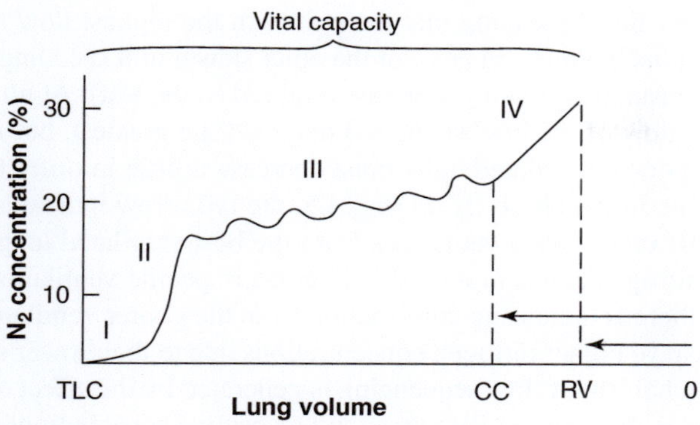

Fig. 4.4 Example of a single-breath nitrogen washout after O_2 inhalation from RV. N_2 nitrogen, CC closing capacity, I phase I, II phase II, III phase III, IV phase IV. The expiration starts from TLC, i.e., exhalation goes from left to right. Phase I gas is pure dead space, i.e., 100% oxygen and therefore 0% nitrogen. The phase II gas is a mix between dead space and alveolar gas. Phase III is alveolar gas and phase IV is gas expired after the onset of airway closure. The arrows indicate the magnitude of the CC and RV. Phase III has bumps to it, which are the cardiogenic oscillations due to heterogeneity of nitrogen concentrations from the heartbeat that intermittently "pushes" gas from higher N_2 regions into the expirate

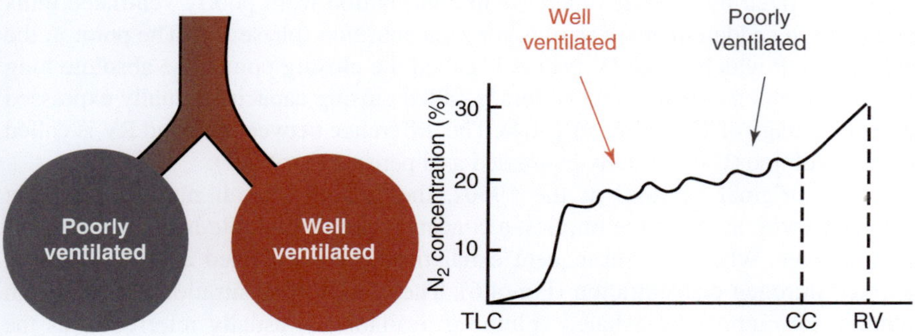

Fig. 4.5 The two-compartment representation of ventilation distribution. Gray indicates slow or poorly ventilating lung units (hence higher N_2 concentrations), and red indicates better or well-ventilated units. The well-ventilated compartment makes a greater contribution to the early part of the phase III (hence lower N_2 concentrations at the start), while the poorly ventilated part contributes more later, explaining the increase in N_2 concentrations as expiration proceeds

phase III slope is always positive, indicating that there must be another mechanism occurring in addition to regional heterogeneity in SV.

The second mechanism that is crucial to understanding the SBNW, and also how ventilation distribution in the lungs translates into a washout curve during exhalation, is that there is sequential emptying of the lung units. That is, not all lung units empty at the same constant rate during the entire exhalation. The best ventilated unit is said to "empty first," meaning that the unit with the highest flow slows down a little as exhalation continues, in favor of the other slower unit speeding up a little (to maintain the constant expiratory flow rate required in the test). At all times during exhalation, the flow of the best ventilated may well be greatest, but its magnitude relative to the poorly ventilated units must decrease a little in order to explain the positive N_2 slope in the phase III. In Fig. 4.5, the red arrow indicates that the first part of phase III represents alveolar gas from the best ventilated lung units, which have a lower nitrogen concentration due to greater specific ventilation. As exhalation proceeds there is increasing contribution from the poorer ventilated units (gray arrow), which have higher nitrogen concentrations due to their lower specific ventilation. One mechanism of flow sequencing is generated by the effect of gravity, due to the curvilinear shape of the PV curve, and respective contributions to ventilation from upper and lower parts of the lungs as the exhalation progresses from TLC to RV. We also know from SBNW experiments in microgravity that there are also non-gravitational effects generating a phase III slope. In summary, irrespective of the potential mechanisms generating a sequence of lung emptying, it is a necessary condition for the SV differences in the lung to produce a non-zero phase III slope. In this way, the magnitude of the phase III slope is a measure of degree of ventilation heterogeneity.

As exhalation proceeds further and below FRC, airway closure can occur which is characterized by a sudden increase in contribution from poorly ventilated units and hence a sudden increase in nitrogen concentration (phase IV). The point in the exhalation at which phase IV occurs is called the closing point. The absolute lung volume at which closing point occurs is called closing capacity (usually expressed as a percentage of TLC – see Fig. 4.4). The difference between CC and RV is called closing volume (CV – usually expressed as a percentage of VC).

In its original version, in the 1950s, the multiple-breath nitrogen washout (MBNW) was, as the name implies, a concatenation of multiple inhaled breaths of pure oxygen, where the subsequent exhalations were collected and analyzed for expired nitrogen concentration (Fig. 4.6). The plot of concentration versus breath number (or cumulative exhaled volume if available) is usually referred to as the washout (concentration) curve; it is also usually expressed in a semi-log plot since perfect dilution would produce a perfectly linear dependence of log(concentration) versus breath number. Even with an added dead space, the washout concentration curve would still be linear in semi-log plot yet with a slower descent versus a washout with same volumes but no dead space. In the original studies, the number of breaths necessary to reach a certain level of overall nitrogen dilution was translated into an index named the lung clearance index (LCI). In more recent studies, the LCI is derived from the nitrogen and volume trace, measured continuously as a MBNW progresses. The number of lung turnovers (tidal volume over lung volume, VT/FRC) needed to reach 1/40th of the pre-test alveolar concentration equals the LCI. Depending on the study, the concentration used to compute LCI may be mean expired N_2 concentration, average alveolar plateau N_2 concentration or end-tidal N_2 concentration. Depending on this choice, typical values of LCI in the normal lungs will range 5–6. The advantage of LCI is that it is simple to compute and relatively

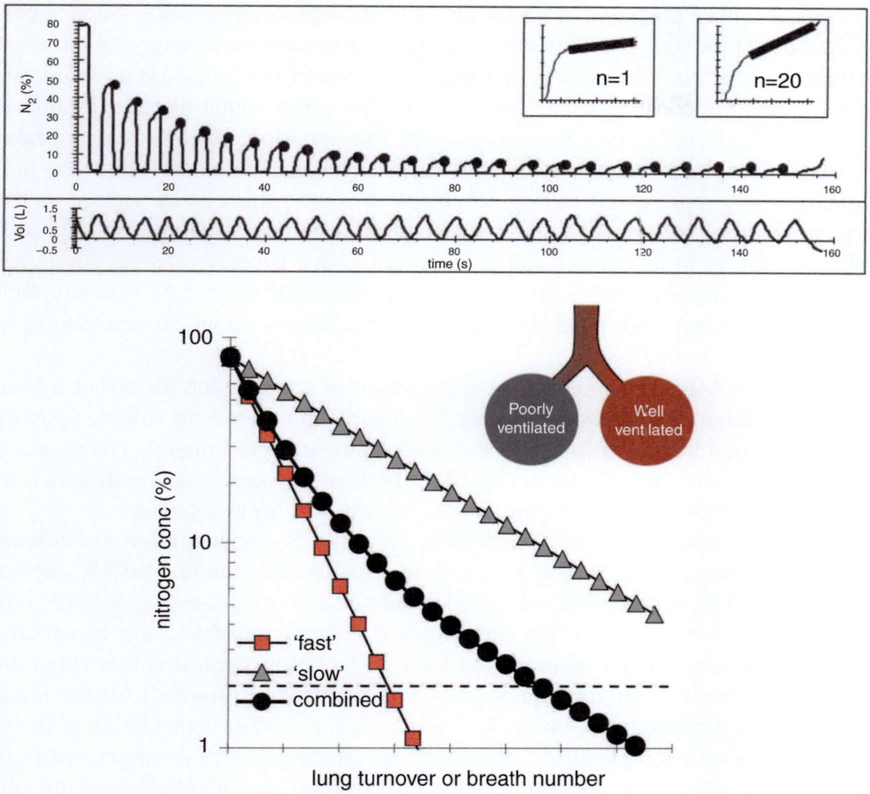

Fig. 4.6 The progressive decrease in nitrogen concentration during a multiple-breath nitrogen washout (MBNW) test (top) and the corresponding semi-log plots of N_2 concentration versus breath number or lung turnover (bottom), conceptually resulting from a combination of a slow and a fast compartment washout curve

independent of the subject's FRC. For example, in a subject with a greater FRC, the unit turnover (VT/FRC in the abscissa) will be smaller, yet the breath-by-breath decrease of N_2concentration due to dilution is also slower because the same O_2 volume is diluted into a greater FRC. This FRC compensation of dilution, by expressing the concentration washout curve versus lung turnover instead of breath number, is the strength of LCI. The weakness of the LCI is that it is determined in a portion of the washout curve where concentrations are very low and thus prone to measurement error.

Other measures of ventilation heterogeneity have been derived from the MBNW washout concentration curves. Moment ratios are simply computed by considering the concentrations measured in each subsequent breath as a distribution of concentrations from which the various moments (average, standard deviation, skewness) can be computed. There is no information about the spatial distribution of differences in concentrations in the lungs in such analyses. Curvilinearity of the semi-log plot has also been proposed as a measure of ventilation heterogeneity, where a perfectly linear plot signals a perfectly homogeneously ventilated lung, and the most extreme case of curvilinearity is that where one part of the lungs has an infinitesimally slow time constant τ and therefore an almost horizontal plateau (infinitesimally small decrease in concentration) in the semi-log plot. A real washout concentration plot in health and disease is somewhat curvilinear in a semi-log plot (schematically represented in Fig. 4.6, black dots) and this can be viewed as the lung functioning as two separate compartments, each one washing out at its own pace (according to its own τ) and generating its own (linear) washout curve. An index of curvilinearity is therefore often computed as the relative N_2 concentration decrease in the fast (early) and slow (late) portion of the washout curve measured at the mouth.

In adults, a MBNW maneuver usually consists of repeated inhalations of a fixed volume of pure oxygen (usually 1 liter) from end-expiratory lung volume (usually FRC) at normal breathing flow (typically 10–12 breaths per minute). The repeated inhalation of 1 liter breaths continues until the final nitrogen concentration is near zero (1/40th of the starting concentration). See Fig. 4.6 for an example.

In a more elaborate analysis of MBNW, the entire N_2 concentration and volume trace can be analyzed as if they were a concatenation of individual SBNW curves, where a phase III slope can be computed in each expiratory phase (see Fig. 4.6, top, where a slope for the 1st and the 20th breath is illustrated in the inset). Based on a large body of computational modeling work, it has been suggested that when the phase III slope in each subsequent breath is normalized (divided) by the mean expired concentration (or alveolar concentration), the relative contribution of large-scale ventilation heterogeneities, also visible on imaging, can be distinguished from ventilation heterogeneity occurring beyond the resolution scale of imaging modalities (at acinar level).

The analysis is somewhat complex, but the principal idea of the test is to partition ventilation heterogeneity generated in the convection-dependent airways and ventilation heterogeneity in the respiratory airways beyond those airways where gas also moves by diffusion; the diffusion-dependent airways. The term used to represent ventilation heterogeneity in the convection-dependent airways is Scond. The corresponding term for ventilation heterogeneity in more peripheral and diffusion dependent airways is Sacin. These abbreviations arise from the specific slopes measured ("S"), while "cond" and "acin" refer to conductive and acinar airways, respectively, since these roughly correspond to the air spaces in the lung where convection and diffusion are predominant. In fact, the actual functional boundary between the convection-dependent and the more peripheral diffusion-dependent lung units is the so-called diffusion front, which is a sigmoid-shaped oxygen profile extending between the entrance and the lung periphery. While the diffusion front is not a sharp scission between the conductive and the acinar airways, it is located at the lung depth where the combined lumen cross-sectional areas of the airways increases rapidly (i.e., where alveolation starts), namely where diffusion takes over from convection as the dominant gas transport mechanism.

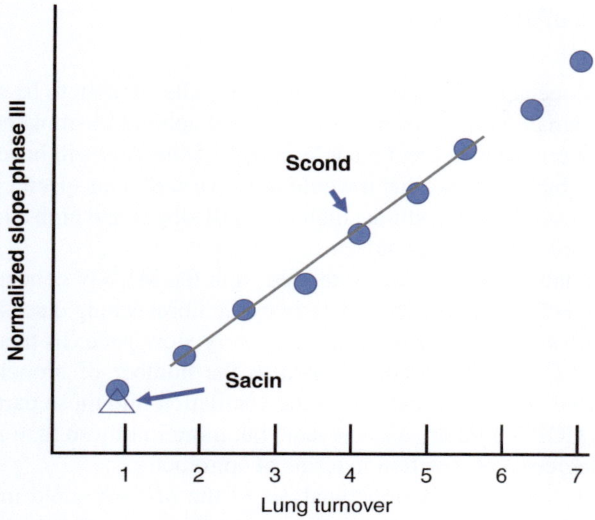

Fig. 4.7 Diagram demonstrating the calculations of Scond and Sacin from the relationship between normalized (for its mean N_2 concentration) Phase III slope of each breath of the washout, plotted against lung turnover (breath volume/FRC). Each blue dot represents each breath during the washout, the number of breaths varying depending on lung size and ventilatory efficiency. The slope of the line fitted to the breaths between turnovers 1.5 and 6 is the value of Scond. The normalized phase III slope of the first breath, with the component of ventilation heterogeneity from Scond subtracted from it (i.e., Scond x lung turnover of the first breath), is the value of Sacin (triangle). Scond and Sacin are calculated from the pooled values of three artifact-free washouts. Therefore, the Sacin calculation will be from the average of three normalized phase III slopes of each of the three washouts and average of their three lung turnovers

The principle of Scond and Sacin computation, both derived from the normalized phase III slope, is as follows (Fig. 4.7). Distribution of oxygen during the first breath of the MBNW is similar to that which occurs in a single-breath washout. The advantage of observing phase III slope in subsequent breaths is that it progressively accentuates concentration differences due to convective gas flow. This principle then allows separation of ventilation heterogeneity due to convection-dependent and diffusion-dependent effects. Ventilation heterogeneity in convection-dependent airways is measured from the rate at which phase III slope increases as the washout progresses. Ventilation heterogeneity in diffusion-dependent airways is measured primarily from the first breath of the washout, since it generates a portion of the phase III that remains almost constant throughout the subsequent breaths; it is calculated as the phase III slope of the first breath from which the calculated (small) contribution of convective ventilation heterogeneity is subtracted. In principle, Scond may represent ventilation heterogeneity in both the large and small conductive airways. Recent four-dimensional CT data in normal man have shown that Scond may be generated between the five lung lobes, whereas during induced bronchoconstriction or in disease, Scond more likely represents ventilation heterogeneity generated between smaller conductive airways.

4.2.5 Clinical Relevance

The phase III slope and CC from SBNW were initially thought to be sensitive indicators of early small airway disease and therefore applied to smokers. However, it appears to be overly sensitive in that at least half of smokers will have an abnormal SBNW index, which suggests that it would not have sufficient specificity to indicate risk of COPD in smokers. In asthma, high phase III slopes and high closing capacity indicate increased risk of severe attacks.

Thus far the lung clearance index derived from the MBNW concentration curve has proven to be clinically useful mostly in cystic fibrosis lung disease, where considerable portions of the lung wash out at a very slow pace. In fact, in adult CF patients, their LCI can be directly linked to the number of bronchial segments affected by bronchiectasis, which slows the ventilation into those parts of the lung. In asthma and COPD, LCI are also elevated but more mildly so than in CF patients for a similar degree of obstruction in terms of spirometry.

Indices from the phase III slope analysis of the MBNW yield insight into the approximate anatomic location of ventilation heterogeneity in the lung, which may be altered by disease (Fig. 4.8).

Scond and Sacin have been shown to correlate strongly with several clinical features of asthma. Scond relates strongly to airway hyperresponsiveness independently of airway inflammation, in subjects under the age of around 50 years. However, in older subjects, Sacin correlates with airway hyperresponsiveness. The

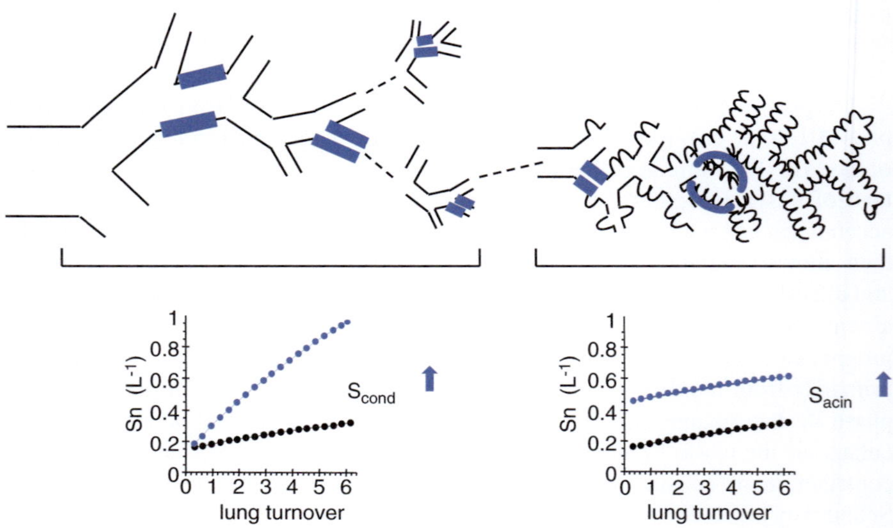

Fig. 4.8 Schematic diagram illustrating how Scond and Sacin are affected by disease. The rate of rise and the offset of the Sn (normalised phase III slope) curves roughly correspond to respectively Scond and Sacin. Scond will typically be affected by structural heterogeneity in the large or conductive small airways. Sacin will typically be affected by structural heterogeneity in the acinar airways

difference was attributed to the age-related changes in lung structure, perhaps with an increasingly important role of the diffusion-dependent airways in older subjects. Interestingly, Scond was also found to predict the magnitude of airway closure that could be induced by methacholine challenge, while Sacin predicted the development of airway narrowing. Both Scond and Sacin relate to symptomatic measures of asthma control, while Sacin predicts the worsening of asthma control when inhaled corticosteroid is reduced in stable asthmatic subjects.

In COPD and smokers, both Sacin and Scond appear to be highly sensitive measures of small airway dysfunction given that they improve following smoking cessation. In smokers with normal spirometry, Sacin relates to smoking history, while Scond relates to bronchitic symptoms. In smokers with overt COPD, where a large number of terminal bronchioles are simply obliterated, Sacin is the most sensitive index to pick up this morphometrical feature. Although the SBNW test has not proven to be clinically useful over time, the MBNW test provides more detailed information and has been shown to have significant clinical correlates in asthma and COPD. The MBNW test is likely to be used in routine clinical practice in the future, although this will be dependent on completion of further informative clinical studies.

Selected References

Bourdin A, Paganin F, Préfaut C, Kieseler D, Godard P, Chanez P. Nitrogen washout slope in poorly controlled asthma. Allergy. 2006;61(1):85–9.

Buist AS, Ross BB. Predicted values for closing volume using a modified single breath nitrogen test. Am Rev Respir Dis. 1973a;107:744–52.

Buist AS, Ross BB. Quantitative analysis of the alveolar plateau in the diagnosis of early airway obstruction. Am Rev Respir Dis. 1973b;108(5):1078–87.

Buist AS, Ghezzo H, Anthonisen NR, Cherniack RM, Ducic S, Macklem PT, Manfreda J, Martin RR, McCarthy D, Ross BB. Relationship between the single-breath N test and age, sex, and smoking habit in three North American cities. Am Rev Respir Dis. 1979;120(2):305–18.

Downie S, Salome C, Verbanck S, Thompson B, Berend N, King G. Ventilation heterogeneity is a major determinant of airway hyperresponsiveness in asthma, independent of airway inflammation. Thorax. 2007;62(8):684–9.

Farah CS, King GG, Brown NJ, Downie SR, Kermode J, Hardaker KM, Peters MJ, Berend N, Salome CM. The role of the small airways in the clinical expression of asthma in adults. J Allergy Clin Immunol. 2012a;129(2):381–7.

Farah CS, King GG, Brown NJ, Peters MJ, Berend N, Salome CM. Ventilation heterogeneity predicts asthma control in adults following inhaled corticosteroid dose titration. J Allergy Clin Immunol. 2012b;130(1):61–8.

Farrow CE, Salome CM, Harris BE, Bailey DL, Bailey E, Berend N, Young IH, King GG. Airway closure on imaging relates to airway hyperresponsiveness and peripheral airway disease in asthma. J Appl Physiol. 2012;113(6):958–66.

Farrow CE, Salome CM, Harris BE, Bailey DL, Berend N, King GG. Peripheral ventilation heterogeneity determines the extent of bronchoconstriction in asthma. J Appl Physiol. 2017;123(5):1188–94.

Fowler WS. Lung function studies: II. The respiratory dead space. Am J Phys. 1948;154(3):405–16.

Fowler WS. Lung function studies: III. Uneven pulmonary ventilation in normal subjects and in patients with pulmonary disease. J Appl Physiol. 1949;2:283.

Hardaker KM, Downie SR, Kermode JA, Farah CS, Brown NJ, Berend N, King GG, Salome CM. The predictors of airway hyperresponsiveness differ between old and young asthmatics. Chest. 2011;139(6):1395–401.
Harris RS, Winkler T, Tgavalekos N, Musch G, Melo MFV, Schroeder T, Chang Y, Venegas JG. Regional pulmonary perfusion, inflation, and ventilation defects in bronchoconstricted patients with asthma. Am J Respir Crit Care Med. 2006;174(3):245–53.
In 't Veen JC, Beekman AJ, Bel EH, Sterk PJ. Recurrent exacerbations in severe asthma are associated with enhanced airway closure during stable episodes. Am J Respir Crit Care Med. 2000;161(6):1902–6.
Jetmalani K, Thamrin C, Farah CS, Bertolin A, Berend N, Salome CM, King GG. Peripheral airway dysfunction and relationship with symptoms in smokers with preserved spirometry. Respirology. 2018;23(5):512–8.
King GG, Eberl S, Salome CM, Meikle SR, Woolcock AJ. Airway closure measured by a Technegas bolus and SPECT. Am J Respir Crit Care Med. 1997;155(2):682–8.
King GG, James A, Wark P. The pathophysiology of severe asthma: we've only just started. Respirology. 2018;23(3):262–71.
Mathew L, Kirby M, Etemad-Rezai R, Wheatley A, McCormack D, Parraga G. Hyperpolarized (3) He magnetic resonance imaging: preliminary evaluation of phenotyping potential in chronic obstructive pulmonary disease. Eur J Radiol. 2011;79(1):140–6.
McDonough JE, Yuan R, Suzuki M, Seyednejad N, Elliott WM, Sanchez PG, Wright AC, Gefter WB, Litzky L, Coxson HO, Paré PD, Sin DD, Pierce RA, Woods JC, McWilliams AM, Mayo JR, Lam SC, Cooper JD, Hogg JC. Small-airway obstruction and emphysema in chronic obstructive pulmonary disease. N Engl J Med. 2011;365(17):1567–75.
Milic-Emili J, Henderson JAM, Dolovich MB, Trop D, Kaneko K. Regional distribution of inspired gas in the lung. J Appl Physiol. 1966;21:749–59.
Milic-Emili J, Torchio R, D'Angelo E. Closing volume: a reappraisal (1967–2007). Eur J Appl Physiol. 2007;99(6):567–83.
Tanabe N, Vasilescu DM, McDonough JE, Kinose D, Suzuki M, Cooper JD, Paré PD, Hogg JC. MicroCT comparison of preterminal bronchioles in centrilobular and panlobular emphysema. Am J Respir Crit Care Med. 2017;195(5):630–8.
Thurlbeck WM, Dunnill MS, Hartung W, Heard BE, Heppleston AG, Ryder RC. A comparison of three methods of measuring emphysema. Hum Pathol. 1970;1(2):215–26.
Tzeng Y-S, Lutchen K, Albert M. The difference in ventilation heterogeneity between asthmatic and healthy subjects quantified using hyperpolarized 3He MRI. J Appl Physiol. 2009;106(3):813–22.
Verbanck S, Paiva M. Gas mixing in the airways and airspaces. Compr Physiol. 2011;1:809–34.
Verbanck S, Schuermans D, Van Muylem A, Melot C, Noppen M, Vincken W, Paiva M. Conductive and acinar lung-zone contributions to ventilation inhomogeneity in COPD. Am J Respir Crit Care Med. 1998;157(5 Pt 1):1573–7.
Verbanck S, Schuermans D, Paiva M, Meysman M, Vincken W. Small airway function improvement after smoking cessation in smokers without airway obstruction. Am J Respir Crit Care Med. 2006;174(8):853–7.
Verbanck S, Van Muylem A, Schuermans D, Bautmans I, Thompson B, Vincken W. Transfer factor, lung volumes, resistance and ventilation distribution in healthy adults. Eur Respir J. 2016;47:166–76.
Verbanck S, King GG, Zhou W, Miller A, Thamrin C, Schuermans D, Ilsen B, Ernst CW, de Mey J, Vincken W, Vanderhelst E. The quantitative link of lung clearance index to bronchial segments affected by bronchiectasis. Thorax. 2018a;73(1):82–4.
Verbanck S, King GG, Paiva M, Schuermans D, Vanderhelst E. The functional correlate of the loss of terminal bronchioles in COPD. Am J Respir Crit Care Med. 2018b. https://doi.org/10.1164/rccm.201712-2366LE.

Chapter 5
Gas Exchange

Brian L. Graham, Neil MacIntyre, and Yuh Chin Huang

5.1 Gas Phase Transport

The gas exchange pathway for a molecule of O_2 is as follows (Fig. 5.1):

1. Transport from the mouth through the airways of the lung to the alveoli by convective and diffusive gas flow and mixing
2. Diffusion across the surfactant layer and the type 1 pneumocytes which form the alveolar wall
3. Diffusion through the interstitium between the alveolar wall and the capillary wall
4. Diffusion across the pulmonary capillary endothelium
5. Diffusion through the plasma to the red blood cell
6. Diffusion across the red blood cell membrane
7. Diffusion through the red blood cell cytoplasm to the Hb molecule
8. Binding with a Hb molecule
9. Transport via the circulatory system to the rest of the body

This section describes the portion of the gas exchange process which occurs in the gas phase from the mouth to the blood-gas barrier.

B. L. Graham (✉)
Division of Respirology, Critical Care and Sleep Medicine, University of Saskatchewan, Saskatoon, SK, Canada
e-mail: brian.graham@usask.ca

N. MacIntyre · Y. C. Huang
Department of Medicine, Division of Pulmonary and Critical Care Medicine, Duke University, Durham, NC, USA
e-mail: neil.macintyre@duke.edu; yuhchin.huang@duke.edu

D. A. Kaminsky, C. G. Irvin (eds.), *Pulmonary Function Testing*,
Respiratory Medicine, https://doi.org/10.1007/978-3-319-94159-2_5

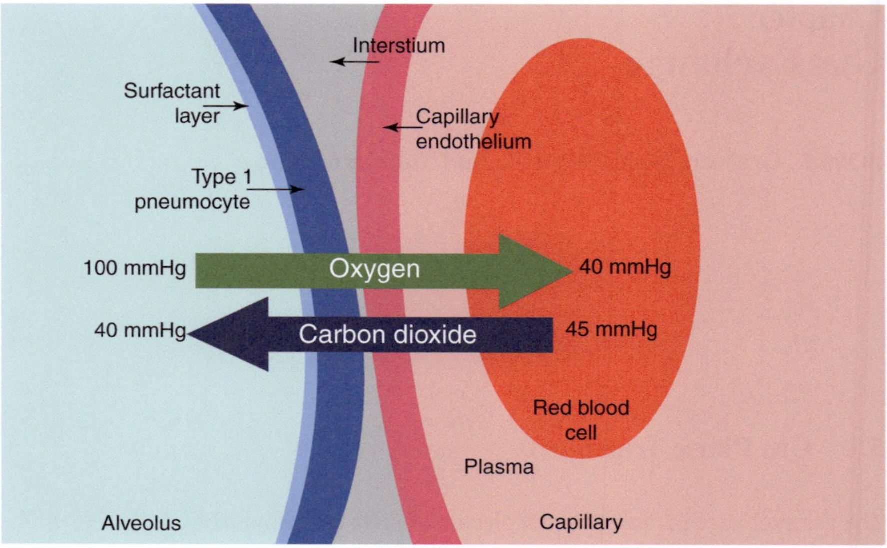

Fig. 5.1 Gas transport from alveolar gas to Hb molecule

The gas exchange pathway for O_2 begins with the inspiration of air at the mouth. In order for the O_2 to reach the alveolar space, it must traverse 18–24 generations of bifurcation in the bronchial tree. With each successive airway generation, the total surface area of the airways increases, and hence the velocity of the inhaled gas is reduced, so that the total amount of airflow remains constant. This affects the manner in which O_2 is transported.

There are two main transport mechanisms in the gas phase – convection and diffusion. Convection refers to the bulk flow of gas driven by gas pressure. Diffusion refers to the movement of individual molecules driven by a partial pressure gradient for that molecule. In the large airways, gas transport is primarily by convection. As the gas moves deeper into the bronchial tree, diffusive transport becomes more and more important. At the level of the peripheral airways, gas transport is primarily by diffusion. Gas mixing at the interface between the inspired gas and the residual gas remaining in the lung at end exhalation occurs by both convection and diffusion as it moves through the airways. It should also be noted that the pores of Kohn and the canals of Lambert (connections between neighboring conducting airways and alveoli) are thought to provide pathways for collateral ventilation which improve gas mixing and transport between adjacent alveoli and adjacent acini.

The distribution of the inspired gas in the lung is not homogeneous. Consider a maximal single-breath maneuver from residual volume (RV) to total lung capacity (TLC) in a subject seated upright. At RV, the alveoli at the base of the lung will have a smaller volume than alveoli at the apex due to the effect of gravity on the lung as it is suspended within the thoracic cavity. The weight of the lung tends to pull the apical regions open and squeeze the basal regions closed. This effect increases as the lung becomes less elastic with age or disease processes. At the end of inhalation, all alveoli tend to be filled to the same volume so that proportionally more inspired gas goes to the basal regions, and they will have a higher O_2 concentration.

In young, healthy subjects, the distribution of ventilation tends to approach uniformity. As the normal lung ages, the distribution of ventilation becomes less uniform, due mainly to the loss of elastic recoil. In people with lung diseases that cause airflow obstruction and/or loss of elastic recoil, the heterogeneity of ventilation can increase markedly. In such cases, the transport of inspired gas to the blood-gas barrier can become a consequential impediment to gas exchange.

The blood-gas barrier is the endpoint of gas phase transport. The blood-gas barrier is formed by the alveolar wall composed of type 1 pneumocytes covered by a film of surfactant, the interstitium (which may be a potential space or may contain interstitial fluid), and the endothelium of the capillaries (Fig. 5.1). There are 200–800 million alveoli in adult humans, depending on the size of their lungs. The blood-gas barrier has been estimated to have an area in the order of 100 m^2 at TLC in a typical adult and a thickness that varies from 200 to 2000 nm. Fick's law states that the mass transfer of a gas across a membrane driven by the partial pressure difference ($P_2 - P_1$) is directly proportional to its surface area (A) and inversely proportional to its thickness (T). Hence, the large area and small thickness of the blood-gas barrier are critically important for gas exchange. The other term in Fick's law is the diffusivity (D) of the gas molecule, which is equal to its solubility divided by the square root of its molecular weight.

$$\text{Fick's law of diffusion: diffusive gas flow } \alpha\, A \cdot D \cdot (P_2 - P_1) / T$$

The alveolar blood-gas barrier is not analogous to a balloon which expands and contracts with inhalation and exhalation, surrounded by a sheet of blood. In such a model, the area for gas exchange would decrease during exhalation proportional to volume to the two-thirds power and the thickness of the membrane through which gas must diffuse would increase. In reality, there are several mechanisms to maintain the effective surface area for gas exchange at lower lung volumes. As the alveolus contracts and expands, there is folding and unfolding of the alveolar wall between the pulmonary capillaries. There is also a bulging of the pulmonary capillaries into the alveoli. Furthermore, there are openings in the alveolar walls (the pores of Kohn), which open as the alveolus expands with inhalation and close during exhalation. These mechanisms help to maintain the surface area available for diffusion across the blood-gas barrier at lower lung volumes, but there remains a decrease in the effective surface area as lung volume decreases. However, the decrease in diffusion at lower lung volumes is less than would be predicted by the balloon model.

Once a gas molecule has crossed the blood-gas barrier, it enters the pulmonary capillaries. The pulmonary capillary blood volume varies with height and sex. It is ~90 mL for an average adult male and ~65 mL for an average adult female.

5.2 Blood Phase Transport

5.2.1 *The Pulmonary Circulation*

Virtually the entire cardiac output is delivered by the right ventricle into the pulmonary vascular bed, which consists of a branching pulmonary arterial system, a pulmonary capillary bed, and a pulmonary venous system draining into the left atrium. Within the pulmonary arterial system, mean pressure is roughly 14 mmHg and mean pulmonary vascular resistance is 1.43 mmHg/L/min. During exercise, the mean pressure increases to 20 mmHg and the resistance falls to 0.62 mmHg/L/min.

The distribution of blood flow through this system is affected by gravitational forces (dependent regions receive more regional blood flow). This has been described by the West three-zone model: zone 1 at the top of the lung where alveolar pressures exceed vascular pressures, zone 2 in the middle of the lung where pulmonary arterial pressure (but not venous pressure) exceeds alveolar pressure, and zone 3 where vascular pressures exceed alveolar pressures. Smooth muscle tone, largely driven by oxygen tension (hypoxia promotes vascular constriction), also affects distribution of blood flow.

The state of inflation also affects vascular resistances and blood flow distribution. Specifically, as inflation increases, peri-alveolar vessels are compressed and extra-alveolar vessels are stretched open. This results in less blood flow/alveolus in non-dependent regions and more blood flow/alveolus to dependent regions as the lung inflates. The net effect of these changes is that pulmonary vascular resistance is at its minimum near functional residual capacity, rising as the lung approaches either residual volume or total lung capacity.

As noted above, the pulmonary capillary bed contains approximately 65–90 mL of blood, and the alveolar-capillary surface area approaches 100 m^2. Oxygen diffusion is driven by an alveolar-capillary O_2 gradient of 60 mmHg (alveolar P_AO_2 of 100 mmHg minus mixed venous $P\bar{v}O_2$ of 40 mmHg) and is virtually complete within 0.25 s, only a fraction of the estimated red blood cell transit time at rest of 0.75–2.5 s. CO_2 diffusion is completed even faster, approximately 20× that of oxygen.

Generally, pulmonary capillary blood leaving each alveolus has about the same PO_2 and PCO_2 as the alveolar gas. However, the ultimate arterial PaO_2 (and to a lesser extent $PaCO_2$) depends upon the relationship of ventilation to perfusion ($\dot{V}_A/\dot{Q}$) in each alveolar-capillary gas exchange unit and the distribution of these relationships. Indeed, in disease states with wide distributions of regional $\dot{V}_A/\dot{Q}$, profound arterial hypoxemia can develop despite overall normal ventilation and perfusion (see $\dot{V}_A/\dot{Q}$ discussion below). Note that even in normal lungs, the ultimate PaO_2 in arterial blood is slightly lower than mean alveolar P_AO_2 because local matching of ventilation and perfusion in normal lungs is imperfect. In addition, a small amount of unoxygenated blood is added to pulmonary capillary blood through anatomic shunts connecting the venous bronchial circulation to the pulmonary venous blood.

5.2.2 Hemoglobin

Oxygen is carried in the blood in two forms: (1) combined with hemoglobin and (2) dissolved O_2 in the plasma. Human hemoglobin (Hb) is a tetramer (four polypeptides) consisting of two α-polypeptides and two β-polypeptides, each containing a heme moiety. The tetramer consists of 547 amino acids and has a molecular weight of 64,800 daltons. The heme and globin interact with each other in a way that determines the O_2-binding characteristics of hemoglobin.

Hb allows blood to carry much more oxygen than would be possible from simply dissolving oxygen in plasma. For example, 15 gm Hb in 100 mL of blood with a PO_2 of 100 mmHg carries 20 mL of oxygen in contrast to 0.3 mL of oxygen dissolved in 100 mL of plasma with a PO_2 of 100 mmHg. Oxygen does not *oxidize* hemoglobin; rather, it *oxygenates* hemoglobin, a reversible process. Combined with oxygen, hemoglobin is called *oxyhemoglobin*, whereas unoxygenated hemoglobin is called *deoxyhemoglobin* or *reduced* hemoglobin.

As oxygen molecules successively bind with heme groups, the hemoglobin molecule physically changes its shape, causing it to reflect and absorb light differently when it is oxygenated than when it is deoxygenated. This phenomenon is responsible for the bright red color of oxygenated hemoglobin and the deep purple color of deoxyhemoglobin. This difference in light absorption and reflection makes it possible to measure the amount of oxygenated hemoglobin present (see Sect. 5.7).

O_2 affinity to hemoglobin increases during progressive oxygenation, a phenomenon called *cooperativity*. The cooperativity is responsible for the sigmoid shape of the oxyhemoglobin equilibrium curve (OEC), which affects how O_2 is loaded and unloaded under physiologic conditions (Fig. 5.2). Its position often is expressed by

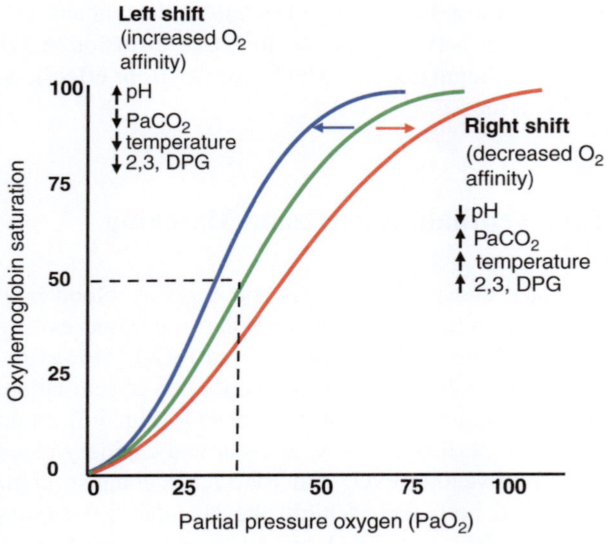

Fig. 5.2 Oxyhemoglobin equilibrium curve (OEC), which reflects Hb saturation as a function of PaO_2. The green curve represents the normal position, where hemoglobin is 50% saturated at a PO_2 of 27 mmHg. Factors that shift the curve to the left (blue curve) and to the right (red curve) are shown and discussed in the text

the P_{50}, or the PO_2 that corresponds with 50% hemoglobin saturation. The normal P_{50} for human hemoglobin is approximately 27 mmHg. When the O_2 affinity increases, the OEC shifts to the left (reduced P_{50}). When the O_2 affinity decreases, the OEC shifts to the right (increased P_{50}).

Several factors affect hemoglobin's affinity for O_2, resulting in either a left (increased affinity) or right (decreased affinity) shift in the OEC position, changing the hemoglobin O_2 saturation for a given PaO_2. Increased 2,3-diglycerophosphate (2,3-DPG) in the erythrocyte, acidemia, increased $PaCO_2$, and hyperthermia decrease hemoglobin affinity for O_2 (right shift of the curve). In contrast, decreased 2,3-DPG, alkalemia, decreased $PaCO_2$, and hypothermia increase hemoglobin affinity for O_2 (left shift of the curve).

When hemoglobin is bound to carbon monoxide (CO), its affinity for O_2 is greatly increased; the binding of CO to one heme site increases O_2 affinity of the other binding sites, causing a leftward shift of the OEC. This effect on hemoglobin O_2 affinity explains why the formation of 50% carboxyhemoglobin causes more severe tissue hypoxia than when various forms of anemia cause the reduction of hemoglobin concentration to half the normal concentration.

The hemoglobin molecule simultaneously carries O_2 and CO_2, but not at the same binding sites. Oxygen combines with the molecule's heme groups, whereas CO_2 combines with the amino groups of the α- and β-polypeptide chains. The presence of O_2 on the heme portions of hemoglobin hinders the combination of amino groups with CO_2 (i.e., it hinders formation of carbaminohemoglobin); thus, the affinity of hemoglobin for CO_2 is greater when it is not combined with oxygen (Haldane effect). Conversely, carbaminohemoglobin has a decreased affinity for O_2 (Bohr effect). Thus, oxygenated blood carries less CO_2 for a given $PaCO_2$ than deoxygenated blood. It should be appreciated that the Haldane and Bohr effects are mutually enhancing. As O_2 diffuses into the tissue cells, it dissociates from the hemoglobin molecule, enhancing its ability to carry CO_2 (Haldane effect). At the same time, CO_2 diffusion into the blood at the tissue level decreases hemoglobin's affinity for O_2 (Bohr effect), enhancing the release of O_2 to the tissues.

5.3 Ventilation/Perfusion Matching

As noted above, alveolar gas and capillary blood rapidly equilibrate across the alveolar-capillary interface such that the blood exiting the pulmonary capillary will equal the alveolar gas P_AO_2 and P_ACO_2. However, the ultimate arterial PaO_2 and $PaCO_2$ will depend on the distribution of ventilation/perfusion ($\dot{V}_A/\dot{Q}$) relationships throughout the lungs and the F_IO_2 (Fig. 5.3). In units where ventilation with respect to perfusion is low, alveolar and capillary blood PO_2 and PCO_2 approach the mixed venous $P\bar{v}O_2$ and $P\bar{v}CO_2$. In contrast, in units where ventilation with respect to perfusion is high, the alveolar and capillary blood PO_2 and PCO_2 approach the inspired P_IO_2 and P_ICO_2. At the extremes, shunts ($\dot{V}_A/\dot{Q} = 0$) and dead space ($\dot{V}_A/\dot{Q}$ = infinity) do not participate in gas exchange but only serve to put

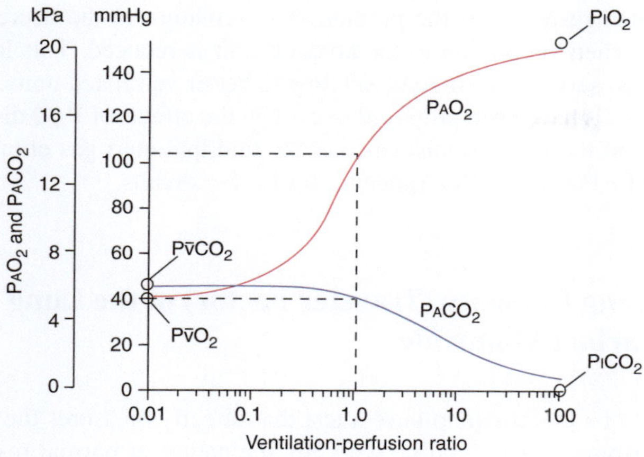

Fig. 5.3 Effect of ventilation/perfusion ratio on gas exchange. Notice how a $\dot{V}_A/\dot{Q}$ ratio less than 1 results in a sharp fall in P_AO_2 but only a slight rise in P_ACO_2, whereas a $\dot{V}_A/\dot{Q}$ ratio greater than 1 results in a rise in P_AO_2 and a fall in P_ACO_2. $P\bar{v}O_2$ and $P\bar{v}CO_2$ represent mixed venous gas values, and P_IO_2 and P_ICO_2 represent inspired gas values. (Reproduced with permission of the © ERS 2018: *European Respiratory Journal.* Oct 2014; 44(4):1023–1041. https://doi.org/10.1183/09031936.00037014)

mixed venous blood into arterial blood and inspired gas into expired gas, respectively.

Note from Fig. 5.3 that at sea level with a P_IO_2 of 150 mmHg, a P_ICO_2 of 0 mmHg, a $P\bar{v}O_2$ of 40 mmHg, and a $P\bar{v}CO_2$ of 45 mmHg, a $\dot{V}_A/\dot{Q}$ of 1 results in a PaO_2 of 80–100 mmHg, which fully saturates Hb. This is what occurs in the vast majority of normal alveolar-capillary units and results in a $PaCO_2$ of 40 mmHg. In disease states producing large numbers of both low and high $\dot{V}_A/\dot{Q}$ units (<1 and >1, respectively), high $\dot{V}_A/\dot{Q}$ units can compensate for low $\dot{V}_A/\dot{Q}$ units in removing CO_2 and keep the $PaCO_2$ near 40 mmHg. However, once pulmonary capillary hemoglobin is fully saturated with oxygen, the higher PaO_2 in high $\dot{V}_A/\dot{Q}$ units results in only a small increase in dissolved oxygen. A high $\dot{V}_A/\dot{Q}$ unit can therefore not compensate for a low $\dot{V}_A/\dot{Q}$ unit for oxygenation. The presence of large numbers of low $\dot{V}_A/\dot{Q}$ units in disease thus has far more effects on oxygenation than carbon dioxide removal and, along with shunts ($\dot{V}_A/\dot{Q} = 0$), is the major cause of abnormal alveolar-arterial oxygen differences ($P_{(A-a)O_2}$).

It has long been recognized that the normal lung has a distribution of $\dot{V}_A/\dot{Q}$ units around one. This distribution is relatively tight in normal subjects, and the differences that do exist are explained by the greater effects of gravity on the vertical distribution of perfusion than on ventilation and the non-gravity dependent heterogeneity in ventilation and perfusion due to the structural asymmetry in the airways and blood vessels. As a consequence only a small alveolar-arterial difference ($P_{(A-a)O2}$) exists in normal subjects.

Vascular smooth muscle modulation is an important mechanism to assist in matching perfusion to ventilation. This is largely controlled by oxygen and is a locally mediated response of the pulmonary vasculature to the decrease in P_AO_2, which occurs when ventilation to the alveolar unit is reduced. This local hypoxic vasoconstriction serves to reroute blood flow to better-ventilated units.

Various models have been proposed to explain the effects of $\dot{V}_A/\dot{Q}$ distributions in the lung. One of the most sophisticated is the multiple inert gas elimination technique (MIGET). Please see the Appendix for further details.

5.4 Diffusing Capacity (Transfer Factor) of the Lung for Carbon Monoxide

While it would be preferable to have a test that directly measures the conductance of O_2 from inspired gas to binding with Hb, the nature of normal respiration precludes such a measurement using noninvasive techniques. Passive diffusion is driven by the difference in O_2 partial pressure (PO_2) across the blood-gas barrier. Consequently, in order to quantify the rate of O_2 diffusion, measurements of the alveolar and pulmonary capillary PO_2 would be required. While estimates of mean P_AO_2 might be made, the pulmonary capillary PO_2 will vary between the $P\bar{v}O_2$ and PaO_2 during the course of blood flow through the pulmonary capillary bed.

In 1915, Marie Krogh published a method to estimate the conductance of gases across the blood-gas barrier using a very low concentration of CO as a proxy for O_2. The transport of a CO molecule is very similar to that of an O_2 molecule. The molecular weight and the solubility of CO are both a little lower than that of O_2, with the net result that Fick's law predicts CO transport across a membrane will be about 83% of O_2 transport at the same driving pressure. Krogh's method is based on the assumption that any CO molecule that diffuses across the blood-gas barrier is immediately tightly bound by Hb and consequently the pulmonary capillary PCO can be assumed to be zero. Hence, the driving pressure for CO is simply P_ACO which can be estimated knowing the CO concentration and volume of the inspired gas and the alveolar volume. The conductance of CO can then be calculated by measuring the uptake of CO over a given interval of breath-holding at TLC and dividing by the driving pressure and breath-hold time. Because the concentration of CO decreases as CO diffuses across the blood-gas barrier, the decay in P_ACO will be exponential, which precludes the use of a simple arithmetic calculation of diffusive flow. In the Krogh equation, an exponential diffusion constant was introduced which has since been modified and named the diffusing capacity of the lung for carbon monoxide (DLCO).

The Krogh equation is applied as follows:

$$\text{DLCO} = V_A \cdot \ln\left(\text{F}_A\text{CO}t_0 / \text{F}_A\text{CO}t_1\right) / \left(t_1 - t_0\right) / \left(P_B - 47\right)$$

where V_A is the alveolar volume; F_ACOt_0 and F_ACOt_1 are the fractional alveolar gas concentrations of CO at time t_0 and time t_1, respectively; t_0 is the time at the beginning of the measurement interval and t_1 is the time at the end of the interval; P_B is the ambient barometric pressure; and 47 mmHg is the partial pressure of water vapor at body temperature.

Diffusing capacity is an unfortunate term since, as we will see, the process includes more than diffusion and it is not a true capacity in the usual pulmonary function use of the term. Outside of North America, the measurement is more appropriately called transfer factor (TLCO).

An important step in translating Krogh's experimental technique to a pulmonary function test was the single-breath maneuver developed by Forster and Ogilvie who introduced the use of helium as a tracer gas to permit the measurement of both V_A and F_ACOt_0. The single-breath maneuver consisted of exhalation to residual volume (RV), rapid inhalation of test gas to TLC, breath-holding at TLC for 10 s, and rapid exhalation back to RV. A sample of alveolar gas was collected during exhalation after discarding a given volume of gas for dead space washout. The Krogh equation is only applicable at a constant lung volume so rapid inhalation and exhalation were used to approximate a pure breath-hold maneuver. The test gas consisted of 0.3% CO, 10% He, 21% O_2, and balance N_2.

Helium was initially chosen as a tracer gas because it is biologically inert and has a very low solubility so that it can be safely assumed that all of the helium remains in the lung with no diffusion. As such, the alveolar He concentration at the end of the inhalation of test gas will remain constant for the duration of breath-holding and exhalation. This concentration is used to estimate the alveolar CO concentration at the beginning of breath-holding by assuming that during a rapid inhalation, the tracer gas (Tr) and CO will be diluted by the same fraction:

$$\frac{F_A COt_0}{F_I CO} = \frac{F_A Trt_0}{F_I Tr}$$

where F_ICO and F_ITr are the fractional concentrations of CO and Tr in the inhaled test gas, respectively. Because the alveolar concentration of Tr remains constant, F_ATrt_0 is the same as the concentration of Tr in the exhaled gas sample, FsTr. Thus

$$F_A COt_0 = FsTr \cdot F_I CO / F_I Tr$$

Using this relationship, the Krogh equation becomes

$$DLCO = V_A \cdot \ln\left(F_I CO / FsCO \cdot FsTr / F_I Tr\right) / t_{BH} / \left(P_B - 47\right) \tag{5.3}$$

where t_{BH} is the breath-hold time and FsCO is the CO concentration in the exhaled gas sample.

Conventional DLCO systems use a simplified mass balance equation to calculate alveolar volume, which assumes that the lung ventilation is homogeneous and there is continuous, complete gas mixing in the alveolar space with no mixing of the dead space. In such a model, the volume of Tr inhaled into the alveolar space is

$F_ITr \cdot (V_I - V_d)$ where V_I is the inhaled volume of test gas and V_d is the dead space. The concentration of Tr in the alveolar space at end inhalation (which will be the same as FsTr) will then be the volume of Tr inhaled divided by the alveolar volume:

$$FsTr = F_I Tr \cdot (V_I - V_d) / V_A \text{ and thus } V_A = (V_I - V_d) \cdot F_I Tr / FsTr$$

However, lung ventilation becomes progressively more heterogeneous in normal adults as age increases and to a greater degree in patients with obstructive lung diseases. In the 2017 ERS/ATS DLCO standards, a more accurate calculation of alveolar volume is recommended for DLCO systems with rapidly responding gas analyzers which measure all of the tracer gas inhaled and all of the tracer gas exhaled to determine how much tracer gas is left in the lung at end exhalation and use the measured tracer gas concentration at end exhalation to determine the end-expiratory alveolar volume.

Many current systems use 0.3% methane (CH_4) as a tracer gas. Although it is not as insoluble or inert as helium, it has been shown to be acceptable for use as a tracer gas for measurement of DLCO. One of the reasons for using CH_4 is that it can be measured using the same nondispersive, infrared gas analyzer technology that is used for measuring CO concentration.

In traditional units, DLCO is measured in mL/min/mmHg. As in other lung volume measurements, alveolar volume is reported under body temperature, saturated with water vapor (BTPS) conditions. While reporting in BTPS units is necessary for measures of lung volumes and flows, because they reflect the actual heated and humidified volumes that occur in the lung, this is not the case for gas exchange variables. In considering gas exchange, it is the number of moles of gas that are available for metabolism that is important rather than the amount of space that the gas takes up in the lung. For this reason, the DLCO calculated using V_A in BTPS must be converted to standard temperature, pressure, and dry gas conditions (STPD). When using traditional units, the conversion factor from BTPS to STPD is $273/310 \cdot (P_B - 47)/P_B \cdot P_B/760$ or $(P_B - 47)/863$. Outside of North America, DLCO (or TLCO) is reported in SI units which are mmol/min/kPa. To convert DLCO in SI units to traditional units, multiply by 2.987.

5.5 Interpretation of DLCO

Before interpreting a DLCO result, a number of non-disease factors that affect CO uptake need to be considered. Besides varying with age, sex, height, and possibly ethnicity, DLCO also changes with Hb, COHb, lung volume, P_IO_2, barometric pressure, and ventilation distribution. Because predicted DLCO values are derived from measurements in normal subjects who are disease-free, have normal Hb, have minimal COHb, are breathing room air, and have normal lung volumes and uniform ventilation distribution, allowances for all of these must be incorporated into an interpretation of a result.

5.5.1 Factors Affecting the Measurement of DLCO

(a) *Pulmonary capillary blood volume and Hb level:* As noted above, gas exchange involves more than the diffusion of gas across the blood-gas barrier. Once a CO molecule has entered the plasma, it must diffuse into a red blood cell and bind with Hb. Roughton and Forster showed that the conductance of CO uptake is equal to the transmembrane conductance (D_m) plus the intra-blood conductance, with both steps of roughly equal importance. The latter term is the product of the reaction rate of CO with oxyhemoglobin (θ) and the volume of blood in the alveolar capillaries (V_c). Knowing that conductances in series add like resistances in parallel, the relationship is:

$$\frac{1}{\text{DLCO}} = \frac{1}{D_\text{m}} + \frac{1}{\theta V_\text{c}}$$

This relationship shows that DLCO will increase as pulmonary capillary blood volume increases. Furthermore, the reaction rate of CO with Hb is dependent on the Hb concentration in the blood such that θ will increase as Hb concentration increases.

$$\text{DLCO}[\text{adjusted for Hb}] = \text{DLCO}[\text{measured}] \cdot \left(1.7\text{Hb} / \left(0.7\text{Hb}_\text{ref} + \text{Hb}\right)\right)$$

where Hb_{ref} is the reference Hb concentration for the subject. While the common values for Hb_{ref} are 13.4 g/L for females and males <15 years old and 14.6 g/L for males >15 years old, studies have found that Hb concentrations in the normal population vary considerably with age and ethnicity as well as gender. A change of 10% in Hb concentration will result in a 4.4% change in DLCO. Anemia reduces DLCO, while polycythemia increases DLCO. Data from NHANES III provide a source of reference values for Hb levels in different age groups and ethnicities.

Pulmonary blood capillary volume will increase with increased cardiac output (e.g., exercise), a Müller maneuver, and the supine position among other mechanisms. A Valsalva maneuver can decrease pulmonary capillary blood volume. Note that the blood volume must be considered independently of blood flow. Static blood in the lung will also increase DLCO.

(b) *Carboxyhemoglobin:* The partial pressure of CO in the pulmonary capillaries is not zero. Although CO is bound very tightly to Hb to form carboxyhemoglobin

(COHb), because the pulmonary capillary PO_2 is much higher than PCO (due to the very low concentration of CO present), some of the CO will be displaced from the COHb by the O_2 and thus present a partial pressure of CO in the capillaries that will act as a back pressure, countering the P_ACO driving pressure. Furthermore, there is a very small amount of CO produced endogenously in the body. Other environmental sources of CO will contribute to higher levels of COHb. Smokers typically have 5–15% COHb depending on the amount of smoking. (Note that subjects are advised not smoke on the day of the DLCO test.) Outdoor and indoor air pollution, occupational exposures, and faulty heating or cooking appliances can all lead to increased COHb levels. Since CO is used in the test gas, repeated measurements of DLCO will also raise COHb levels. The inhalation of 0.3% CO in the single-breath maneuver typically causes COHb to increase by 0.6–0.7% for each maneuver.

The presence of COHb compromises the assumption that the CO driving pressure across the blood-gas barrier is simply the P_ACO and causes DLCO to be underestimated by about 1% for each 1% increase in COHb concentration. DLCO systems with rapid gas analyzers meeting the 2017 ERS/ATS standards can measure the CO concentration in the alveolar gas exhaled just prior to the inhalation of test gas in order to estimate the back pressure of CO in the pulmonary capillaries, which can then be used in the calculation of DLCO to offset the CO back pressure.

COHb has an additional effect on DLCO. The COHb in the pulmonary capillaries prior to testing is not available for binding leaving a reduced amount of Hb for further CO uptake. This so-called anemia effect will reduce DLCO measurements, but DLCO can be compensated for this effect using the CO back pressure measurement and equations provided in the 2017 ERS/ATS DLCO technical standards.

(c) *Alveolar O_2 partial pressure:* The reaction rate of CO with Hb is dependent on the P_AO_2. The affinity of Hb for CO is about 230 times the affinity of Hb for O_2, and the competition for Hb-binding sites swings even more in favor of CO as the P_AO_2 decreases with a consequential increase in DLCO. In normal subjects tested at a barometric pressure of 760 mmHg (sea level), P_AO_2 is typically 100 mmHg. When barometric pressure is reduced, either by the presence of an atmospheric low pressure cell or an increase in altitude, P_AO_2 decreases and DLCO will increase by about 0.53% for each 100 m of increase in altitude. Note that the 2017 reference values for DLCO provided by the Global Lung Function Initiative are corrected to 760 mmHg and the 2017 ERS/ATS standards recommend correcting DLCO measurements to 760 mmHg. If other reference values are used and the measured DLCO is corrected to 760 mmHg, then the reference values should also be corrected to 760 mmHg using the altitude of the center in which the reference values were obtained as a proxy for P_B, using the formula provided in the 2017 ERS/ATS standards.

The subject should not breathe supplemental oxygen for at least 10 min prior to a DLCO maneuver. However, if P_AO_2 has to be increased during the DLCO test for patients requiring supplemental O_2, the resulting DLCO measurement will be reduced, and an adjustment for the change in P_AO_2 will be required as described in the 2017 ERS/ATS DLCO technical standards.

(d) *Lung volumes:* As the lung inflates, D_m increases (due to unfolding membranes and increasing surface area), while V_c effects are variable (due to differential stretching and flattening of alveolar and extra-alveolar capillaries). The net effect of these changes is that DLCO tends to increase as the lung inflates. However, the relationship between DLCO and lung volume is complex and certainly not 1:1 with DLCO changes substantially less than lung volume changes. Thus, in a normal subject with a reduced inspired volume, the ratio DLCO/V_A will rise.

The ERS/ATS recommends using the inspired volume (V_I) as an index of test quality (Grade A requires V_I to be >90% of the vital capacity (VC) and Grade F would be a V_I/VC < 85%). This is based on two rationales: (a) a small V_A resulting from a suboptimal inspiration from RV will variably reduce DLCO as described above; (b) a reduced V_I will reduce the alveolar P_AO_2 from what would be expected, and this can increase DLCO as described above.

(e) *Ventilation distribution:* CO uptake will primarily reflect gas exchange in lung units which contribute most to inhalation and exhalation. This is particularly important in diseases such as emphysema, where the inhaled CO will preferentially go to the better-ventilated regions of the lung and the subsequently measured CO uptake will be determined mainly by uptake properties of those regions. Under these conditions, the tracer gas dilution used to calculate V_A will also reflect mainly regional dilution and underestimate the lung volume as a whole (a low V_A/TLC ratio (eg <0.75–0.85)) especially when a small alveolar gas sample is used. There are no good ways to adjust for this other than to comment that DLCO in the setting of a low V_A/TLC ratio is reflecting mainly the CO uptake properties of the better-ventilated regions of the lung.

5.5.2 Interpreting the Results

Once the DLCO measurement has been determined to be accurate and the appropriate adjustments have been made, the results need to be assessed in relation to a reference value. Many reference sets have been reported over the years with age, gender, and height being the most common prediction parameters. Race/ethnicity is also likely important, but data on these are limited. Unfortunately, there is considerable disparity among these data sets, and recommendations have been made to use the reference equation that best fits a normal population in your laboratory. More recently, the Global Lung Function Initiative (GLI) has taken a large number of these data sets, and using complex statistical procedures has produced a single set of reference equations. This is likely to become a worldwide standard. An abnormal

Table 5.1 Effect of pathologic processes on DLCO

Pathologic process	DLCO	KCO (actual/reference)
Obstructive diseases		
Bronchitis (asthma)	Normal	1
Emphysema	<LLN[a]	<1 to 1
Restrictive diseases		
Interstitial disease	<LLN	<1 to 1
Alveolar inflammation/edema	<LLN	<1 to 1
Extra-pulmonary	<LLN	>1
Lobectomy/pneumonectomy	<LLN	>1
Vascular disease	<LLN	<1
Neuromuscular weakness/effort	<LLN	>1

[a]Low V_A/TLC common

DLCO is a value below the lower limit of normal (LLN) of the reference equation. Severity of the abnormality can be addressed by either reporting a percent predicted value or a Z score based on the number of standard deviations that the observed DLCO is below the predicted value.

Interpretation of the DLCO should be guided by the concept that CO uptake is driven largely by alveolar-capillary interface surface properties (D_m, which is affected by area and, to a lesser extent, thickness) and alveolar-capillary blood volume (V_c). Diseases that reduce either D_m or V_c (or both) can thus be expected to reduce DLCO. In practice this means a variety of disease states including interstitial diseases, pulmonary vascular diseases, alveolar inflammatory diseases, chronic capillary hypertension from left heart failure, and emphysema all are associated with a low DLCO (Table 5.1). Progressive loss of DLCO in these diseases implies worsening of either D_m or V_c (or both). In normal subjects, maneuvers that decrease V_c (Valsalva maneuver, high vertical G-forces) will also decrease DLCO.

DLCO can be expressed as DLCO with respect to alveolar volume (essentially the rate of CO concentration change during the breath-hold, often expressed as KCO). This is commonly reported as DLCO/V_A, but it is important to remember that this expression does not represent DLCO "corrected" for V_A. Since predicted values for KCO were obtained in normal subjects with normal V_A, using this predicted KCO to infer normality when the V_A is low is misleading.

KCO, however, can help further characterize the processes underlying a low DLCO. A high KCO (actual/reference ratio>1) implies a preserved D_m and V_c in the face of a loss of lung volume. As noted above, this is what occurs with a suboptimal inspired volume. In practice, this may also reflect an inability to fully inspire due to chest wall abnormalities or neuromuscular issues. A large lobectomy or pneumonectomy may also produce a low DLCO with a high KCO because the remaining capillary bed volume is increased by increased perfusion. A low DLCO with a KCO near the reference value (actual/reference ratio near 1), as noted above, does NOT imply normal D_m and V_c properties in the lung. Instead it means that loss of D_m and/or V_c roughly parallels the loss of V_A, a situation reflecting many parenchymal lung diseases. Finally a low DLCO with a low KCO (actual/reference ratio <1) usually suggests a loss of V_c out of proportion to any loss in V_A as would occur in predominant pulmonary vascular disease (Table 5.1).

DLCO can also be elevated, usually by mechanisms that increase V_c. For example, increasing the perfusion pressure of the pulmonary circulation can increase DLCO substantially because higher perfusion pressure recruits and distends pulmonary capillaries (increasing V_c). Exercise, the supine position, and Müller maneuvers (inspiratory efforts against a closed glottis) can all recruit and dilate alveolar capillaries, thereby increasing V_c and DLCO. Finally, acute alveolar hemorrhage with its large volume of hemoglobin in the lungs has also been noted to increase DLCO. To differentiate a high DLCO from alveolar hemorrhage from a high DLCO due to increased V_c, one needs to inspect serial measurements of DLCO made during the DLCO maneuver. In alveolar hemorrhage, subsequent measurements of DLCO will decrease, while in increased V_c, subsequent measurements of DLCO will remain elevated.

5.6 Blood Gas Assessment

An important measure of pulmonary gas exchange is the amount of O_2 and CO_2 in the blood. An arterial blood sample, typically drawn from the radial artery, is analyzed to determine the partial pressures of O_2 (PaO_2) and CO_2 ($PaCO_2$) and the pH in blood leaving the lungs. Blood gases can also be analyzed in mixed venous blood. Details regarding the techniques for this measurement are available in the American Thoracic Society Pulmonary Function Laboratory Management and Procedure Manual.

5.6.1 *Arterial and Venous PO_2*

Arterial and venous PO_2 are the partial pressures of oxygen in arterial and mixed venous blood, respectively. In normal subjects at sea level, arterial PaO_2 is 80–100 mmHg, enough to easily fully saturate normal Hb (Fig. 5.2). Arterial hypoxemia is generally defined by values less than this, and severe arterial hypoxemia is generally defined as less than 55 mmHg, levels resulting in pulmonary vasoconstriction and the potential to compromise tissue oxygen delivery (see below).

Arterial hypoxemia can be a consequence of a low inspired oxygen concentration, alveolar hypoventilation, or $\dot{V}_A/\dot{Q}$ mismatching (including shunts). Diffusion impairments due to thickened membranes are generally not responsible for reduced arterial PaO_2 *at rest.* During exercise, however, blood flow velocity in patients with thickened alveolar-capillary membranes may increase enough to prevent equilibration between alveolar gas and capillary blood during the short transit through the lung, causing arterial hypoxemia. Thus, exercise can unmask diffusion defects that are not apparent at rest. A falling PaO_2 with exercise indicates that a diffusion defect may be an important contributing factor for hypoxemia.

The difference between alveolar and arterial PO_2 ($P_{(A-a)O_2}$) can be used to separate these mechanisms (a widened gradient suggests $\dot{V}_A/\dot{Q}$ mismatch and/or shunt). $P_{(A-a)}O_2$ is calculated as the difference between the PaO_2 and the PaO_2. PaO_2 is computed from the alveolar gas equation:

$$P_AO_2 = P_IO_2 - (PaCO_2 / RQ)$$

where RQ is the respiratory quotient ($\dot{V}CO_2/\dot{V}O_2$). The $P_{(A-a)O_2}$ is more sensitive and specific than the arterial PaO_2 alone as an indicator of $\dot{V}_A/\dot{Q}$ abnormalities. The $P_{(A-a)O_2}$ in healthy adults breathing room air increases with age. As a general rule, the $P_{(A-a)O_2}$ for an individual should be no more than half the chronologic age and no more than 25 mmHg while breathing room air. Thus, the upper normal limit of $P_{(A-a)O_2}$ for a 30-year-old person is 15 mmHg, whereas the upper normal limit of $P_{(A-a)O_2}$ for a 60-year-old individual is 25 mmHg. The $P_{(A-a)O_2}$ in normal adults is the result of the combination of mild $\dot{V}_A/\dot{Q}$ mismatch and a small anatomic right-to-left shunt. Each of these mechanisms is responsible for about half the total $P_{(A-a)O_2}$.

The $P_{(A-a)O_2}$ increases with increasing alveolar P_AO_2. In lungs with severe nonuniform $\dot{V}_A/\dot{Q}$ distribution, the $P_{(A-a)O_2}$ reaches a maximum at F_IO_2 of 0.6–0.7 and then decreases at higher F_IO_2 values. The decline in $P_{(A-a)O_2}$ at higher F_IO_2 is caused by more uniform rises in PaO_2, which overcome the nonuniform distribution of $\dot{V}_A/\dot{Q}$ ratios. This nonlinear relationship between the $P_{(A-a)O_2}$ and F_IO_2 makes reference $P_{(A-a)O_2}$ values obtained with supplemental O_2 difficult to use in critically ill patients, whose F_IO_2 values vary frequently.

The PaO_2/F_IO_2 ratio is a simple, bedside index of O_2 exchange when $\dot{V}_A/\dot{Q}$ mismatch is the primary cause of hypoxemia. However, this ratio loses reliability when hypoventilation contributes to hypoxemia. The PaO_2/P_AO_2 ratio is another easily calculated index of oxygenation. It has advantages and disadvantages similar to that of the PaO_2/F_IO_2 ratio. In addition, the PaO_2/P_AO_2 ratio can be misleading if $P\bar{v}O_2$ fluctuates. For example, when cardiac output decreases, the $P\bar{v}O_2$ falls because the tissues extract more O_2 from the arterial blood. Thus, more profoundly hypoxemic mixed venous blood decreases PaO_2, resulting in lower PaO_2/P_AO_2, but the decrease is not because of worsening gas exchange in the lungs; rather, it is because of low cardiac output. The PaO_2/P_AO_2 ratio is also affected by P_ACO_2 (e.g., hypoventilation).

The presence of right-to-left shunt can be differentiated from low $\dot{V}_A/\dot{Q}$ causes of hypoxemia by breathing 100% O_2. While the individual breathes pure O_2, the alveolar P_AO_2 in different lung units differs according to differences in alveolar P_ACO_2. Lung units with low $\dot{V}_A/\dot{Q}$ ratios increase their P_AO_2 values maximally with elevation of the inspired PO_2, but shunt does not. The amount of the shunt can be calculated with the following equation:

$$\frac{\dot{Q}_s}{\dot{Q}_t} = \frac{(Cc'O_2 - CaO_2)}{(Cc'O_2 - C\bar{v}O_2)}$$

where $\dot{Q}_s/\dot{Q}_t$ is the shunt ($\dot{Q}_s$) as a fraction of cardiac output ($\dot{Q}_t$), $Cc'O_2$ is end-capillary O_2 concentration, CaO_2 is arterial O_2 concentration, and $C\bar{v}O_2$ is mixed venous O_2 concentration. Healthy individuals have a small shunt that amounts to 2–5% of the cardiac output. This shunt or venous admixture occurs because some venous blood normally drains into the pulmonary veins, left atrium, or left ventricle from bronchial and myocardial (Thebesian) circulation.

Breathing 100% O_2 increases the arterial PaO_2 to greater than 600 mmHg in normal adults. If PaO_2 only rises to 250 mmHg during 100% O_2 breathing, the shunt is about one-fourth the cardiac output (25%). This procedure does not determine the anatomic location of a shunt, which may be intracardiac or intrapulmonary, but the calculation can help the clinician focus the differential diagnosis for causes of hypoxemia that develop predominantly by shunt mechanisms. Furthermore, because PaO_2 shows little response to variations in F_IO_2 at shunt fractions that exceed 25%, the clinician may be encouraged to reduce toxic and marginally effective concentrations of O_2. However, the shunt calculation frequently overestimates the true shunt because alveoli with very low $\dot{V}_A/\dot{Q}$ ratios (<0.1) may collapse completely during O_2 breathing.

Oxygen delivery to the tissue (DO_2) is determined by arterial oxygen content (CaO_2) × cardiac output ($\dot{Q}$) and is normally 1000 mL/min (200 mL O_2/L × 5 L/min). Tissues extract oxygen at different rates, but overall, under normal conditions, total body extraction is 25% of the oxygen delivered resulting in mixed venous oxygen content of 150 mL/L (75% Hb O_2 saturation, venous $P\bar{v}O_2$ near 40 mmHg). When oxygen delivery is compromised (hypoxemia or depressed cardiac output) or oxygen demands are high (e.g., exercise), total body tissue oxygen extraction can increase and mixed venous content will fall. In disease states where oxygen extraction is compromised, mixed venous oxygen and mixed venous $P\bar{v}O_2$ will be high.

5.6.2 *Arterial and Venous PCO_2 and HCO_3^-*

Arterial $PaCO_2$ is the partial pressure of CO_2 in arterial blood and is determined by the relationship between CO_2 production in the tissues ($\dot{V}CO_2$) and alveolar ventilation in the lungs ($\dot{V}_A$):

$$PaCO_2 = \left(\dot{V}CO_2 / \dot{V}_A\right) \cdot K$$

where $\dot{V}CO_2$ is carbon dioxide production in mL/min, $\dot{V}_A$ is alveolar ventilation in mL/min, and K is a constant accounting for CO_2 content and its relationship to $PaCO_2$ (described below) and is approximately 800 mmHg. Normal values for arterial $PaCO_2$ are 35–45 mmHg, a value reflecting the alveolar ventilation required to bring the alveolar P_AO_2 to 100 mmHg breathing room air at sea level (P_IO_2 = 150 mmHg). Because of the relationship of $PaCO_2$ with pH and

HCO_3^- described below, a normal arterial $PaCO_2$ results in a pH of 7.38–7.42. Hypercapnia usually results from reductions in $\dot{V}_A$ necessary for a given $\dot{V}CO_2$ and creates an acidosis; hypocapnia usually results from excess $\dot{V}_A$ for a given $\dot{V}CO_2$ and results in an alkalosis.

The transport pathway of CO_2 begins with the diffusion of CO_2 from tissues into the capillary blood and ends at the alveolar-capillary interface where CO_2 rapidly diffuses along a concentration gradient into alveolar gas. Under normal conditions, the mixed venous $P\bar{v}CO_2$ is 45 mmHg and the resulting gradient in the alveolus with a $PaCO_2$ of 40 mmHg is 5 mmHg.

About 90% of the CO_2 that enters the blood diffuses into the RBCs, where it undergoes one of three chemical reactions: (1) it remains as dissolved CO_2, (2) it combines with the NH_2 groups of hemoglobin to form carbaminohemoglobin, or (3) it combines with water to form H_2CO_3, which dissociates into H^+ and HCO_3^-. The remaining 10% of the CO_2 in the plasma exists as dissolved CO_2 and carbamino compounds after reacting with NH_2 groups of plasma proteins.

The amount of CO_2 that dissolves in plasma at 37 °C is about 0.03 mmol/L for every mmHg of PCO_2; thus, for a normal $PaCO_2$ of 40 mmHg, the normal amount of dissolved CO_2 in arterial blood is 40×0.03, or 1.2 mmol/L. Although the amount of dissolved CO_2 is relatively small, it is in equilibrium with the plasma $PaCO_2$, which in turn determines the direction and rate of CO_2 diffusion at body tissue and alveolar levels.

In plasma, CO_2 undergoes the following reaction:

$$CO_2 + H_2O \rightarrow H_2CO_3 \rightarrow HCO_3^- + H^+$$

The rate of this reaction is relatively slow in plasma, and the amount of carbonic acid (H_2CO_3) in the plasma is extremely small; even so, plasma H_2CO_3 is a major determinant of the blood's H^+ concentration (i.e., the pH). The reaction rate of CO_2 with H_2O in the erythrocyte is about 13,000 times faster than in the plasma due to the influence of carbonic anhydrase, an intracellular catalytic enzyme. As a result H^+ is rapidly generated, but it is immediately buffered by hemoglobin and thus removed from solution. Consequently, the reaction keeps moving to the right, continually drawing more CO_2 into the erythrocyte, generating HCO_3^- in the process. As HCO_3^- accumulates in the erythrocyte, its intracellular concentration rises; HCO_3^- then diffuses down its concentration gradient into the plasma. This mechanism is responsible for nearly all of the HCO_3^- in the plasma.

When negatively charged HCO_3^- ions diffuse out of the erythrocyte, an electropositive environment develops inside the erythrocyte. In response, Cl^-, the most abundant anion in the plasma, diffuses into the erythrocyte (the so-called *chloride shift,* a process governed by the anion exchange protein 1 (AE or band 3) on the RBC membrane), which maintains intracellular electrical neutrality. Some movement of water inward occurs simultaneously with the chloride shift to maintain osmotic equilibrium, resulting in a slight swelling of erythrocytes in venous blood relative to those in arterial blood.

The CO_2 hemoglobin equilibrium curve is essentially linear over the physiologic range of $PaCO_2$, in contrast to the S-shaped oxyhemoglobin equilibrium curve. This means a change in alveolar ventilation is much more effective in changing arterial CO_2 content than O_2 content; for example, a doubling of the alveolar ventilation in the healthy lung cuts the blood CO_2 content in half but changes arterial O_2 content very little because hemoglobin is already nearly 100% saturated with normal ventilation. The steepness of the CO_2 hemoglobin equilibrium curve also permits continued excretion of CO_2 even in the presence of significant mismatching of pulmonary ventilation and blood flow.

5.7 Noninvasive Measurement of the Hemoglobin Oxygen Saturation

Pulse oximetry provides a quick, noninvasive measure of the hemoglobin O_2 saturation (SpO_2) which can be a useful indicator of problems with gas exchange. It is sometimes called the fifth vital sign. The measurement is based on the change in color of Hb that occurs when reduced Hb is oxygenated. Oxyhemoglobin is red, while reduced Hb (deoxyhemoglobin) is bluish-purple. The different colors affect the absorption of different wavelengths of light. Oxyhemoglobin absorbs more infrared light and transmits more red light. Conversely, reduced hemoglobin absorbs more red light and transmits more infrared light. A pulse oximeter has bright sources of red and infrared light that are shone through a thin area of skin with good perfusion such as the fingertip, toe, or earlobe. A detector on the opposite side monitors the change in light transmission that occurs with pulsatile blood flow. The ratio of red to infrared transmission during the arterial surge of blood is used to calculate the percentage of arterial Hb that is O_2Hb.

A limitation of standard pulse oximetry is that COHb, being a cherry red color, is not distinguished from O_2Hb and so that the reported SpO_2 includes both O_2Hb and COHb. This limitation can be overcome by using CO-oximetry which uses additional light sources with different wavelengths to detect COHb.

A normal, healthy person at altitudes less than 1 km should have $SpO_2 > 95\%$. A resting $SpO_2 \leq 88\%$ is often an indication of the need for continuous supplemental O_2 therapy with the goal of increasing SpO_2 above 92%. Similarly, if SpO_2 falls below 88% during exercise or for a significant portion of a night's sleep, supplemental O_2 therapy may be indicated during exercise or sleep.

The correlation between PaO_2 and SpO_2 is nonlinear and is affected by temperature, pH, and P_ACO_2. However, SpO_2 measurements can complement the information obtained from arterial blood gas measurements. While PaO_2 is the preferred measure of gas exchange from the lung to the bloodstream, arguments have been made that SpO_2 is a better measure of oxygenation of the tissues. Arterial blood gas measurements provide data from a single time point, while SpO_2 can be continuously monitored, including in ambulatory patients.

5.8 Example Cases

1. A 63-year-old man has known COPD. There is very severe airway obstruction and substantial air trapping on spirometry and volume testing (Fig. 5.4). His arterial blood gases reveal a PaO_2 of 61 mmHg, a $PaCO_2$ of 49 mmHg, and a pH of 7.37. His hypercapnia is typical for severe COPD with a high work of breathing and his hypoxemia reflects both hypoventilation and ventilation/perfusion mismatching. The DLCO is dramatically reduced likely reflecting emphysematous destruction of alveoli. However, V_I during the DLCO maneuver was only 65% of the FVC and 70% of the slow VC measured during volume testing – typical of bad airway obstruction where the longer expiratory time of the FVC maneuver (>12 s) and the longer time allowed for the "slow" VC produce larger vital capacities than the V_I inhaled during the rapid inspiratory time of the DLCO maneuver. The impact of this low V_I on such a markedly reduced DLCO, however, is likely small. More

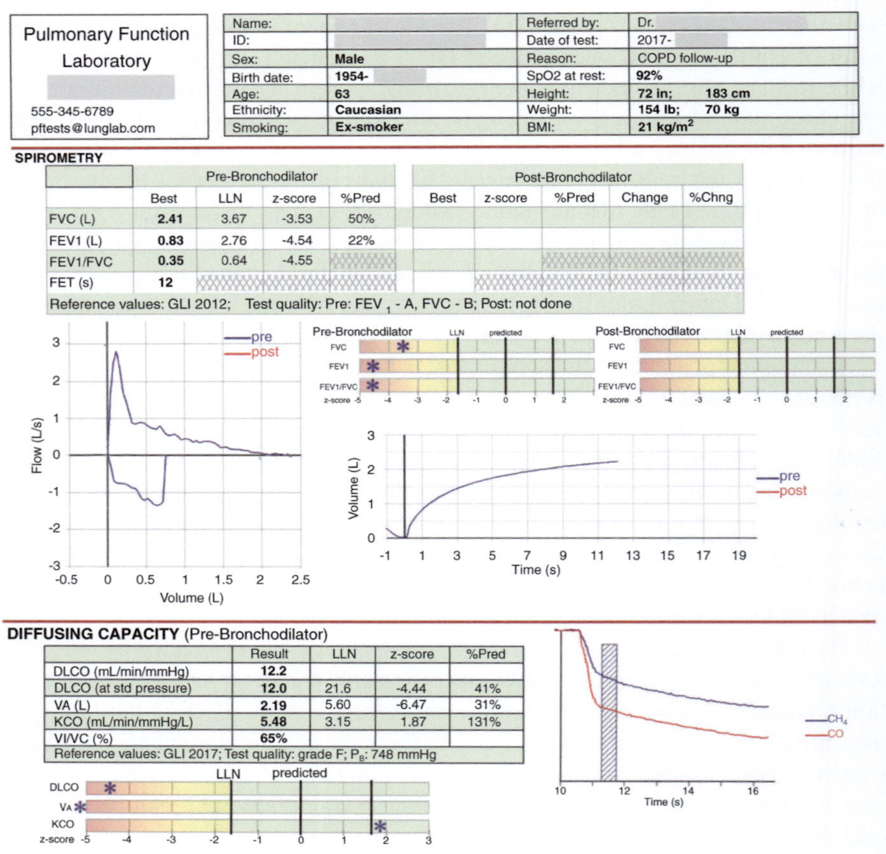
Pulmonary Function Laboratory
555-345-6789
pftests@lunglab.com

Name:		Referred by:	Dr.
ID:		Date of test:	2017-
Sex:	Male	Reason:	COPD follow-up
Birth date:	1954-	SpO2 at rest:	92%
Age:	63	Height:	72 in; 183 cm
Ethnicity:	Caucasian	Weight:	154 lb; 70 kg
Smoking:	Ex-smoker	BMI:	21 kg/m²

SPIROMETRY

	Pre-Bronchodilator				Post-Bronchodilator				
	Best	LLN	z-score	%Pred	Best	z-score	%Pred	Change	%Chng
FVC (L)	2.41	3.67	-3.53	50%					
FEV1 (L)	0.83	2.76	-4.54	22%					
FEV1/FVC	0.35	0.64	-4.55						
FET (s)	12								
Reference values: GLI 2012; Test quality: Pre: FEV 1 - A, FVC - B; Post: not done									

DIFFUSING CAPACITY (Pre-Bronchodilator)

	Result	LLN	z-score	%Pred
DLCO (mL/min/mmHg)	12.2			
DLCO (at std pressure)	12.0	21.6	-4.44	41%
VA (L)	2.19	5.60	-6.47	31%
KCO (mL/min/mmHg/L)	5.48	3.15	1.87	131%
VI/VC (%)	65%			
Reference values: GLI 2017; Test quality: grade F; P_B: 748 mmHg				

Fig. 5.4 Pulmonary function test results for case 1 fix VA = 2.19 (not = 12.0)

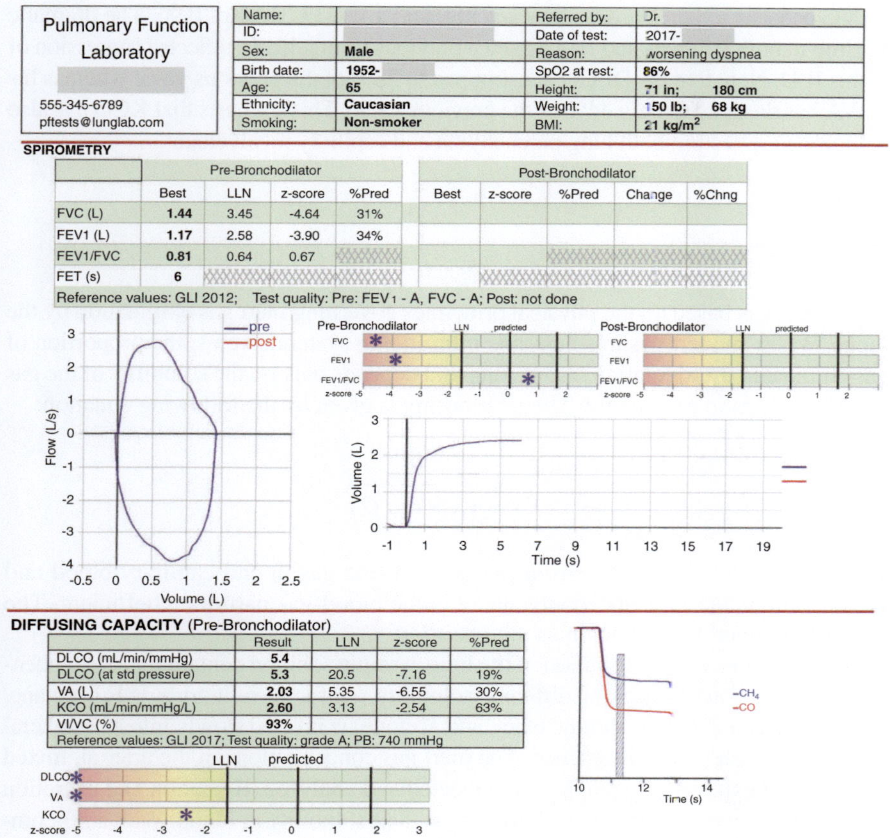
Pulmonary Function Laboratory

555-345-6789
pftests@lunglab.com

Name:		Referred by:	Dr.
ID:		Date of test:	2017-
Sex:	**Male**	Reason:	worsening dyspnea
Birth date:	**1952-**	SpO2 at rest:	**86%**
Age:	**65**	Height:	**71 in; 180 cm**
Ethnicity:	**Caucasian**	Weight:	**150 lb; 68 kg**
Smoking:	**Non-smoker**	BMI:	**21 kg/m²**

SPIROMETRY

	Pre-Bronchodilator				Post-Bronchodilator				
	Best	LLN	z-score	%Pred	Best	z-score	%Pred	Change	%Chng
FVC (L)	**1.44**	3.45	-4.64	31%					
FEV1 (L)	**1.17**	2.58	-3.90	34%					
FEV1/FVC	**0.81**	0.64	0.67						
FET (s)	**6**								

Reference values: GLI 2012; Test quality: Pre: FEV1 - A, FVC - A; Post: not done

DIFFUSING CAPACITY (Pre-Bronchodilator)

	Result	LLN	z-score	%Pred
DLCO (mL/min/mmHg)	**5.4**			
DLCO (at std pressure)	**5.3**	20.5	-7.16	19%
VA (L)	**2.03**	5.35	-6.55	30%
KCO (mL/min/mmHg/L)	**2.60**	3.13	-2.54	63%
VI/VC (%)	**93%**			

Reference values: GLI 2017; Test quality: grade A; PB: 740 mmHg

Fig. 5.5 Pulmonary function test results for case 2

importantly, the slope of the exhaled CH_4 over time curve is markedly downward consistent with poor gas mixing (consistent with the significant air trapping). This is also reflected in the V_A/TLC ratio of only 29%. Both of these markers of poor gas mixing essentially mean that the observed DLCO is likely reflecting gas exchange properties in only a small portion of better-ventilated lung regions. The high KCO is interesting and may suggest that this better ventilated region has good gas transfer properties but a low DLCO from either a reduced inspired volume and/or regional volume compression from adjacent hyperinflated lung units.

2. A 65 year-old man with known interstitial lung disease reports worsening dyspnea over last 3 months. Arterial blood gases reveal a PaO_2 of 53 mmHg (breathing room air), a $PaCO_2$ of 36 mmHg, and a pH of 7.46. His hypoxemia reflects ventilation/perfusion mismatching due to his interstitial lung disease and should be treated with supplemental O_2. His $PaCO_2$ and pH reflect mild hyperventilation in response to his hypoxemia. His PFTs show marked loss of lung volumes over last 5 months (Fig. 5.5). His hemoglobin adjusted DLCO is very low. Testing looks good with a V_I/

VC of 93%, a flat CH_4 over time tracing, and a V_A/TLC ratio of 0.96. The dramatic drop in both volumes and DLCO since previous testing likely reflects progression of his ILD. Note that his DLCO has dropped to 28% of the previous value whereas his VA has dropped to only 44% of the previous value. This suggests that KCO has also dropped reflecting both lung parenchyma and capillary involvement.

Appendix

The MIGET is based on the physical principles governing inert gas elimination by the lungs. When an inert gas in solution is infused into systemic veins, the proportion of gas eliminated by ventilation from a lung unit depends only on the solubility of the gas and the $\dot{V}_A/\dot{Q}$ ratio of that unit. The relationship is given by the following equation:

$$\frac{Pc'}{P\overline{v}} = \frac{\lambda}{\left(\lambda + \dot{V}_A / \dot{Q}\right)}$$

where Pc' and $P\overline{v}$ are the partial pressures of the gas in end-capillary blood and mixed venous blood, respectively, and λ is the blood-gas partition coefficient. The ratio of Pc' over $P\overline{v}$ is known as the *retention.*

To obtain the $\dot{V}_A/\dot{Q}$ distribution of the lung, a saline solution containing low concentrations of six inert gases of different solubility (sulfur hexafluoride [SF_6], ethane, cyclopropane, isoflurane, diethyl ether, and acetone) is infused slowly into a peripheral vein until a steady state is reached. The inert gas concentrations in the arterial, mixed venous, and expired gas samples are collected and analyzed. Retention and excretion values for the inert gases are graphed against their solubility in blood. With a 50-compartment model, the retention-solubility plots can be transformed to obtain the distribution of $\dot{V}_A/\dot{Q}$ ratios in the lung. A lung containing shunt units ($\dot{V}_A/\dot{Q} = 0$) shows increased retention of the least-soluble gas, SF_6. Conversely, a lung having large amounts of ventilation-to-lung units with very high $\dot{V}_A/\dot{Q}$ ratios and dead space ($\dot{V}_A/\dot{Q}$ = infinity) shows increased retention of the high-solubility gases (such as ether and acetone).

In healthy subjects, the distributions for both ventilation and blood flow (dispersion) are narrow and span only one log of $\dot{V}_A/\dot{Q}$ ratios. Essentially, no ventilation or blood flow occurs outside the range of approximately 0.3–3.0 on the $\dot{V}_A/\dot{Q}$ ratio scale, and no significant intrapulmonary shunt is detected. With aging, the dispersion of ventilation and perfusion increases. In older subjects, as much as 10% of the total blood flow may go to lung units with $\dot{V}_A/\dot{Q}$ values of less than 0.1, but still no shunt is detected. The increased low $\dot{V}_A/\dot{Q}$ regions adequately explain the decreased Pao_2 and increased $P_{(A-a)O_2}$ difference with aging. The cause of such age-related $\dot{V}_A/\dot{Q}$ mismatch often is attributed to degenerative processes in the small airways with aging.

Various abnormal patterns of $\dot{V}_A/\dot{Q}$ distributions measured by the MIGET method adequately explain gas exchange abnormalities in diseased lungs. For example, Fig. 5.6 shows the distribution of $\dot{V}_A/\dot{Q}$ ratios from an individual with chronic obstructive lung disease. The $\dot{V}_A/\dot{Q}$ distribution is bimodal, and large amounts of ventilation go to lung units with extremely high $\dot{V}_A/\dot{Q}$ ratios. This $\dot{V}_A/\dot{Q}$ pattern can be seen in individuals with predominant emphysema (Fig. 5.6, top). Presumably the high $\dot{V}_A/\dot{Q}$ regions represent lung units in which many capillaries have been destroyed by the emphysematous process. In some patients, there are regions of low $\dot{V}_A/\dot{Q}$ (Fig. 5.6, middle), as is commonly seen in patients with predominant chronic bronchitis. Finally, some patients have combinations of both high and low $\dot{V}_A/\dot{Q}$ units (Fig. 5.6, bottom). Note that the main modes of $\dot{V}_A$ and $\dot{Q}$ in the middle and the bottom graphs center on units with $\dot{V}_A/\dot{Q}$ ratio greater than 1 (high $\dot{V}_A/\dot{Q}$ units).

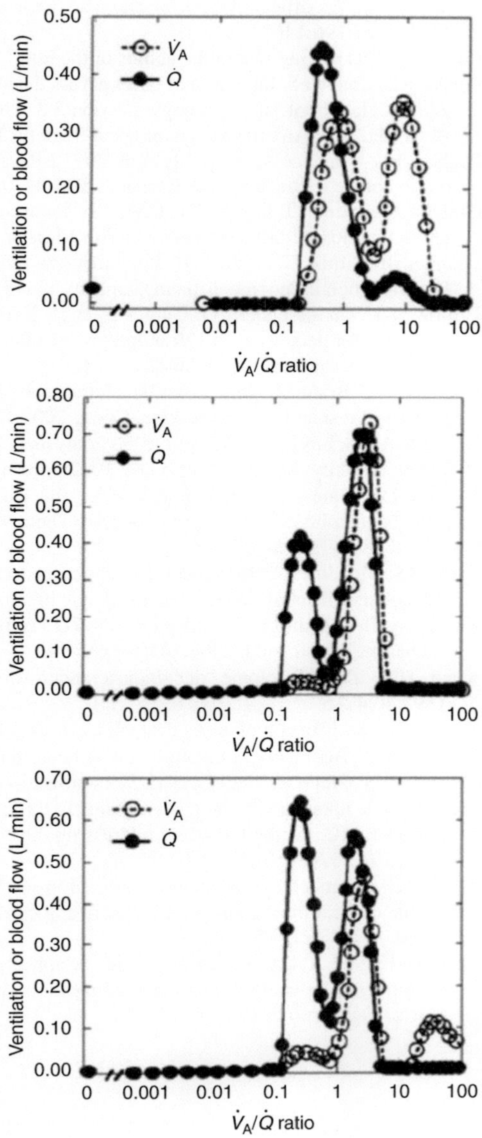

Fig. 5.6 Distribution of $\dot{V}_A/\dot{Q}$ ratios in different patients with COPD, illustrating predominant emphysema, with high $\dot{V}_A/\dot{Q}$ units (top), predominant chronic bronchitis, with low $\dot{V}_A/\dot{Q}$ units (middle), and a mixture of both high and low $\dot{V}_A/\dot{Q}$ units (bottom). (Reproduced with permission from Springer)

Selected References

Bachofen H, Schurch S, Urbinelli M, Weibel ER. Relations among alveolar surface tension, surface area, volume, and recoil pressure. J Appl Physiol. 1987;62:1878–87.

Butler JP, Tsuda A. Transport of gases between the environment and alveoli – theoretical foundations. Compr Physiol. 2011;1(3):1301–16.

Chan ED, Chan MM, Chan MM. Pulse oximetry: understanding its basic principles facilitates appreciation of its limitations. Respir Med. 2013;107:789–99.

Cotes JE, Chinn DL, Miller MR. Lung function. 6th ed. Oxford: Blackwell Scientific Publications; 2006.

Culver BH, Graham BL, Coates AL, et al. Recommendations for a standardized pulmonary function report. An official American Thoracic Society technical statement. Am J Respir Crit Care Med. 2017;196:1463–72.

Engel LA. Gas mixing within the acinus of the lung. J Appl Physiol. 1983;54:609–18.

Forster RE. Chapter 5. Diffusion of gases across the alveolar membrane. In: Farhi LE, Tenney SM, editors. Handbook of physiology. Section 5.3. The respiratory system. Vol IV. Gas exchange. Bethesda, MD: American Physiological Society; 1987. p. 71–88.

Graham BL, Brusasco V, Burgos F, et al. 2017 ERS/ATS standards for single-breath carbon monoxide uptake in the lung. Eur Respir J. 2017;49:1600016.

Graham BL, Mink JT, Cotton DJ. Effects of increasing carboxyhemoglobin on the single breath carbon monoxide diffusing capacity. Am J Respir Crit Care Med. 2002;165:1504–10.

Graham BL, Mink JT, Cotton DJ. Implementing the three equation method of measuring single breath carbon monoxide diffusing capacity. Can Respir J. 1996;3:247–57.

Hollowell J, Van Assendelft O, Gunter E, et al. Hematological and iron-related analytes—reference data for persons aged 1 year and over: United States, 1988–94. National Center for Health Statistics. Vital Health Stat. 2005;11:1–156.

Huang YC, O'Brien SR, MacIntyre NR. Intrabreath diffusing capacity of the lung in healthy individuals at rest and during exercise. Chest. 2002;122(1):177–85.

Huang YC, MacIntyre NR. Real-time gas analysis improves the measurement of single-breath diffusing capacity. Am Rev Respir Dis. 1992;146(4):946–50.

Hughes JM, Bates DV. Historical review: the carbon monoxide diffusing capacity (DLCO) and its membrane (DM) and red cell (Theta.Vc) components. Respir Physiol Neurobiol. 2003;138(2–3):115–42.

Jones RS, Meade F. A theoretical and experimental analysis of anomalies in the estimation of pulmonary diffusing capacity by the single breath method. Q J Exp Physiol. 1961;46:131–43.

Kaminsky DA, Whitman T, Callas PW. DLCO versus DLCO/VA as predictors of pulmonary gas exchange. Respir Med. 2007;101(5):989–94.

Kohn HN. Zur Histologie der indurierenden fibrinösen Pneumonie. Münch Med Wschr. 1893;40:42–5.

Krogh M. The diffusion of gases through the lungs of man. J Physiol. 1915;49:271–300.

Lambert MW. Accessory bronchiole-alveolar communications. J Pathol Bacteriol. 1955;70:311–4.

MacIntyre N, Crapo R, Viegi G, et al. Standardisation of the single-breath determination of carbon monoxide uptake in the lung. Eur Respir J. 2005;26:720–35.

McCormack MC. Facing the noise: addressing the endemic variability in D(LCO) testing. Respir Care. 2012;57(1):17–23.

Ogilvie CM, Forster RE, Blakemore WS, Morton JW. A standardized breath holding technique for the clinical measurement of the diffusing capacity of the lung for carbon monoxide. J Clin Invest. 1957;36:1–17.

Paiva M, Engel LA. Gas mixing in the lung periphery. In: Chang HK, Paiva M, editors. Respiratory physiology. An analytic approach. Lung biology in health and disease, vol. 40. New York: Marcel Dekker, Inc; 1989. p. 245–76.

Piiper J, Scheid P. Chapter 4. Diffusion and convection in intrapulmonary gas mixing. In: Farhi LE, Tenney SM, editors. Handbook of physiology. Section 5.3. The respiratory system. Vol IV. Gas exchange. Bethesda, MD: American Physiological Society; 1984. p. 51–69.

Roughton FJW, Forster RE. Relative importance of diffusion and chemical reaction rates in determining rate of exchange of gases in the human lung, with special reference to true diffusing capacity of pulmonary membrane and volume of blood in the lung capillaries. J Appl Physiol. 1957;11:290–302.

Sikand RS, Magnussen H, Scheid P, Piiper J. Convective and diffusive gas mixing in human lungs: experiments and model analysis. J Appl Physiol. 1976;40:362–71.

Smith TC, Rankin J. Pulmonary diffusing capacity and the capillary bed during Valsalva and Muller maneuvers. J Appl Physiol. 1969;27:826–33.

Stanojevic S, Graham BL, Cooper BG, et al. Official ERS technical standards: Global Lung Function Initiative reference values for the carbon monoxide transfer factor for Caucasians. Eur Respir J. 2017;50:1700010.

Wanger J. ATS Pulmonary Function Laboratory Management and Procedure Manual. 3rd ed: American Thoracic Society, New York, NY, USA; 2016. https://www.thoracic.org/professionals/education/pulmonary-function-testing/

West JB, Dollery CT, Naimark A. Distribution of blood flow in isolated lung; relation to vascular and alveolar pressures. J Appl Physiol. 1964;19:713–24.

West JB, Wagner PD. Pulmonary gas exchange. Am J Respir Crit Care Med. 1998;157:S82–7.

West JB. Respiratory physiology: the essentials. 9th ed. Philadelphia, PA: Lippincott Williams & Wilkins; 2012.

Chapter 6
Breathing Out: Forced Exhalation, Airflow Limitation

James A. Stockley and Brendan G. Cooper

6.1 Expiratory Mechanics

Spirometry requires that a subject exhales fully at maximal speed from the starting point of full inspiration total lung capacity (TLC). The speed at which the subject can expire is governed by the many mechanical properties of the pulmonary system, including the elastic recoil of the lungs and the compliance of the chest wall and airways, as well as the physical properties of air itself.

At the point of full inspiration (itself determined by respiratory muscle strength), the glottis is open, and there is no airflow. Therefore, the intraluminal pressure throughout the respiratory tract from the mouth (P_{MO}) to the bronchi (P_{BR}) to the alveoli (P_A) is universally equal to barometric pressure (P_{BAR}). Due to the stretching of the lungs, the elastic recoil of the lungs (P_{EL}) is opposing inflation, resulting in small, negative intrapleural pressure (P_{PL}) (Fig. 6.1a).

At the start of the maximal exhalation, an additional force is applied to the thoracic cavity by the contraction of the accessory expiratory muscles. This causes the pleural pressure (P_{PL}) and alveolar pressure (P_A) to increase far beyond atmospheric pressure (P_{BAR}), which results in expulsion of air from the lungs. The intraluminal pressure (P_{BR}) is now gradated throughout the respiratory tract, from the maximum in the alveoli (P_A) to the minimum at the mouth (P_{MO}). The point at which P_{PL} is equal to P_{BR} is referred to as the "equal pressure point", above which airway compression occurs (as P_{PL} is greater than P_{BR}). At the beginning of a forced expiration, airway compression first occurs in the trachea (Fig. 6.1b), where the dorsal membrane allows for the cartilaginous rings to bend, forming a slit-like aperture. As the

J. A. Stockley (✉) · B. G. Cooper
Lung Function and Sleep Department, Queen Elizabeth Hospital Birmingham, Birmingham, UK
e-mail: James.Stockley@uhb.nhs.uk; Brendan.Cooper@uhb.nhs.uk

D. A. Kaminsky, C. G. Irvin (eds.), *Pulmonary Function Testing*, Respiratory Medicine, https://doi.org/10.1007/978-3-319-94159-2_6

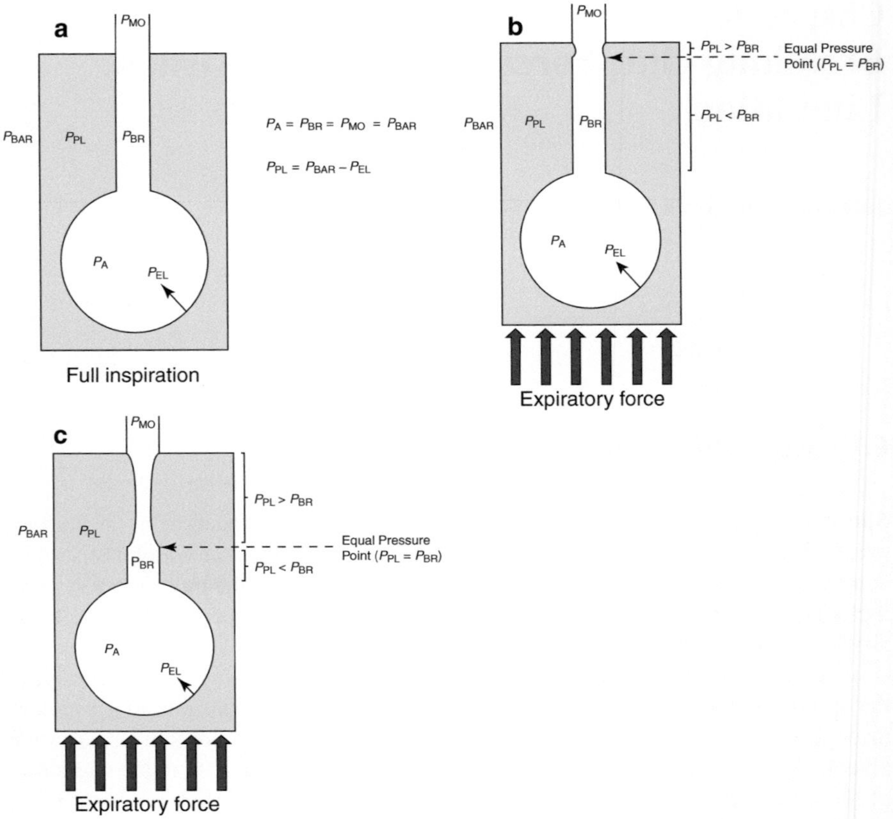

Fig. 6.1 A model of the respiratory tract, showing the relationship of intraluminal and intrapleural pressures (**a**) at full inspiration. Intraluminal pressures are equal, although the respiratory system is not at rest. (**b**) At the beginning of a forced expiration, where the equal pressure point is in the trachea; (**c**) towards the end of a forced expiration, where the equal pressure point has progressed to the peripheral airways

lungs continue to empty, the equal pressure point moves further away from the mouth, through the larger airways, and into the peripheral airways (Fig. 6.1c). The end of expiration is determined by the point at which small airway closure ("residual volume") finally occurs and airflow ceases.

While the equal pressure point mechanism explains expiratory flow limitation on the basis of the viscous properties of a gas flowing through a collapsible tube, another mechanism invokes flow limitation on the basis of the Bernoulli effect, which depends on the density of the gas. By this mechanism, the flow ($\dot{V}$) of air through a collapsible tube can never exceed the speed at which a wave can be propagated through it, regardless of the driving force ($P_A - P_{MO}$) behind it. This is referred to as "wave speed theory" and is dependent on the cross-sectional area of the airways (*A*), the collapsibility of the airway under pressure (*dA*/*dP*), and the density of the gas (*r*):

$$\dot{V} = \sqrt{\left[A \times \left(dA / dP\right) / r\right]}$$

This formula indicates that maximal flow varies (1) directly with the area (*A*) of the tube, such that narrowing of the tube results in reduced flow (as occurs in asthma); (2) directly with the stiffness (*dA*/*dP*) of the tube, such that a more collapsible tube results in reduced flow (as occurs in emphysema); and (3) inversely with the density of the gas, such as occurs with a mixture of helium and oxygen, which results in higher flow due to the lower density of the gas mixture. During wave propagation, the sides of the tube would oscillate inward and outward to accommodate the wave of pressure, and at some point, the inward oscillation would result in a narrowing, or choke point, that would limit flow. This is analogous to the equal pressure point explained above.

6.2 The Measurement of Forced Expiration

A spirometry test involves a full inspiration followed by a complete expiration. The expiration is performed in either in a relaxed manner for a vital capacity (VC) or at maximum speed for a forced vital capacity (FVC). The first spirometers able to measure an FVC did so directly, producing a time/volume "spirogram" (Fig. 6.2a), integral to which is the forced expiratory volume in 1 s (FEV_1). Modern systems more commonly measure flow, which yield a flow-volume loop (Fig. 6.2b) and derive volume parameters indirectly via integration. Flow-volume loops also include various flow parameters at stages throughout the expiration, including the peak expiratory flow (PEF), MEF_{75} (maximal expiratory flow when 75% of FVC remains), MEF_{50} (when 50% of FVC remains), MEF_{25} (when 25% of FVC remains), and the maximal mid-expiratory flow (MMEF) (average flow between 25% and 75% of FVC). However, the clinical usefulness of these additional flow parameters for general clinical management is not well supported. Many modern spirometers also allow for the measurement of a forced inspiratory vital capacity (FIVC) after an FVC, which includes the MIF_{50} (maximal inspiratory flow when 50% of FVC remains). Both of these inspiratory measurements can be useful in certain respiratory disorders (e.g. upper airway obstruction – see later). The ratio of MEF_{50}:MIF_{50} is approximately 1.0 in healthy subjects, but it can vary with different types of airflow obstruction. Visual pattern (shape) recognition of the flow-volume loop is important when interpreting spirometry, and a flow/volume aspect ratio of 1:2 in equivalent units (i.e. L/s vs. L) is recommended.

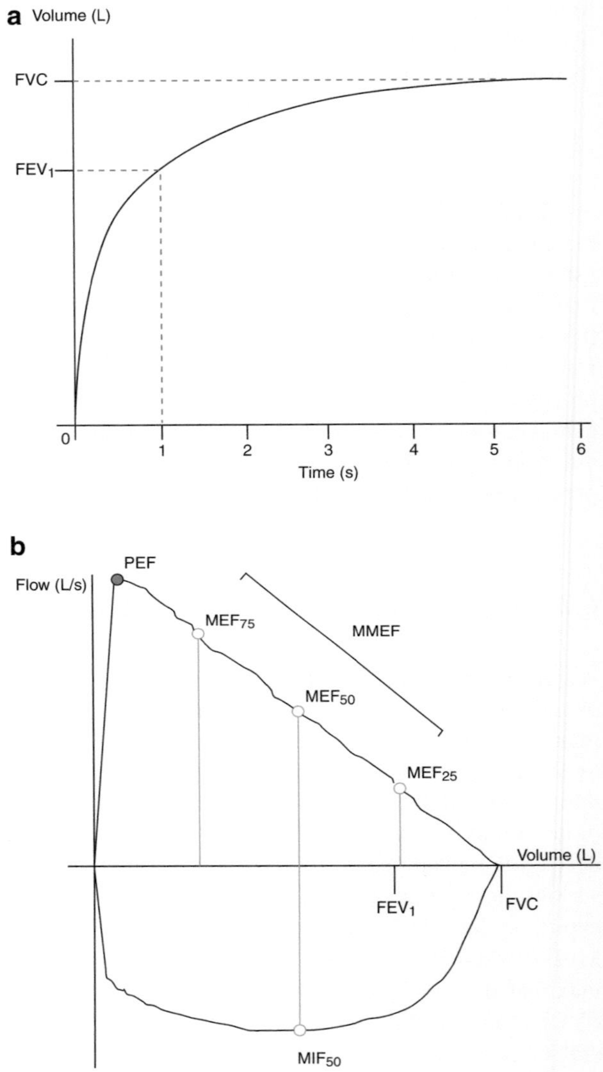

Fig. 6.2 (**a**) A classical expiratory "spirogram" from a healthy individual, showing the FEV_1 (volume expired at 1 s) and FVC (total volume expired). (**b**) A typical flow-volume loop from a healthy individual, showing the expiratory loop (above the *x*-axis) and inspiratory loop (below the *x*-axis). Highlighted are all flow parameters (measured directly) and volume parameters (derived by the integration of flow)

6.2.1 Indications and Contraindications

The most common symptom that patients present with in respiratory clinics is dyspnoea (shortness of breath), which may be present only on exertion or even at rest. There are many causes of dyspnoea (both respiratory and non-respiratory) and spirometry is a good starting point for physiological assessment to determine if there may be a respiratory cause. It is also a useful tool for determining the severity of disease and monitoring progressive pathology or the response to treatment. There are also a number of other indications for spirometry, all of which are listed below:

- To determine the presence or absence of ventilatory dysfunction
- To determine the severity of lung disease
- To monitor lung function changes over time
- To assess short-term and long-term effects of interventions
- To determine the effects of occupational/environmental factors
- To assess the potential risk for surgical procedures ("pre-operative assessment")
- Pre-lung transplant assessment (as part of full lung function assessment)
- To assess disability
- For legal reasons or insurance evaluation
- As an outcome measure for clinical research

As spirometry involves a sustained forced expiratory manoeuvre, it increases intrathoracic, intra-abdominal, and intracranial pressure. Therefore, there are a number of reasons when it may be inappropriate for a patient to perform spirometry, which have been primarily designed to protect the patient from potential discomfort/pain/death but also abolish any risk of cross infection and to ensure results are representative of clinical stability. Most common contraindications are relative and include:

- Recent thoracic, abdominal, or ocular surgery
- Pneumothorax
- Thoracic, abdominal, or cerebral aneurysm (exceptions may be made for smaller aneurysms, e.g. <9 mm)
- Haemoptysis
- Active respiratory infection (exceptions may be made in cases of chronic infective diseases such as bronchiectasis)
- Unstable cardiovascular status
- Recent myocardial infarction or pulmonary embolism
- Nausea and vomiting
- Any other condition that may affect the ability to perform the test (e.g. inability to sit upright, cognitive dysfunction)

6.2.2 *Pre-test Instructions*

There are a number of pre-test recommendations for spirometry to optimise test performance and ensure that a true baseline measurement is recorded. The patient should be aware of these at least 24 h prior to testing. Ideally, patients should:

- Stop smoking for 24 h before the test (although, realistically, this may have to be shortened to ensure patient compliance)
- Not consume alcohol for at least 4 h before testing

- Avoid vigorous exercise for at least 30 min before testing
- Avoid eating a substantial meal for at least 2 h before testing
- Stop taking bronchodilators for the duration of their action (this may not be necessary for COPD monitoring, where post-bronchodilation spirometry may be preferable)

Therefore, any relevant clinical information that is likely to impair the performance of a spirometry test should be checked and noted when the patient arrives before testing commences.

6.2.3 Test Performance

Spirometry can be a physically and technically demanding test. Furthermore, patients who have never performed lung function tests before may understandably be anxious. Therefore, before attempting spirometry, the physiologist should take time to explain clearly to the patient what they will be required to do. It is also often useful to physically demonstrate a forced manoeuvre, so the patient appreciates how forceful the expiration will need to be. It is often necessary for the physiologist to adopt different styles of explanation and coaching for different patients.

The test procedure for performing spirometry is as follows:

- The patient should then be seated in an upright position in a chair with armrests with the chin level and both feet flat on the floor.
- Nose clips are recommended to minimise the chance of leak from the nose.
- Both relaxed VC and FVC manoeuvres start with a full inspiration. Some spirometers will require this before the mouthpiece is inserted ("open circuit"), whereas others will require tidal breathing through the spirometer first ("closed circuit").
- Following a full inspiration, the patient must expire fully and continually in either a relaxed manner (for VC) or as forcibly as possible (for an FVC) while maintaining an upright position and an airtight seal around the mouthpiece with the lips.
- For an FVC manoeuvre, it is recommended that expiration commence within 1 s of reaching full inspiration.
- The person performing the test should continually encourage and coach the patient during expiration to ensure maximal effort and good technique.

6.2.4 Normal Ranges

Clinical interpretation of lung function data requires the comparison of obtained results to reference equations based on an individual's height, age, sex, and race. These equations allow for the derivation of percent predicted values and standardised residuals (or "*z*-scores").

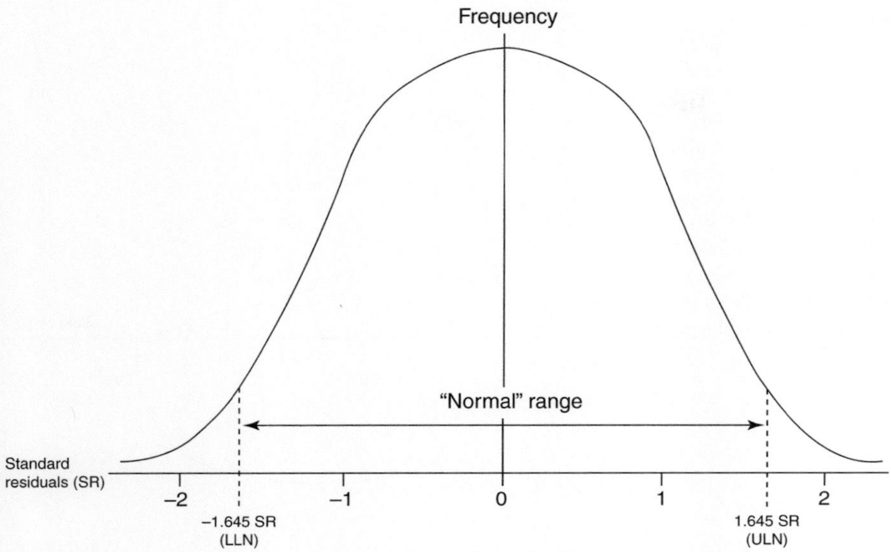

Fig. 6.3 A normal distribution curve with standardised residuals. The normal range only includes 90% of this population, which ranges from the lower limit of normal (LLN) at −1.645 SR to the upper limit of normal (ULN) at 1.645 SR. The probability of a value outside this range being "normal" is less than 5% ($p < 0.05$)

Traditionally, a threshold of 80% predicted was used to define normality. Although this may be comparatively easy to understand, it is now generally considered outdated as standardised residuals (SRs) can more accurately define the normal range. The normal range using SRs includes 90% of the population within the normal distribution curve, with the "lower limit of normal" (LLN) at −1.645 SR (Fig. 6.3). This method is not without limitations, although the probability of a measured value below the LLN being normal is less than 5% which, statistically, is considered non-significant (i.e. $p < 0.05$).

Recently, the European Respiratory Society Global Lung Function Initiative (GLI) has developed new reference equations, derived from lung function data from 74,187 healthy individuals. Importantly, this initiative included 3–95-year-old male and female never-smokers from multiple ethnic groups. Consequently, there is now a robust set of worldwide spirometry reference equations available for the first time.

Reference equations are discussed in greater detail in Chap. 14.

6.3 Patterns of Ventilation

Spirometry can identify both obstructive and restrictive ventilatory defects. Obstructive defects occur due to a narrowing of the airways. As mentioned, the cross-sectional area of the airways is a defining factor in airflow, and the result of

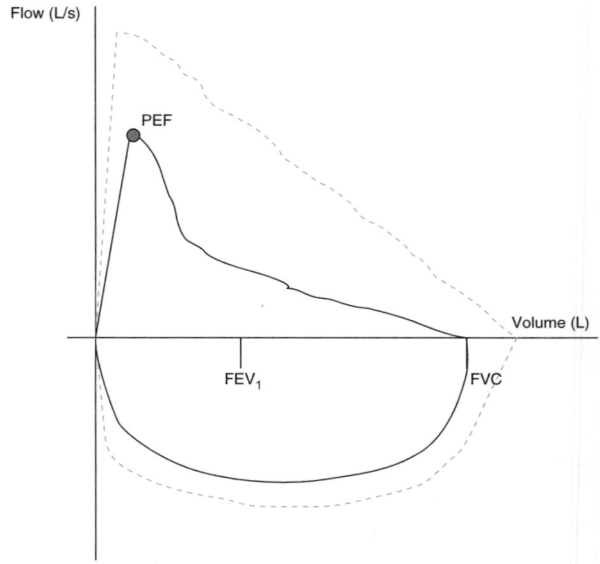

Fig. 6.4 A typical flow-volume loop from a patient with peripheral airflow obstruction. FEV_1 is considerably more reduced than FVC (which is often normal until more severe disease develops), leading to an FEV_1/FVC ratio below the normal range. For reference, a normal flow-volume loop is represented by the grey dotted line

airflow obstruction is decreased airflow due to increased airway resistance. Most obstructive defects affect the peripheral airways, leading to airflow obstruction predominantly on exhalation and a reduction in FEV_1 relative to the FVC (i.e. an FEV_1/FVC ratio below the normal range). Traditionally, the presence of airflow obstruction has been defined as an FEV_1/FVC ratio below 70%. However, the LLN is likely to be more appropriate at defining what is normal for an individual, as it accounts for natural age-related decline in lung function (e.g. emphysema can develop naturally in old age). Common diseases that cause peripheral airflow obstruction include chronic obstructive pulmonary disease (COPD), asthma, bronchiectasis, and cystic fibrosis. A typical flow-volume loop from a patient with airflow obstruction is shown in Fig. 6.4.

Following diagnosis of airflow obstruction from the FEV_1/FVC ratio, it may be further categorised into different severities based on the FEV_1% predicted. While the use of % predicted over SRs is contentious, it unfortunately remains the most widely accepted method of stratifying the severity of airflow obstruction. However, the use of SRs can easily replace % predicted once practitioners accept and remember their importance (Table 6.1). In addition to spirometry, it is also important to consider other factors such as breathlessness, cough, exercise capacity, and exacerbation frequency to give a more robust assessment of the impact of the disease as a whole.

The ratios between other volume parameters have also been suggested as a more accurate measure of airflow obstruction than FEV_1/FVC. These include FEV_1/VC (as patients can often expire more when doing so in a relaxed VC manoeuvre), FEV_3/FVC (which may be a better marker of early disease), and FEV_3/FEV_6 (FEV_6 is more repeatable than FVC and FEV_3/FEV_6 has also been shown as a marker of early small airway disease). However, these ratios are yet to be implemented in general clinical practice, and the FEV_1/FVC ratio remains the current standard.

Table 6.1 The most widely accepted methods of stratifying the severity of airflow obstruction in current use (GOLD and ERS/ATS), which are based in the FEV_1 expressed as a percentage of the predicted value

Severity of airflow obstruction	Global Initiative for Obstructive Lung Disease (GOLD)	European Respiratory Society (ERS)/American Thoracic Society (ATS)	Proposed SR range
	FEV_1	FEV_1	FEV_1
Mild	>80% predicted	>70% predicted	> −2
Moderate	50–80% predicted	60–70% predicted	−2.5 to −2
Moderately severe	n/a	50–60% predicted	−3 to −2.5
Severe	30–50% predicted	35–50% predicted	−4.0 to −3.0
Very severe	<30% predicted	<35% predicted	< −4

An example SR range (based on the ERS/ATS guidelines) to more accurately stratify airflow obstruction is included alongside

Larger obstructions (e.g. goitre, stenosis, tumour) can occur within the larger airways, which may impede expiratory airflow, inspiratory airflow, or both. This is dependent on whether the upper airway obstruction is intra- or extrathoracic and whether it is fixed (non-moveable) or variable (moveable). This is best determined physiologically by assessing the shape of the flow-volume loop, where truncation (flattening) of the expiratory/inspiratory curves indicates upper airway obstruction. A fixed extrathoracic obstruction will lead to flattening (often severe) of both the expiratory and inspiratory curves. A fixed intrathoracic airway obstruction will also cause a truncation of both the expiratory and inspiratory curves, but it may be less pronounced if the obstruction is in one of the bronchi rather than the trachea (as the degree of obstruction in relation to the total cross-sectional area of the airways is less). A variable extrathoracic obstruction will only impede inspiratory flow due to the negative intraluminal pressure on forced inspiration, whereas the positive intraluminal pressure in the upper airway on forced expiration effectively "pushes" the obstruction away from the airway lumen. The reverse is true in cases of variable intrathoracic upper airway obstruction, where obstruction only occurs on forced expiration due to an effective "amplification" of the dynamic airway compression at the site of obstruction. These are best understood from visual pattern recognition of the flow-volume loops (Fig. 6.5).

Therefore, the flow-volume loop has a number of advantages over the more basic spirogram in airflow obstruction. Visual assessment of the shape can itself be indicative of pathology (e.g. upper airway obstruction). Comparison of the maximal expiratory flow-volume curve (MEFVC) to a partial expiratory flow-volume curve (PEFVC) has been used to demonstrate the effect of a deep inhalation on airflow. In addition, volume-dependent changes in airflow that occur with differing degrees of gas compression on forced exhalation may be demonstrated by comparing flow measured at the same volume ("iso-volume") using a body plethysmograph vs. flow at the mouth, where mouth flow is typically less due to increased gas compression. This difference is generally more pronounced in airflow obstruction (Fig. 6.6) than in health, but this method has predominantly been a research tool rather than a clinical outcome.

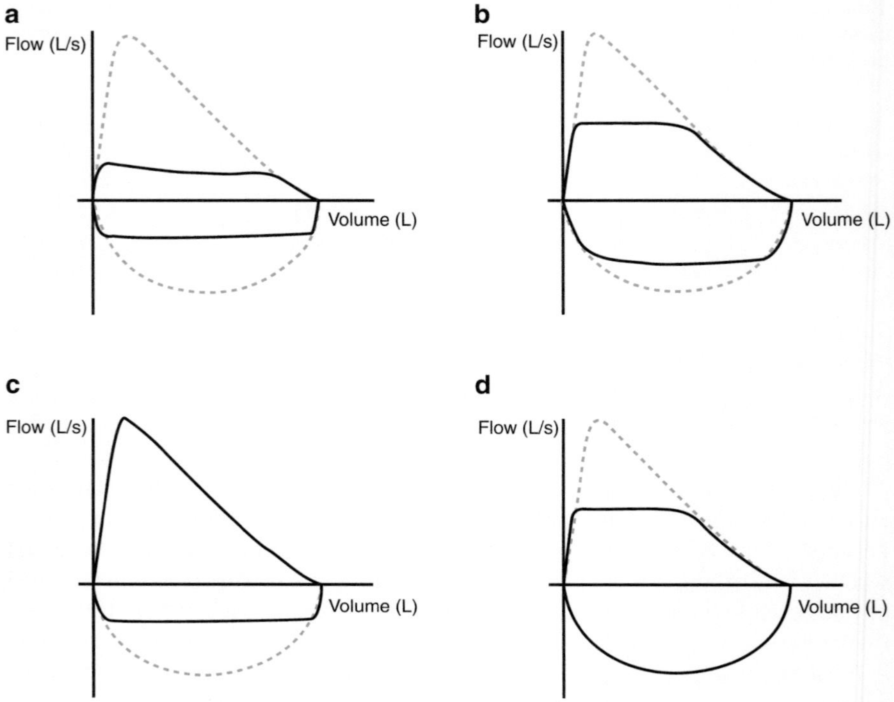

Fig. 6.5 Typical flow-volume loops from patients with various forms of upper airway obstruction. (**a**) Fixed thoracic obstruction (truncation of both expiratory and inspiratory curves); (**b**) fixed intrathoracic obstruction (truncation of both expiratory and inspiratory curves, which *may* be less pronounced as shown here), depending on the location of the obstruction); (**c**) variable extrathoracic obstruction (severe truncation of the inspiratory curve only); (**d**) variable intrathoracic obstruction (truncation of expiratory curve only, which may also be less pronounced, depending on the location of the obstruction)

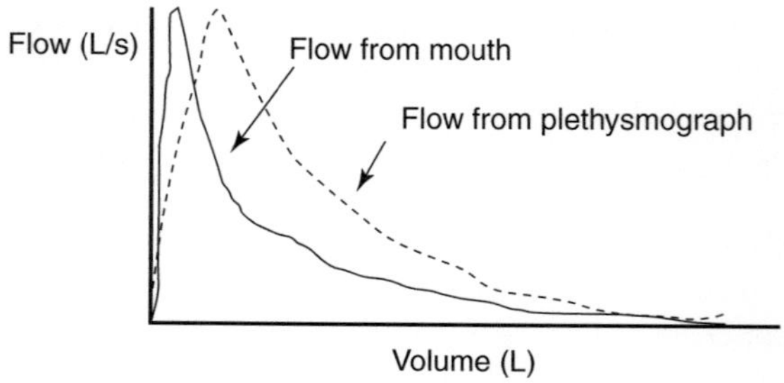

Fig. 6.6 Typical maximal expiratory flow-volume curves from a patient with emphysema. Isovolumetric analysis shows a marked difference in expiratory flow due to a greater degree of gas compression on forced exhalation when measured from volume changes in a body plethysmograph (dashed line) than volume changes expired at the mouth (solid line)

Restrictive ventilatory defects may be defined as a reduced ability of the lungs to expand, which can result from different pathophysiological processes. The pathology may be intrapulmonary, where fibrotic changes can lead to reduced compliance and the lungs themselves cannot expand as easily (e.g. pulmonary fibrosis, systemic lupus erythematosus, sarcoidosis). Alternatively, the pathology may be extrapulmonary, where the lungs are healthy but pathology outside the lungs restricts their expansion. This could be within the pleura (e.g. where plaques may form, making the pleura less compliant), the thoracic cage (e.g. skeletal abnormalities such as kyphoscoliosis, ankylosing spondylitis), or the muscles driving lung expansion (e.g. neuromuscular disease, inflammatory/metabolic myopathies). Obesity can also result in extrapulmonary restriction due to the excessive weight limiting thoracic expansion. In isolated ventilatory restriction, there is a concurrent and relative reduction on both FVC and FEV_1 with a preserved FEV_1/FVC ratio, which may actually increase in severe disease when patients can inspire so little, the vast majority (if not all) is expired within 1 s. On most cases, the shape of the flow-volume loop resembles that of a healthy individual but with an overall reduction in size and, in some instances (particularly advanced fibrotic lung disease), a partly convex expiratory loop due to reduced compliance (Fig. 6.7a). In cases of respiratory muscle weakness, there may be a rounding of the expiratory loop, a more abrupt end to expiration, and an abnormally slow inspiratory flow near full inflation (Fig. 6.7b).

There may also be cases where patients develop a mixed obstructive/restrictive defect, which occurs in approximately 1% of patients. This could either be due to two separate pathologies (e.g. COPD with fibrosis) or one pathology that causes both effects (e.g. sarcoidosis). In these cases, the FEV_1/FVC ratio will be below the normal limit together with an FVC below the normal range. However, it is worth noting that, in cases of severe airflow obstruction alone, FVC may also be below the normal limit. Therefore, a mixed defect would most likely demonstrate a reduced FVC that is disproportionately large compared to the degree of airflow obstruction. To confirm a true mixed defect, TLC should be measured. If TLC is normal, then the low FVC is solely due to severe obstruction, whereas if TLC is reduced, a true mixed defect is present. When this is the case, the severity of airflow obstruction can be more accurately assessed by adjusting the decrement in the FEV_1% predicted by the degree to which the TLC is reduced (i.e. adjusted FEV_1% predicted = measured FEV_1% predicted/measured TLC % predicted).

An interesting pattern that is described is a low FVC in the setting of a normal FEV_1/FVC, thus suggesting restriction, but a normal TLC, thus ruling against restriction. This has been called the "non-specific" pattern and appears to include patients with obstruction, restriction, chest wall disease, and neuromuscular weakness. Another recently described pattern has been called "complex restriction", which describes the situation where the FVC is disproportionally reduced compared to the reduction in TLC, with a relatively normal or elevated RV/TLC and normal FEV_1/FVC. This has been found to occur in about 4% of patients. Typically these patients had problems with impaired lung emptying such as neuromuscular disease, chest wall restriction, or subtle air trapping.

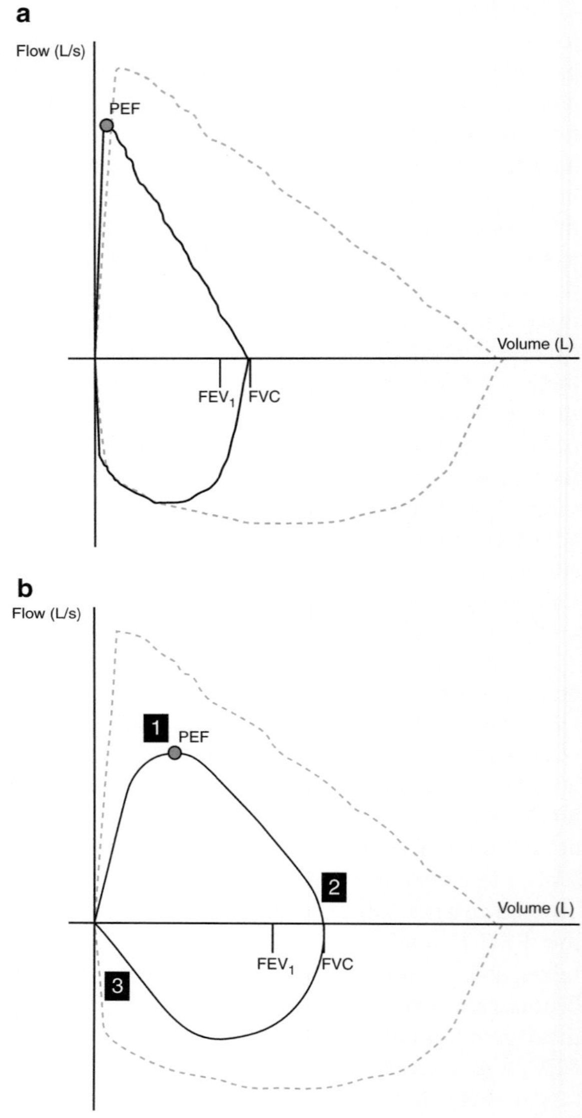

Fig. 6.7 Typical flow-volume loops from patients with ventilatory restriction. FVC and FEV_1 are reduced in proportion. (**a**) General restriction (including fibrotic lung disease, pleural disease, and skeletal abnormalities), (**b**) respiratory muscle weakness (common features are labelled and may include (1) a rounding of the expiratory curve, (2) an abrupt end to expiration, and (3) a slower inspiratory flow near full expansion)

6.4 Technical Performance

There are three components of an FVC manoeuvre; (i) a maximal inspiration followed immediately by (ii) the sharp "blast" at the start of a forced expiration, continuing on to (iii) complete exhalation. Therefore, the achievement of accurate spirometry is highly effort-dependent and requires good technical performance at all stages of the test. Consequently, poor technique/effort at any stage can affect the measurements. For instance, submaximal effort at the start of expiration will not only underestimate PEF but, due to a smaller degree of dynamic airway compression, can actually overestimate FEV_1 (so-called "negative effort dependence"). Achievement of a full FVC can also be physically demanding, particularly for patients with advanced lung disease. The European Respiratory Society (ERS)/ American Thoracic Society (ATS) 2005 guidelines outline recommendations for the achievement of technically acceptable spirometry. It is important that the time between maximal inspiration and the start of the forced expiration is minimal (2 s maximum), as a long delay may reduce expiratory power and affect PEF and FEV_1 (likely due to stress relaxation of elastic elements). Furthermore, the PEF at the start of the forced expiration must be achieved almost immediately following commencement of exhalation, and guidelines recommend an expiratory "extrapolation volume" less than 5% of FVC or 150 ml (whichever is greater) (Fig. 6.8).

Continued effort to achieve a true maximum exhalation without pause or intermittent inhalation is also difficult, particularly for patients with severe airflow obstruction. Guidelines recommend a minimum exhalation time of 6 s and an expiratory plateau (<0.025 L change in >1 s) denote a technically acceptable FVC endpoint. However, it is worth noting that patients with airflow obstruction, who can

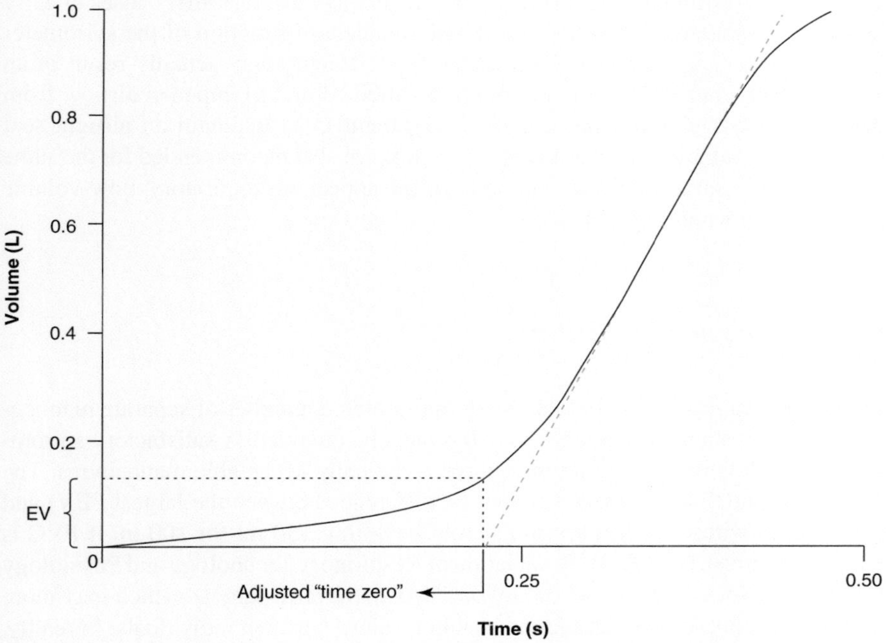

Fig. 6.8 An expanded view of the start of a spirogram. A line (grey dashed) through the steepest part of the expiratory curve (which equates to PEF) yields an adjusted "time zero" at the intersect of the time axis. The extrapolation volume (EV) is the volume at which a vertical line from the adjusted time zero intersects the expiratory curve. Guidelines recommend that EV should not exceed 5% of FVC

often expire for far longer than 6 s, may not achieve an expiratory plateau. In all cases, it is the responsibility of the physiologist to encourage patients to achieve their maximum, and it is generally at the very start and towards the end of forced expiration that most encouragement is needed.

It is also the operator's responsibility to recognise and attempt to correct any technical errors. As mentioned, a submaximal effort at the start will adversely influence PEF and FEV_1 measurements, although it should be noted that flow-volume loops from patients with respiratory muscle weakness may look "submaximal" despite maximum effort on their part (Fig. 6.7). A cough may also occur during forced expiration, which may either be a "cough-like" PEF due to brief glottis closure after full inspiration (this may overestimate PEF, but the manoeuvre may still be technically acceptable) or a true cough later in the forced expiratory manoeuvre. If a true cough occurs before 1 s, it will render the attempt unacceptable, as FEV_1 will be affected. If it occurs after 1 s, the attempt may still be acceptable (FEV_1 will certainly be valid), providing expiration is continuous and the end of test criteria are met. Patients also often strain too hard during a forced expiration, which not only makes it more difficult to expire and could lead to cough or even syncope but may also underestimate results due to increased upper airway resistance. Glottis closure (a Valsalva manoeuvre) is also relatively common (which may occur due to straining) and will underestimate FVC due to premature airway closure. Other causes of early termination include unsustained effort and complete obstruction of the spirometer tube by the tongue. A partial obstruction by the tongue may actually result in an accurate FVC, but FEV_1 will commonly be affected due to impeded airflow from the lungs into the spirometer. Finally, the patient must maintain an airtight seal around the mouthpiece to avoid leak (nose clips are also recommended for the same reason). How some of these common errors appear on expiratory flow-volume curves are shown in Fig. 6.9.

6.4.1 Repeatability Criteria

In order for spirometry to be accurately interpreted, a number of separate manoeuvres with repeatability at a single session must be obtained. A satisfactory spirometry session requires a minimum of three technically acceptable manoeuvres. The ATS/ERS guidelines recommend that the difference between the largest FEV_1 and FVC values within the test session should be within 150 ml (or 100 ml if FVC is <1 L). In contrast, the ARTP (Association of Respiratory Technology and Physiology (UK)) guidelines recommend 100 ml or 5% (whichever is larger), which may more robustly account for the variation in absolute values between individuals. In reality, many good respiratory physiology departments can achieve <70 ml repeatability in 80% of subjects tested. Both guidelines recommend that the maximum for each parameter be reported, even if they are not from the same attempt. Neither

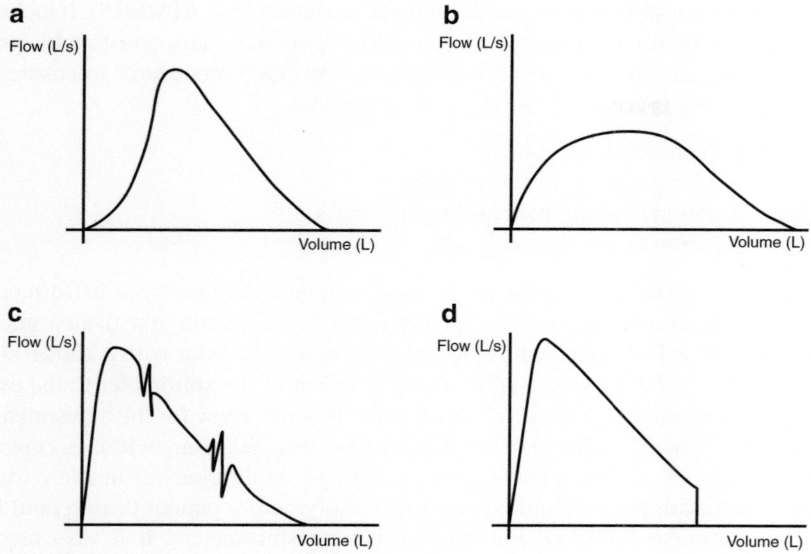

Fig. 6.9 Examples of how common technical errors appear on expiratory flow-volume curves, including (**a**) a slow start, (**b**) poor effort (at the start of forced expiration), (**c**) cough, and (**d**) glottis closure

guidelines propose a repeatability criterion for PEF as part of an FVC manoeuvre (even though it can influence FEV_1), although the ATS/ERS guidelines address this indirectly by suggesting that the "shape" of the expiratory flow-volume curve should be repeatable. These guidelines also recommend that, as a stand-alone measurement, PEF should be repeatable within 0.67 L/s. It should be noted that poor repeatability can sometimes be a clinical feature (e.g. bronchoconstriction on repeated attempts or fatigue due to muscle weakness).

A maximum of eight FVC manoeuvres should be attempted, and, in cases where repeatability acceptability criteria are not met, the best results may still be reported (providing they are technically acceptable) with an interpretative note. Over time, patients can often learn how to perform more technically acceptable spirometry through practice with repeat testing.

6.4.2 *Quality Assurance*

Spirometry is a biomedical diagnostic procedure and should, consequently, have appropriate quality assurance (QA) standards to ensure the measurements and their interpretation are both accurate. QA is a set of procedures implemented to guarantee that spirometry testing adheres to international standards (e.g. ATS/ERS). It includes both assessment of the patient's performance of spirometry during testing by qualified physiologists and also separate quality control (QC) procedures to ensure the equipment itself is accurate. QC procedures include:

- Equipment calibration/verification
- A log of calibration/verification results
- Documentation of equipment faults and repairs
- Documentation of software upgrades

Calibration is different from verification, although they are both performed in the same manner using a precision syringe (usually a 3-L syringe with an accuracy of less than 15 ml). Calibration is the checking of a spirometer with a known standard (e.g. 3-L volume), followed by the adjustment of the spirometer to the exact value of that standard. In contrast, verification does not allow for the adjustment of the spirometer but is, rather, a check that the device is measuring within acceptable limits (e.g. +3% of the known value). Syringe calibration/verification (often termed "physical QC") should be performed daily before patient testing (and following equipment transfer). For flow-measuring spirometers, it is also recommended that calibration/verification be performed using variable flows (to represent the different flows at which patients may expire/inspire). Older volume-measuring devices (e.g. wedge-bellows spirometer) may instead require daily verification with a 3-L syringe together with leak checks and quarterly time checks (with a stopwatch) to ensure the carriage moves at an accurate speed. In addition, it is important that every syringe is checked for accuracy by the manufacturer (usually annually).

An additional simple QC procedure is to perform regular tests on healthy subjects (e.g. physiology staff). This biological (or "physiological") QC is usually performed weekly and matched to an individual's expected range (determined from previous repeat testing) but may also be used as a robust and full assessment of equipment performance that allows for the differentiation of patient and equipment error in instances where acute technical issues are suspected.

6.5 Bronchodilator Reversibility Assessment

As spirometry is a physiological test of airway ventilation, it is often used to assess the short-term effects of pharmacological agents that aim to improve airway calibre and, hence, ventilation. Bronchodilators may be categorised into two general types: (i) beta-2 agonists and (ii) antimuscarinic agents. These drugs are inhaled either as an aerosol or dry powder (via a handheld inhaler device) or nebulised.

Beta-2 agonist act on the beta-2 adrenergic receptors which, in turn, produce cyclic adenosine monophosphate (cAMP) through the coupled G-protein, adenylyl cyclase. In the lungs, cAMP has a number of downstream signalling effects, including decreased intracellular calcium, inactivation of myosin light chain kinase, and increased potassium conductance. These effects lead to the relaxation of the smooth muscle surrounding the airways and concordant bronchodilation (increased airway calibre). The effect of beta-2 agonists is direct and rapid, with peak bronchodilation occurring within 20 min. Inhaled antimuscarinic agents achieve bronchodilation via a different signalling pathway. These are anticholinergic drugs that block acetylcholine activity by binding to muscarinic acetylcholine receptors. Acetylcholine is a neurotransmitter released by neurones into the neuromuscular junction to activate muscles. Therefore, inhibition of this pathway in the lungs inhibits contraction of the smooth muscle around the airways, leading to bronchodilation. The mode of action is indirect and, hence, less rapid than a beta-2 agonist, with peak bronchodilator effect occurring after approximately 45 min.

Bronchodilation reversibility assessments include the assessment of baseline spirometry followed by bronchodilator administration and, after the recommended time for peak effect (20 min for beta-2 agonists and 45 min for antimuscarinic agents), repeat "post-bronchodilator" spirometry. Therefore, it is essential that patients withhold their bronchodilators for up to 24 h (depending on the duration of the bronchodilator effect) prior to baseline spirometry.

Determining a positive bronchodilator response is not straightforward. There are a number of published guidelines (Table 6.2), where the definition of a positive response is based either on absolute change (ml), a percentage change, or both. A percentage change may be more appropriate than an absolute change, as it expresses the change more accurately in terms of the baseline value. Moreover, a percentage change is also independent of demographic factors (particularly height) that influence the natural variability of an individual's measurement. For instance, 160 ml could be within the natural variability of the FEV_1 from an individual who is very tall, whereas a very short individual may struggle to increase their FEV_1 by over 160 ml following bronchodilation, particularly if they have severe airflow obstruction and a very small baseline FEV_1 (e.g. <50 ml). It has recently been shown that a bronchodilator response expressed as change in % predicted is a good predictor of mortality in patients with suspected respiratory disorders. Another strategy for determining a bronchodilator response is to measure the change in FEV_1 and/or FVC after bronchodilator in relation to the individual's intratest variability in these parameters when measured at baseline. If the change after bronchodilator statistically exceeds this intratest variability, then one might conclude that there has been a statistically significant response. Whether or not such a change is clinically significant would still need to be determined.

Table 6.2 Published guidelines from four sources stating the criteria that define a positive bronchodilator response

Guidelines	Criteria
Association of Respiratory Technology and Physiology (ARTP)	160 ml in FEV_1 and/or 330 ml in FVC
British Thoracic Society (BTS)	200 ml and 15% in FEV_1
Global Initiative for Obstructive Lung Disease (GOLD) and ERS/ATS 2005	200 ml and 12% in FEV_1
National Institute for Health and Care Excellence (NICE) (2010)	400 ml in either FEV_1 or FVC

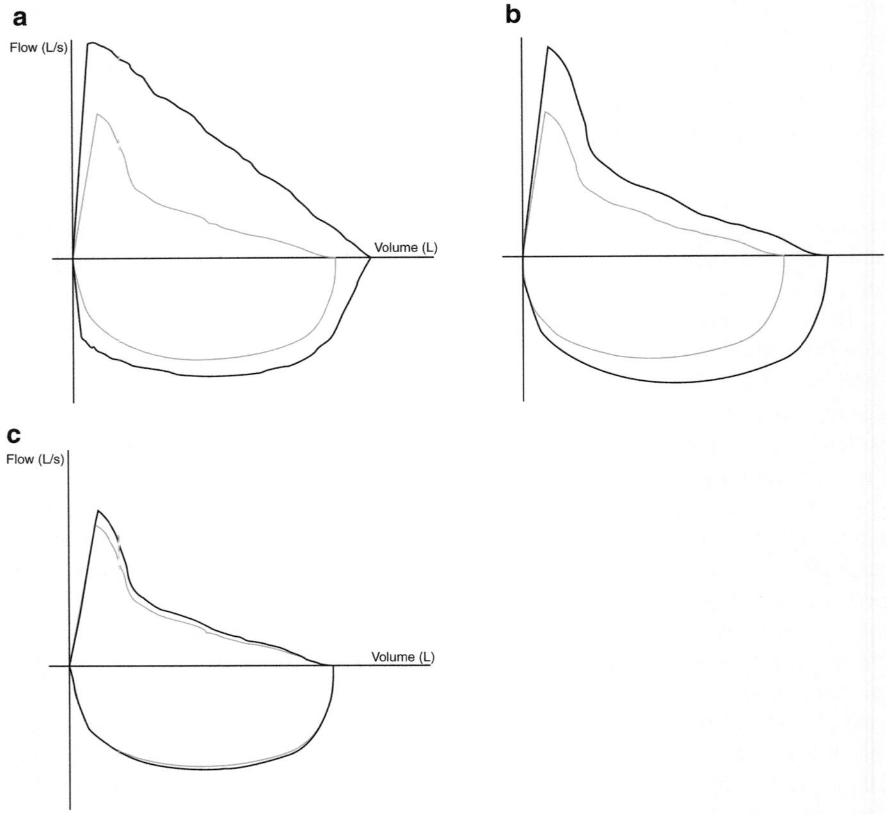

Fig. 6.10 Typical flow-volume loops representing pre-bronchodilator (grey) and post-bronchodilator (black) spirometry from patients with (**a**) full reversibility, (**b**) partial reversibility, and (**c**) no reversibility ("fixed" obstruction)

Following bronchodilation, patients will either demonstrate full reversibility (with post-bronchodilator spirometry within normal limits), partial reversibility (with a positive bronchodilator response but post-bronchodilator spirometry still showing airflow obstruction), or no significant reversibility ("fixed" airflow obstruction) (Fig. 6.10). Full reversibility is generally only seen in asthma in response to a beta-2 agonist, where the diagnosis is further supported if the patient is young and has never smoked (or has minimal smoking history). Partial or no reversibility is common in COPD, bronchiectasis, and chronic severe asthma, and it is well recognised that these conditions can occur concurrently. It is important to note that the lack of a significant bronchodilator response does not mean that bronchodilators are not clinically useful as, for many patients (particularly those with COPD), bronchodilators can improve airway calibre over the tidal breathing range, reduce hyperinflation and the work of breathing, and lead to an improvement in symptoms. Common clinical differences between asthma and COPD (which should be elucidated during clinical consultation to support diagnostic spirometry) are listed in Table 6.3.

Table 6.3 Common clinical features that may help differentiate asthma and COPD in developed countries

Clinical feature	Asthma	COPD
Smoker/ex-smoker	Possibly	Nearly all
Symptoms in younger age (<35 years)	Common	Rare
Dyspnoea	Variable	Chronic and progressive
Chronic, productive cough	Rare	Common
Diurnal and day-to-day symptom variation	Significant	Uncommon
Nighttime waking with dyspnoea + wheeze	Common	Rare

It is worth noting that each can occur in both conditions but are usually far more common in one. It is also possible to have asthma with COPD (sometimes referred to as "asthma-COPD overlap syndrome"). Combining clinical history with diagnostic spirometry (and sometimes other tests, such as imaging) is more likely to give an accurate diagnosis

6.5.1 Bronchial Challenge Testing

Normal spirometry does not exclude a diagnosis of asthma where, in many cases, bronchoconstriction and airflow obstruction may only develop in response to certain triggers (e.g. an allergen). Therefore, if a patient with normal spirometry presents with symptoms and clinical signs of asthma, it may be beneficial to perform a bronchial challenge test to support the diagnosis.

There are various means by which the airways can be provoked to induce bronchoconstriction, which may be classified as direct or indirect. Direct stimuli act directly on the effector cells (e.g. smooth muscle cells, bronchial capillary endothelial cells, and secretory cells in the airway epithelium), and the most common of these in clinical practice is methacholine, although histamine has also been used. Indirect stimuli induce bronchoconstriction by acting on intermediate cells (e.g. inflammatory cells, epithelial cells) that then stimulate effector cells. Common indirect stimuli include mannitol, hypertonic saline, exercise, and eucapnic voluntary hyperpnoea (hyperventilation of cold, dry air). The physiological effects of the stimulus are assessed by comparing pre- and post-stimulus spirometry (particularly FEV_1), with a decrease of 10–20% (depending on the test) indicating a positive response. In cases where a pharmacological agent is used, a "provocative dose" (PD) or "provocative concentration" (PC) is calculated, which may be cumulative if the protocol uses increasing doses (e.g. mannitol).

Mannitol is a good example of an indirect agent that is now widely used for bronchial challenge testing. It is inhaled as a dry powder (housed within small capsules) through a small handheld device. Once inhaled, it increases the osmolarity of the bronchial mucosa and induces the release of inflammatory mediators (including histamine, prostaglandins, and leukotrienes) from mast cells and eosinophils. Spirometry is performed 1 min after each dose, and a positive response is defined as a 15% fall in FEV_1 compared to baseline within a total cumulative mannitol dose of 645 mg.

The mannitol challenge test has a reasonable sensitivity but will only detect around 60% of asthma cases (i.e. 40% of asthmatics will not respond to mannitol).

However, it has very high specificity, meaning that, if a mannitol test shows a positive response, a diagnosis of asthma can be made with confidence.

As the aim of a challenge test is to induce bronchoconstriction, it is important that patients withhold all treatments that are known to influence bronchial responsiveness for sufficient time to render their effects negligible (e.g. bronchodilators, antihistamines, and leukotriene modifiers such as montelukast).

6.5.2 Assessment of Airway Sensitivity to Inhaled Antibiotics

Patients with obstructive lung disease often have acute exacerbations, which may be defined as a sustained worsening of symptoms beyond natural day-to-day variability and may require a change in treatment (e.g. short course of oral antibiotics +/- steroids). In many cases, exacerbations are caused by bacterial colonisation, and a proportion of patients may even be chronically colonised and exacerbate frequently (most commonly those with bronchiectasis, cystic fibrosis, or COPD). For such patients, prophylactic nebulised antibiotic therapy may be indicated. However, some patients may experience adverse and allergic reactions to certain inhaled antibiotics. Therefore, it is essential to perform an assessment of airways sensitivity to a proposed antibiotic to ensure that it does not induce bronchospasm.

The assessment should be performed in a clinically stable state and involves the measurement of baseline spirometry followed by nebulised antibiotic administration and repeat spirometry at 15 and 30 min post-antibiotic (this is a recommended minimum, and it may also be useful to assess at 45 and 60 min post-antibiotic). Due to the possibility of bronchospasm, a beta-2 agonist (e.g. salbutamol 2.5 mg) should be made available. It is also important to monitor the patient to ensure symptoms (e.g. wheeze, dyspnoea) do not manifest or worsen following antibiotic administration. If FEV_1 does not decrease by >15% and >200 ml from baseline and the patient does not experience symptomatic side effects, the antibiotic may be safely prescribed. If FEV_1 does decrease by >15% and >200 ml from baseline or the patient experiences symptoms of bronchospasm, the patient has had an adverse reaction. Testing should be terminated and the beta-2 agonist administered immediately. It may then be useful to reassess the patient 20 min after the beta-2 agonist to ensure spirometry and symptoms have returned to baseline.

6.5.3 Peak Flow Monitoring

PEF when measured as part of an expiratory flow-volume curve is far less informative then FEV_1 and FVC. However, as a stand-alone measurement, it can be a useful domiciliary monitoring tool for suspected asthma (where diurnal variability of symptoms is common). It may be particularly useful in patients who do not have an accurate perception of symptoms when their asthma is worsening (so-called "poor perceivers"). PEF monitoring may also be useful to diagnose occupationally-related asthma. PEF meters are cheap and easy to use and do not require a power supply, making them ideal for home monitoring. As the patient will be monitoring their own PEF, it is important that they are correctly educated on the performance of a technically acceptable PEF manoeuvre prior to issue.

To monitor diurnal variation accurately, it is necessary for the patient to measure their PEF at three intervals throughout the day: in the morning, around noon, and in the evening. Generally, the patient will perform three or four PEF measurements in each of these sessions and select the best of a consistent group. It is also useful for monitoring purposes that the patient keep the session times consistent day-to-day and also ensure that any bronchodilators they are prescribed are used at the same time every day (e.g. to measure their morning PEF before taking bronchodilators every day). Measuring PEF three times daily in this manner (usually for a 2-week period) is necessary for detecting variations in lung function throughout the day that asthmatics often experience. For instance, asthmatics often have worse lung function early in the morning and later in the evening, with improvement in the middle of the day. In contrast, patients whose asthma only occurs when exposed to an occupational allergen are more likely to have lower PEF when at work.

In addition to a diagnostic aid, PEF monitoring can also be used to demonstrate therapeutic benefits. For example, an asthmatic patient may show a gradual but sustained improvement in PEF following the prescription of an inhaled corticosteroid. In this case, it may not be necessary to perform PEF three times per day. Monitoring PEF only twice per day is often sufficient (Fig. 6.11), with a minimum

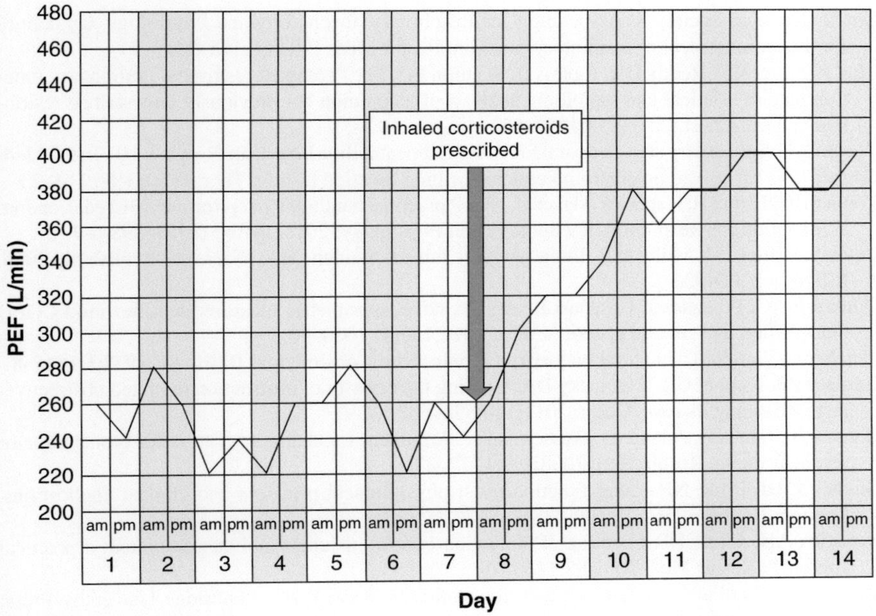

Fig. 6.11 A typical daily PEF diary showing improvement in PEF following the prescription of an inhaled corticosteroid at day 8. Patients may not demonstrate a therapeutic response to PEF within 7 days of treatment, so the post-treatment monitoring period may need to be extended to 2 or 3 weeks

of 1 week before and after the prescription of medication. However, noticeable therapeutic benefit may not occur until 3 weeks, so post-treatment monitoring may need to be extended.

6.6 Summary

The measurement of expiratory flows provides robust information about pulmonary ventilation, which may become compromised in a variety of respiratory disorders. Spirometry can be performed on small, portable devices, making it one of the most common and readily available lung function tests. It is ideal for use in both primary and secondary care as a diagnostic aid and monitoring tool. However, due to the maximal effort required from the patient and the associated technical issues, spirometry should only be performed and interpreted by fully trained and certified healthcare practitioners.

Selected References

Anderson SD, Brannan J, Spring J, et al. A new method for bronchial-provocation testing in asthmatic subjects using a dry powder of mannitol. Am J Respir Crit Care Med. 1997;156(3 Pt 1):758–65.

British Thoracic Society & Association for Respiratory Technology and Physiology. Guidelines for the measurement of respiratory function. Respir Med. 1994;88:165–94.

Clay RD, Iyer VN, Reddy DR, Siontis B, Scanlon PD. The "complex restrictive" pulmonary function pattern: clinical and radiologic analysis of a common but previously undescribed restrictive pattern. Chest. 2017;152:1258–65.

Cooper BG. Spirometry standards and FEV_1/FVC repeatability. Prim Care Respir J. 2010;19:292–4.

Cooper BG. An update on contraindications for lung function testing. Thorax. 2011;66:714–23.

Cooper BG, Hunt JH, Kendrick AH, et al. ARTP practical handbook of spirometry. 3rd ed. London: Association for Respiratory Technology and Physiology; 2017. ISBN: 0-9536898-6-7

Cotes JE, Chinn DJ, Miller MR. Lung function. 6th ed. Malden, MA: Blackwell Publishing; 2006. ISBN: 0632064935

Dilektasli AG, Porszasz J, Casaburi R, et al. A novel spirometric measure identifies mild COPD unidentified by standard criteria. Chest. 2016;150(5):1080–90.

Fletcher C, Peto R. The natural history of chronic airflow obstruction. Br Med J. 1977;1:1645–8.

Gardner ZE, Ruppel GL, Kaminsky DA. Grading the severity of obstruction in mixed obstructive-restrictive lung disease. Chest. 2011;140:598–603.

Hansen JE, Sun XG, Adame D, Wasserman K. Argument for changing criteria for bronchodilator responsiveness. Respir Med. 2008;102:1777–83.

Hughes JMB, Pride NB. Lung function tests: physiological principle and clinical applications. London: Bailliere Tindall; 1999. ISBN: 0702023507

Kendrick AH, Johns DP, Leeming JP. Infection control of lung function equipment: a practical approach. Respir Med. 2003;97:1163–79.

Laszlo G. Pulmonary function: a guide for clinicians. New York: Cambridge University Press; 1994. ISBN: 0521446791

Mannino DM, Diaz-Guzman E. Interpreting lung function using 80% predicted and fixed thresholds identifies patients at increased risk of mortality. Chest. 2012;141:73–80.
Miller MR, Crapo R, Hankinson J, et al. General considerations for lung function testing. Eur Respir J. 2005;26:153–61.
Miller MR, Hankinson J, Brusasko V, et al. Standardisation of spirometry. Eur Respir J. 2005;26:319–38.
Miller MR, Quanjer PH, Swanney PM, et al. Interpreting lung function data using 80% predicted and fixed thresholds misclassifies more than 20% of patients. Chest. 2011;139:52–9.
Miller MR. Does the use of per cent predicted have any evidence base? Eur Respir J. 2015;45(2):322–3.
Morris ZQ, Coz A, Starosta D. An isolated reduction of the FEV3/FVC ratio is an indicator of mild lung injury. Chest. 2013;144(4):1117–23.
Pellegrino R, Viegi G, Brusasco V, et al. Interpretive strategies for lung function tests. Eur Respir J. 2005;26:948–68.
Quanjer PH, Stanojevic S, Cole TJ, et al. Multi-ethnic reference values for spirometry for the 3-95 year age range: the global lung function 2012 equations. Eur Respir J. 2012;40(6):1324–43.
Quanjer PH, Brazzale DJ, Boros PW, et al. Implications of adopting the Global Lungs Initiative 2012 all-age reference equations for spirometry. Eur Respir J. 2013;42(4):1046–54.
Quanjer PH, Pretto JJ, Brazzale DJ, et al. Grading the severity of airflow obstruction: new wine in old bottles. Eur Respir J. 2014;43(2):505–12.
Quanjer PH, Cooper B, Ruppel GL, et al. Defining airflow obstruction. Eur Respir J. 2015;45:561–2.
Schilder DP, Roberts A, Fry DL. Effect of gas density and viscosity on the maximal expiratory flow-volume relationship. J Clin Invest. 1963;42(11):1705–13.
Seed L, Wilson D, Coates AL. Children should not be treated like little adults in the PFT lab. Respir Care. 2012;57:61–74.
Vogelmeier CF, Criner GJ, Martinez FJ, et al. Global strategy for the diagnosis, management, and prevention of chronic obstructive lung disease 2017 report: GOLD executive summary. Eur Respir J. 2017;195:557–82.
Ward H, Cooper BG, Miller MR. Improved criterion for assessing lung function reversibility. Chest. 2015;148(4):877–86.

Chapter 7
Breathing In and Out: Airway Resistance

David A. Kaminsky and Jason H. T. Bates

7.1 Introduction

In order to fully appreciate the complexities of pulmonary airflow, one must consider all of the pressures necessary to move air into and out of the lung. These pressures are required to overcome the elastic stiffness of the lung and chest wall, the frictional resistance to airflow offered by the airways and parenchymal tissues, and the inertia of the gas within the central airways. Considering the respiratory system as a single expansible unit served by a single airway conduit, these pressures add to give the so-called equation of motion:

$$P(t) = EV(t) + R\dot{V}(t) + I\ddot{V}(t) \quad (7.1)$$

where P is the total pressure across the respiratory system, V is the volume of gas in the lungs (referenced to some initial volume, usually functional residual capacity – FRC), $\dot{V}$ is flow entering the airways, and $\ddot{V}$ is volume acceleration. The constants E, R, and I are termed elastance, resistance, and inertance, respectively. This chapter will focus on the component of R that is due to flow of air through the pulmonary airways. This component, known as airway resistance, can be measured in several different ways and is of major clinical significance.

D. A. Kaminsky (✉)
Pulmonary Disease and Critical Care Medicine, University of Vermont Larner College of Medicine, Burlington, VT, USA
e-mail: david.kaminsky@med.uvm.edu

J. H. T. Bates
University of Vermont Larner College of Medicine, Burlington, VT, USA
e-mail: Jason.h.bates@med.uvm.edu

D. A. Kaminsky, C. G. Irvin (eds.), *Pulmonary Function Testing*,
Respiratory Medicine, https://doi.org/10.1007/978-3-319-94159-2_7

7.2 What Is Resistance?

By definition, resistance, R, is the pressure required to produce a unit flow through a system. It is convention in the field of lung function measurement to express pressure in units of cmH_2O and gas flow in liters per second (L/s). The unit of resistance is thus cmH_2O/L/s, or cmH_2O.s/L. The resistance of a conduit, or tube, is simply the difference in pressure, ΔP, between the two ends of the conduit divided by the flow through it. That is,

$$R = \frac{\Delta P}{\dot{V}} \tag{7.2}$$

R is thus a measure of function, but it can be related to structure: a high value of R is indicative of a long and/or narrow conduit, and vice versa. The precise link between structure and function reflected in R depends on many factors, but under certain ideal circumstances this link can be stated in relatively straightforward mathematical terms based on the laws of physics.

Qualitatively, there are two steady flow situations that are important to understand. When flow is sufficiently low, the flow streamlines, observable from the behavior of a very thin stream of smoke injected into the flow at some point, move along parallel with the bulk flow in an orderly fashion. This is known as *laminar flow* (Fig. 7.1a). At the other extreme, when flow is sufficiently rapid, the streamlines cannot be visualized at all because the injected smoke stream immediately swirls around to quickly encompass the entire diameter of the tube. This is known as *turbulent flow* (Fig. 7.1b). Most real flow situations are neither perfectly laminar nor completely turbulent, but rather sit within a transition region between these two extremes. Nevertheless, it is useful to consider how R is linked to tube geometry under the ideal condition of laminar flow through a rigid cylindrical conduit, because here it is possible to derive an equation for R from first physical principles. The result is known as the Poiseuille equation given by

$$\Delta P = 8\mu L\dot{V} / \pi r^4 \tag{7.3}$$

where L is the length of the conduit, μ is gas viscosity, and r is the radius of the conduit. An equivalently precise formula for turbulent flow does not exist, but empirically R still varies inversely with r to the fourth power and linearly with l, similar to Eq. 7.3. An important difference between laminar and turbulent flow, however, is that while R is constant during laminar flow, as shown by Eq. 7.3, R increases roughly linearly with increasing flow when flow is turbulent. Also, whereas R is proportional to the viscosity of the gas when flow is laminar, R is determined by the density of the gas when flow is turbulent.

Of course, airflow through the pulmonary airways is not precisely steady because it reverses direction with every breath. In addition, the airways themselves are not perfectly rigid or perfectly cylindrical, and they branch frequently over a range of

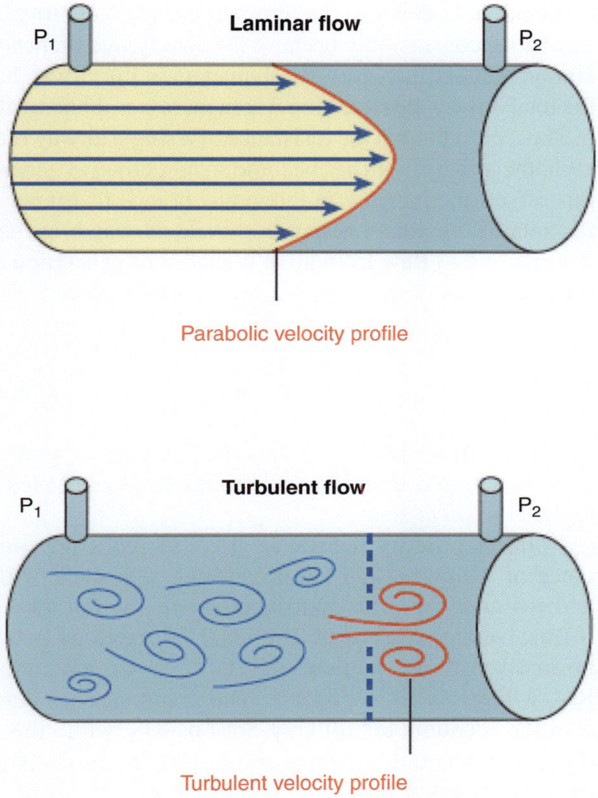

Fig. 7.1 (**a**) Illustration of laminar flow through a rigid tube, where the resistance to flow is constant with flow. (**b**) Illustration of turbulent flow through a rigid tube, where the resistance to flow varies roughly linearly with flow. (From Bossé, Riesenfeld, Paré, and Irvin 2010, with permission from Annual Review of Physiology)

angles, so the flow through them is neither laminar nor turbulent. Accordingly, the relationship between Raw and flow can only be stated empirically. An expression that has been widely used in pulmonary physiology and medicine is the so-called Rohrer equation

$$\text{Raw} = K_1 + K_2\dot{V} \tag{7.4}$$

where K_1 and K_2 are constants that have no particular physical interpretation but nevertheless serve as useful empirical quantifiers of airway pressure-flow characteristics.

Thus, to the extent that the pulmonary airways can be viewed as behaving like a single conduit, the above discussion provides an understanding of the key factors that influence airway resistance, Raw. Most importantly, it illustrates the incredibly powerful effect of airway radius on function; if airway radius decreases by 50%, for example, then Raw increases by 16 times!

Of course, the airways are not a single conduit, but rather comprise a branching tree structure that can be viewed as having multiple generations from the trachea (generation 1) down to the terminal bronchioles (roughly generation 23, although this varies considerably because the airway tree branches asymmetrically). As generation number increases, the diameters of the airway branches decrease. However, the total airway cross-sectional area increases dramatically beyond about generation 6. Thus, even though the resistance of a single airway branch at generation *n* may be high, the airway branches become so numerous as generation number increases that this offsets the increase in individual branch resistance. This can be seen from the formula for the total resistance of many airway branches in parallel. If Raw_n is the contribution to Raw from all *m* branches of generation *n*, and Rn_1, Rn_2, …, Rn_n are the resistances of the *m* individual branches, then

$$\frac{1}{\mathrm{Raw}_n} = \frac{1}{\mathrm{Raw}_1} + \frac{1}{\mathrm{Raw}_2} + \ldots + \frac{1}{\mathrm{Raw}_n} \tag{7.5}$$

The result of this is that the distal airways in a normal lung make a negligible contribution to overall Raw, a phenomenon that has led to the lung periphery being termed the *silent zone*.

Total respiratory resistance (Rrs) includes not only Raw but also the resistance of the chest wall (Rcw) and the resistance of the lung tissues (Rti). Rcw and Rti arise from dissipative processes within the chest wall and lung tissues themselves as a result of frictional interactions between their constituents. At normal breathing frequencies (10–12 bpm), Rti contributes about 40% to total Rrs, while Rcw is negligible. The component of Raw due to the large central airways accounts for roughly 50% of Rrs, while the small airways (< 2 mm in diameter) account for only about 10% because of their very large combined cross-sectional area.

Airflow is determined by airway resistance in normal lungs at the modest flows associated with breathing at rest. However, during maximally forced expiration or in severe obstructive disease, flow is limited by dynamic airway collapse, which itself is strongly influenced by transpulmonary pressure. During the resulting flow limitation (see Chap. 6), the conventional concept of resistance as developed above does not apply.

7.3 The Importance of Lung Volume

The relationship of Raw to the fourth power of radius reflects the critical importance of the caliber of an airway on the ease with which air can move through it. Accordingly, the factors that are most important for increasing Raw are those that cause radius to decrease. These factors include transpulmonary pressure (Ptp), airway smooth muscle contraction, airway inflammation and mucus secretion that may either thicken the airway wall or partially occlude the airway lumen, and dynamic airway compression. Of these, Ptp is particularly potent because of its effect on the ability of the airway smooth muscle to shorten when stimulated. Ptp is transmitted across the intrapulmonary airway walls by the alveolar walls that are attached to their outside borders. These alveolar walls exert an outward tethering effect on the airway wall that opposes smooth muscle shortening and hence limits the degree to which the airways can narrow. Ptp decreases with decreasing lung volume, which results in increased airway narrowing from smooth muscle constriction, with an inverse dependence on volume that becomes particularly strong as volume descends below normal FRC. Conversely, at high lung volumes, the radial traction from tethering increases, and a greater opposing load is presented to airway smooth muscle, which reduces airway narrowing from smooth muscle constriction. For this reason, increasing Ptp through a deep lung inflation is one of the most effective ways of reversing bronchoconstriction in normal lungs. Interestingly, bronchoconstriction becomes worse after a deep inflation in some asthmatic subjects, but the reasons for this remain controversial and poorly understood.

Lung volume is often altered in disease and thus has a direct effect on Raw. For example, in obstructive disease, airway closure and hyperinflation may raise FRC and thus reduce Raw. In restrictive lung disease, patients breathing at low lung volumes may have increased Raw, but if associated with increased elastic recoil of the lung parenchyma, such as in pulmonary fibrosis, any tendency for Raw to increase is offset by increased radial traction of the surrounding lung. Of note, obesity commonly results in increased Raw due to the reduced lung volumes that result from mass loading by the adipose tissues of the chest wall and abdomen. Any such reduction in volume has the potential to substantially increase airways responsiveness, which may at least partly explain why asthma is so common in obese individuals.

7.4 Measurement of Airway Resistance by Body Plethysmography

Traditionally, airway resistance has been measured by relating airflow and driving pressure through the use of body plethysmography, providing measures of Raw, specific airway resistance (sRaw), and specific airway conductance. In 1956, Dubois and colleagues described the plethysmographic method that we still use today. The principle of measuring Raw through body plethysmography is based on *Boyle's law*, which expresses how the pressure in a gas is related to the amount by which its volume has been compressed (see Chap. 3).

To calculate airway resistance, one needs to know flow and alveolar pressure; the former can be measured directly, but the latter cannot. What Dubois realized was that under conditions of no-flow, mouth pressure would approximate alveolar pressure. Therefore, resistance is calculated by combining two measurements: one of flow vs. box pressure, and the other of mouth pressure vs. box pressure (from which TGV is measured, see Chap. 3) (Fig. 7.2). In this way, flow vs. mouth pressure (as a surrogate for alveolar pressure) can be inferred at equal box pressures, allowing the calculation of airway resistance, Raw. For a more detailed explanation, see the Appendix A.

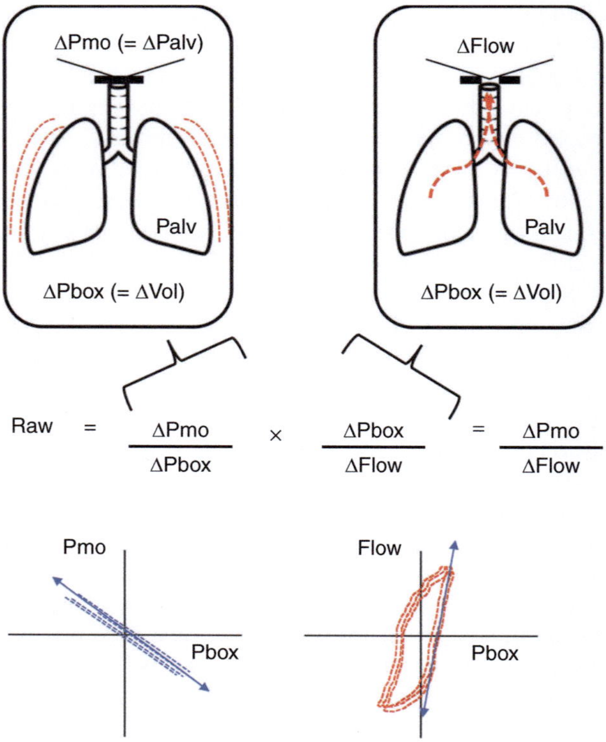

Fig. 7.2 Relationship of mouth pressure and box pressure by body plethysmography under closed-loop panting conditions (left) and open-loop panting conditions (right). Under conditions of no-flow (left), mouth pressure (P_{mo}) would approximate alveolar pressure (P_{alv}), so the relationship of alveolar pressure to change in lung volume (Vol) (as determined by change in box pressure, P_{box}) is measured. When the shutter is opened (right), the relationship between flow and lung volume (change in box pressure) is measured. Airway resistance (Raw) is calculated as the change in alveolar pressure (~P_{mo}) divided by flow, which is derived by multiplying the slope of the closed-shutter maneuver (bottom left) and the inverse slope of the open-shutter maneuver (bottom right), with the P_{box} (volume) terms canceling out

A few technical details are important to keep in mind. During the measurement of flow vs. box pressure, the patient breaths with rapid, shallow panting breaths through the circuit at a frequency of 1.5–2.5 Hz (90–150 breaths per minute) for 1–2 s (Fig. 7.3). The rapid shallow panting is designed to optimize the signal-to-noise ratio and increase the accuracy of measurement by (1) minimizing thermal shifts and gas exchange, (2) maintaining glottic opening, (3) minimizing flow turbulence and gas compression, and (4) ensuring a measureable difference between P_A and Pao. During the measurement of mouth pressure vs. box pressure, a shutter is closed occluding the mouthpiece, and the patient is asked to pant at a rate of 0.5–1.0 Hz (30–60 breaths per minute) for 1–2 s (Fig. 7.3). This relatively slower rate is meant to allow adequate time for equilibration of mouth and alveolar pressure.

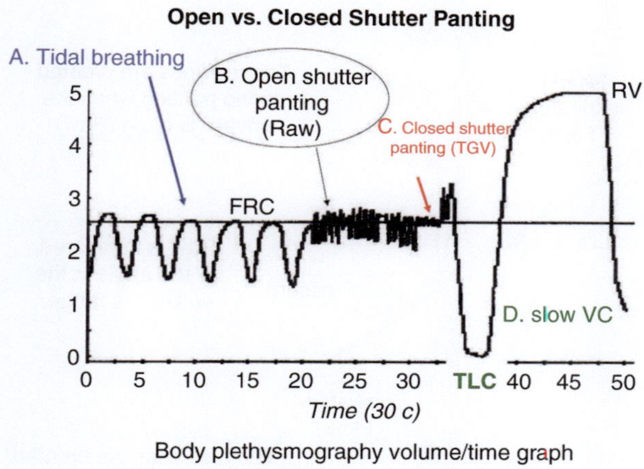

Fig. 7.3 Tracing of volume vs. time in a patient having Raw measured. Following tidal breathing (A), there is a brief period of open-shutter panting (B), followed immediately by closed-shutter panting (C). Patient then typically performs a slow vital capacity maneuver (D)

Once the open- and closed-shutter panting maneuvers are complete, the slope of the relationship between mouth pressure and box pressure is determined. The slope is conventionally taken at the transition between the end of inspiration and the beginning of expiration between +0.5 and – 0.5 L/s flow (Fig. 7.4). This low flow range is chosen to mimic the normal range of flow during quiet breathing and ensure that flow is mostly laminar to allow the principles of Poiseuille's law to apply. However, measuring the slope may be difficult because of the potentially complicated configurations of these curves. Multiple technical issues can influence the shape and size of the open-panting loops (Fig. 7.5). Airway resistance as measured by body plethysmography is usually expressed as Raw defined by Eq. 7.6. However, Raw varies inversely with lung volume because bigger airways have a smaller resistance than smaller airways. Consequently, Raw is usually normalized to lung volume to become *specific airway resistance*, sRaw, defined as

$$\mathrm{sRaw} = \mathrm{Raw} \times V_{\mathrm{TG}} \tag{7.6}$$

or its inverse known as *specific airway conductance*, sGaw (Fig. 7.7)

$$\mathrm{sGaw} = \frac{1}{\mathrm{sRaw}} \tag{7.7}$$

Both sRaw and sGaw are thus independent of changes in lung volume that may occur between different measurement conditions in a given subject and so are useful for studies involving serial measurements of lung function separated by significant time intervals. The increased sensitivity of sGaw for airway resistance compared to FEV1 is especially useful in pharmacological studies that involve normal healthy

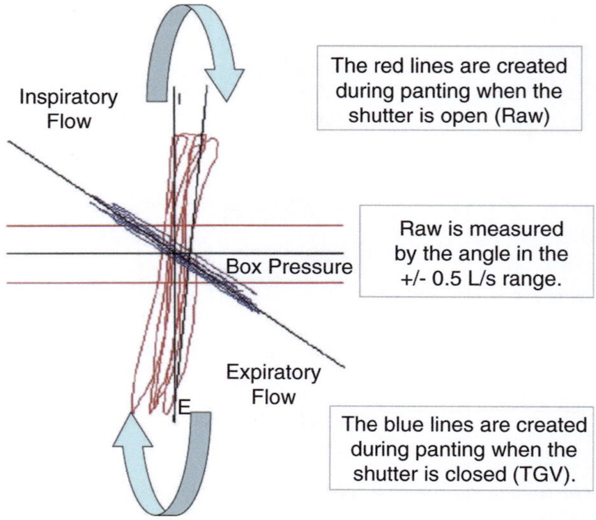

Fig. 7.4 Close-up of open- and closed-shutter panting loops. Open-shutter panting is shown in red, and the loops move clockwise during shallow panting including inspiration (positive *y*-axis) and expiration (negative *y*-axis). The slope of flow vs. box pressure (angled black line) is conventionally measured at the end of the inspiratory loop between +0.5 and – 0.5 L/S (horizontal red lines). Closed-shutter panting is shown in blue where the *y*-axis is now mouth pressure and the *x*-axis remains box pressure

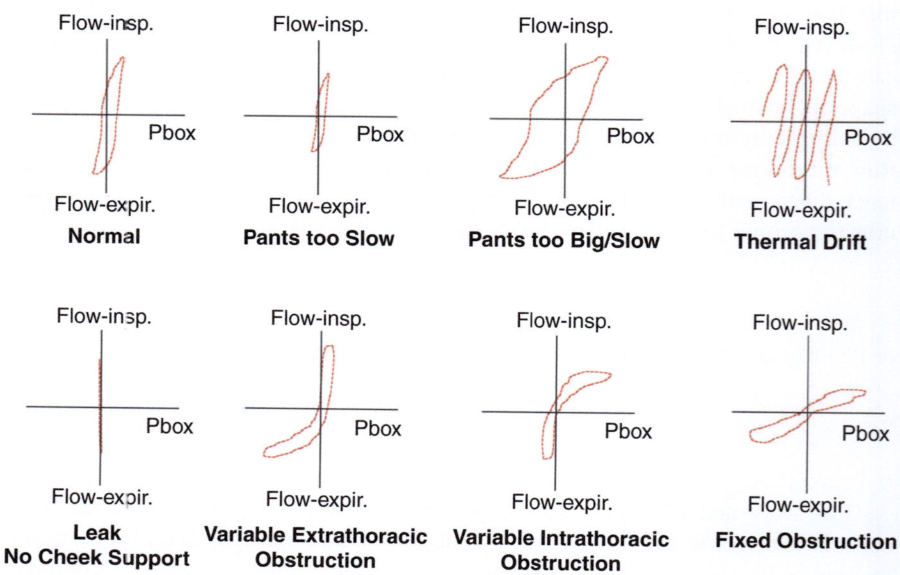

Fig. 7.5 Examples of normal and abnormal open-shutter loops, plotted on *y*-axis of inspiratory (negative *y*-axis) vs. expiratory flow (positive *y*-axis) versus *x*-axis of box pressure (P_{box})

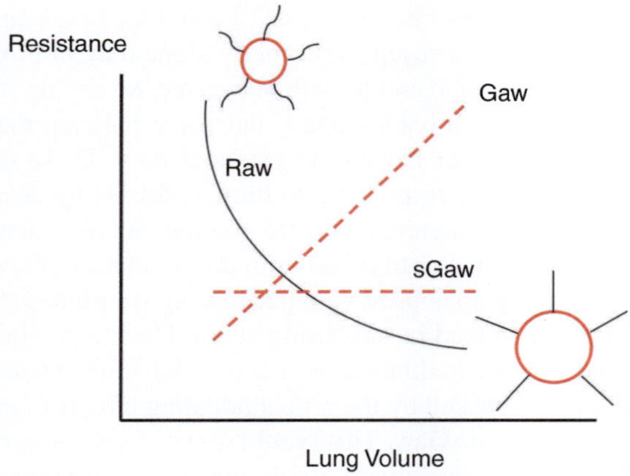

Fig. 7.6 Relationship between Raw and lung volume (hyperbolic), with increased tethering of airways (circles) resulting in increased airway diameter and lower Raw at higher lung volumes. Notice the relationship of the reciprocal of Raw (Gaw) to lung volume (linear, but still dependent on lung volume) and Gaw/TGV (sGaw) to lung volume (horizontal, independent of lung volume)

subjects. However, sGaw is less reproducible than FEV1, and thus it must be measured repeatedly to determine an accurate mean value. Furthermore, there are limited studies establishing normal values for sGaw.

In children, the closed-shutter panting maneuver may be difficult to achieve, so V_{TG} cannot be measured. Instead, flow is related to the small shifts in box pressure (which correspond to changes in lung volume) that occur during tidal breathing to determine sRaw directly, which is calculated as flow divided by changes in box pressure. Multiple different slopes of the flow versus box pressure relationship may be measured, each of which results in a different value of sRaw. The exact slope used in the calculation of sRaw should be specified in the reporting of the results.

7.5 Clinical Utility of sRaw and sGaw

Because the total cross-sectional area of the airways decreases dramatically as one moves from the peripheral to the central regions of the lung, any measure of overall airway resistance, such as sGaw, will be very sensitive to central airway pathology but less sensitive to peripheral changes. Thus, sGaw may pick up changes in large central airways that may be missed by spirometry. Indeed, sGaw has been shown to be sensitive to upper airway involvement in vocal cord dysfunction and vocal cord paralysis. However, sGaw may also be more sensitive to peripheral airway involvement as well, such as what occurs in bronchiolitis obliterans syndrome. This may relate to the loss of sensitivity of FEV1 due to the deep inhalation involved (see below).

Theoretically, sGaw should be sensitive to changes in resistance anywhere along the airway tree, whereas FEV1 will be sensitive to only those changes occurring upstream from the equal pressure point (see Chap. 6). Thus, depending on the location of airway narrowing or dilation in response to a bronchoconstrictor or bronchodilator, FEV1 may change without a significant change in sGaw, and vice versa (see cases illustrated in Figs. 7.7 and 7.8). In the case of airway narrowing, hyperinflation might result. Spirometry alone may fail to find bronchodilator reversibility in 15% of patients with suspected reversible airway obstruction and clinical responses to bronchodilator, but these patients may be identified by changes in sGaw or V_{TG} or isovolume maximal flow. These results suggest that the patients involved were responding to bronchodilator by changes in clinically relevant lung function parameters related to volume, but not changes in spirometry.

Another factor to consider in differentiating sGaw from FEV1 is the deep breath necessarily associated with performing spirometry, but which is not part of the procedure involved in measuring sGaw. Healthy subjects and those with mild asthma tend to bronchodilate after a deep inhalation. Therefore, mild bronchoconstriction could be masked by the bronchodilating effects of measuring FEV1 but should still be evident in sGaw. This would make sGaw a more sensitive test to detect airflow limitation, especially in mildly obstructed patients. Many studies have investigated the relative response in FEV1 versus sGaw during bronchial challenge tests. For example, the provocative concentration causing a 40% drop in sGaw (PC40 sGaw) was found to be more sensitive than the PC20 FEV1 at detecting bronchoconstric-

Gender: Male Age: 62 years Race: Caucasian

Height: 175 cm. Weight: 99 kg. BMI: 32 (kg/m^2)

Clinical Notes: dyspnea on exertion

	Pre-Bronchodilator			Post-Bronchodilator			
Spirometry	**Best**	**%Pred**	**LLN**	**Best**	**%Pred**	**Change**	**%Change**
FVC (L)	3.96	87	3.59	3.92	87	-0.04	0
FEV1 (L)	2.94	87	2.61	3.12	92	+0.18	+5
FEV/FVC	0.74		0.65	0.80			
Lung Volumes	**Actual**	**%Pred**		**Actual**	**%Pred**	**Change**	**%Change**
TLC (L)	7.30	107		6.93	102	-0.37	-5
FRC (L)	3.14	88		2.82	79	-0.32	-10
RV (L)	2.88	128		2.47	110	-0.41	-14
Airway Resistance	**Actual**	**%Pred**		**Actual**	**%Pred**	**Change**	**%Change**
Raw (cm H20/L/s)	2.31	159		1.20	82	-1.11	-37
sGaw (1/cmH20-s)	0.14	70		0.25	124	+0.11	+79

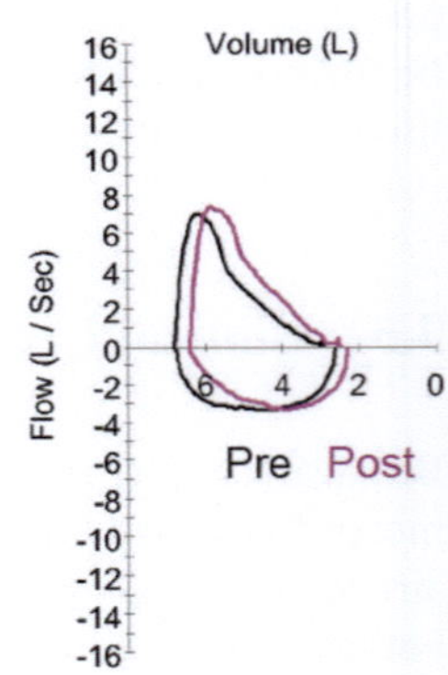

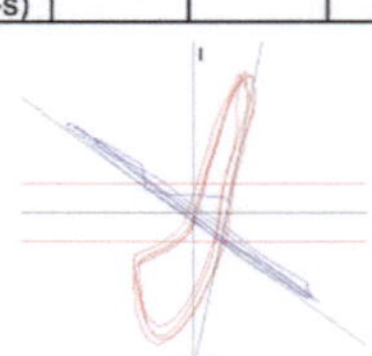

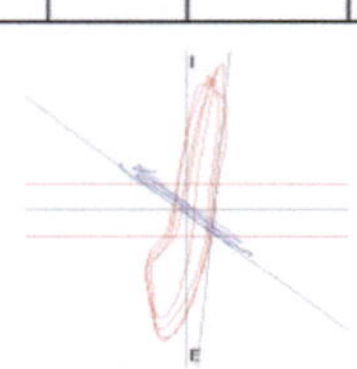

Fig. 7.7 Example of pulmonary function tests performed at baseline and after bronchodilator. Notice that despite no change in FEV1 or FVC after bronchodilator, there has been a 79% increase in sGaw, which was clinically associated with improvement in dyspnea on exertion. Interestingly, there was also a slight drop in FRC and RV, suggesting a beneficial lung volume response to bronchodilator as well

Gender: Male Age: 33 years Race: Caucasian

Height: 173 cm. Weight: 84 kg. BMI: 28 (kg/m²)

Clinical Notes: intermittent cough, shortness of breath

	Diluent			Post-Methacholine (4 mg/ml)	
Spirometry	**Best**	**%Pred**	**LLN**	**Best**	**%Change**
FVC (L)	4.92	94	4.21	4.59	-6
FEV1 (L)	3.77	95	3.14	3.30	-12
FEV/FVC	0.77		0.67	0.72	
Lung Volumes	**Actual**	**%Pred**		**Actual**	**%Change**
TLC (L)	7.34	100		7.56	+3
FRC (L)	2.99	78		3.75	+25
RV (L)	2.23	100		2.86	+28
Airway Resistance	**Actual**	**%Pred**		**Actual**	**%Change**
Raw (cm H20/L/s)	1.65	113		3.82	+131
sGaw (1/cmH20-s)	0.18	90		0.06	-67

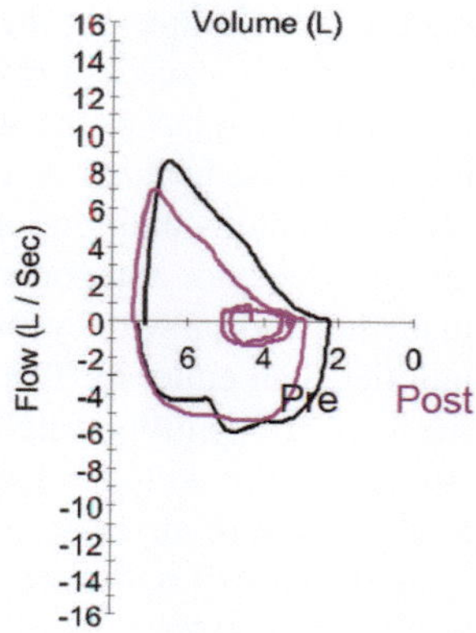

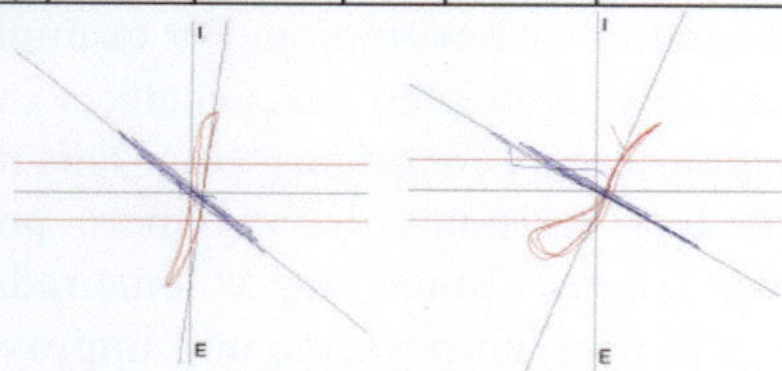

Fig. 7.8 Example of pulmonary function tests performed at baseline and at 4 mg/ml of methacholine during a methacholine challenge test. Notice that despite no significant change in FEV1 at 4 mg/ml (i.e., >/= 20% drop), there has been a substantial decrease in sGaw, which was associated with symptoms of chest tightness and shortness of breath. In addition, there was an increase in FRC and RV, suggesting the development of hyperinflation as well

tion to inhaled histamine, but the PC20 was a more reproducible measure (coefficient of variation = 2.6% vs. 10%). Indeed, combining non-FEV1 parameters, such as sGaw, with FEV1 during a methacholine challenge test increases the sensitivity of the test. Recently, a receiver-operator characteristic analysis demonstrated that the optimal cutoff for change in sGaw corresponding to a 20% fall in FEV1 was 52%. However, the cost of a test with high sensitivity is typically loss of specificity. Indeed, many years ago sGaw was shown to be less specific than FEV1 at distinguishing normal from asthmatic subjects. Another study demonstrated that when the methacholine challenge test was negative, small changes in FEV1 but not in sGaw were predictive of future development of asthma, suggesting again that the FEV1 is a more specific measure for asthma. The differences in response of sGaw versus FEV1 may also reflect underlying differences in anatomy. For example, patients who responded to methacholine with changes in sGaw but not in FEV1 were found to have smaller lung volumes, higher FEV1, and higher FEF25–75/FVC, compared to patients who responded by FEV1 only, indicative of relatively larger airway to lung size, a mismatch referred to as lung dysanapsis. Patients with smaller airway to lung size (lower FEF25–75/FVC) have been found to be more hyperresponsive than those with larger airways in the Normative Aging Study. Thus, comparing responses in FEV1 and sGaw may lend insight into the basic physical relationship between airway size and lung size.

sRaw is commonly used in children and is sometimes used in adults. Details regarding techniques of measurement, quality control, and interpretation are available in recent, excellent reviews. sRaw has been measured in children as young as 2 years old and has been used in the assessment of bronchodilators and responses to methacholine, histamine, and cold air. Other studies have included measuring the effects of short- and long-acting bronchodilators, inhaled corticosteroids, and leukotriene receptor antagonists in asthmatic children. Serial measurements have been made in children with cystic fibrosis and have demonstrated more consistent abnormalities than either FOT or Rint. Since sRaw is primarily used in children, normative data are mainly limited to pediatrics. As most of the children involved in these studies would likely not have been able to perform reliable spirometry, using sRaw as a measure of airways disease is a valuable tool in pediatric lung disease.

In the case of both Raw and sRaw, there may be circumstances where it is useful to differentiate resistance between inspiration and expiration. For example, inspiratory resistance was shown to be inversely associated with changes in FEV1 in patients following lung volume reduction surgery for emphysema. This may be due to patients with less elevated inspiratory resistance having more predominant emphysema rather than intrinsic airway disease. Since lung volume reduction surgery is thought to work, in part, by removing emphysema and improving elastic recoil, these findings suggest that patients with more emphysema are more likely to have less elevated inspiratory resistance and show improvement following surgery.

7.6 Measurement of Airway Resistance by the Forced Oscillation Technique (FOT)

Although body plethysmography remains a gold standard method for measuring Raw, its use requires patient cooperation and some rather cumbersome equipment that is typically only found in hospital pulmonary function laboratories. These limitations are avoided to a large extent by the forced oscillation technique (FOT) that measures the *impedance* of the respiratory system (Zrs) from which a measure of Raw can be derived, and a related method known as the interrupter technique that provides an interrupter resistance (Rint) approximating Raw.

The FOT was first described by Dubois in 1956 and involves applying controlled oscillations in flow to the lungs via the mouth, while the resulting pressure oscillations at the same location are measured (Fig. 7.9). These oscillations are typically applied while the patient continues to breathe quietly, although they can also be applied during a brief period of apnea. A variety of different oscillatory flow signals have been used for the FOT including white noise, sums of individual sine waves (referred to as composite signals), and trains of brief square pulses. All such signals have the property that they contain multiple frequency components, which allows

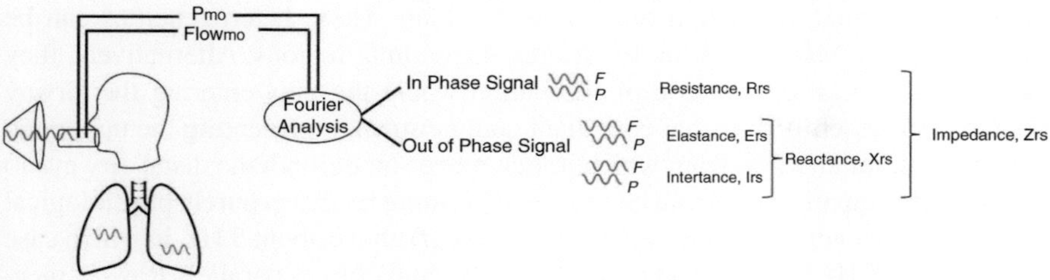

Fig. 7.9 Basic illustration of the forced oscillation technique. The patient breathes through a mouthpiece through which a forced oscillatory flow is produced and transmitted into the airways and lungs. Flow (F) and pressure (P) are recorded at the mouth and processed in the Fourier domain to produce a complex function of frequency (i.e., one having both real and imaginary parts). This function is known as respiratory system impedance (Zrs). The component of P that is in phase with F reflects energy dissipation and gives rise to the real part of Zrs, which is known as respiratory system resistance (Rrs). The component of P that is out of phase with F reflects energy storage and gives rise to the imaginary part of Zrs, which is known as respiratory system reactance (Xrs). The out-of-phase component of P is itself composed of two parts; one lags F by 90° and reflects the elastic stiffness of the respiratory tissues, while the other leads F by 90° and reflects respiratory system inertia

Zrs to be determined simultaneous at each of the frequencies using the fast Fourier transform algorithm. Zrs is thus a function of frequency, f, written as Zrs(f). In fact, Zrs(f) is a *complex function* of frequency, which means it consists of two independent components, a *real part* and an *imaginary part*. The real part is commonly known as *resistance*, Rrs(f), while the imaginary part is known as *reactance*, Xrs(f). Rrs(f) determines how much of the measured pressure oscillations are in phase with the applied oscillations in flow and reflects resistance of the respiratory system. Xrs(f) determines how much of the measured pressure oscillations are out of phase with flow and reflects the elastance (E) (flow leads pressure) and inertance (I) (flow lags pressure) of the system.

During the measurement of Zrs(f) by the FOT, an individual sits and breathes quietly on a mouthpiece while wearing a noseclip and supporting the cheeks and floor of the mouth with their hands, similar to the method used in body plethysmography. Once steady tidal breathing is established, the forced oscillations in flow are applied on top of the breathing pattern. Most FOT systems collect oscillatory pressure and flow data for periods of about 16 s of measurement, after which the patient is free to come off the mouthpiece. The pressure, flow, and volume measurements obtained are then processed to produce calculations of Rrs(f) and Xrs(f) as well as any derivatives of these quantities, such as resonant frequency (f_{res}) and area under the reactance curve (A_X); see below. Subjects may be asked to repeat a FOT measurement 3 to 5 times to provide average values for the final PFT Lab report. For additional interpretation of Zrs(f)by the FOT, see the Appendix A.

Rrs(f) has a marked negative dependence on f below about 2 Hz in normal lungs due to the viscoelastic properties of the respiratory tissues. In obstructive diseases, such as asthma and COPD, Rrs(f) becomes elevated due to the decrease in airway caliber (Fig. 7.10). In addition, the negative frequency dependence of Rrs(f) often becomes accentuated and may extend well above 2 Hz due to mechanical heterogeneities in regional ventilation throughout the lung. These heterogeneities can be distributed in a parallel fashion to different distal lung regions. Alternatively, they can reflect a serial distribution of ventilation where the flow entering the airway opening first enters a proximal compliant compartment, representing the upper and possibly central airways, from which it then moves on through the distal airways to an alveolar compartment. Serial heterogeneity is more likely, on purely physiological grounds, to explain frequency dependence in Rrs(*f*) above about 5 Hz, in which case Rrs(*f*) above 5 Hz likely reflects central airways and closely parallels Raw as measured by body plethysmography. Meanwhile, parallel heterogeneity is more likely to be relevant below 5 Hz, in which case Rrs(*f*) below 5 Hz can be thought of as pertaining to the distal airways. Xrs(*f*) takes a negative hyperbolic form at low frequencies but then becomes linear as it crosses zero at f_{res}, which is about 8–10 Hz in a normal adult subject. Xrs (*f*) can be thought of as an overall measure of respiratory system stiffness, in which below f_{res} is dominated by the elastance of the system (due to actual lung stiffness, loss of lung volume, or airway heterogeneities) and above

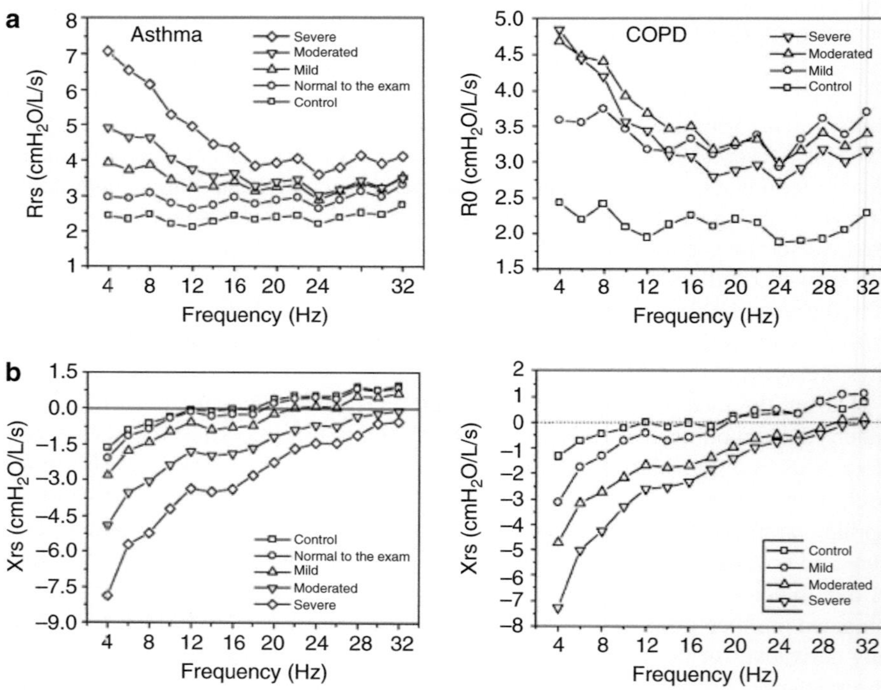

Fig. 7.10 Impedance data from patients with asthma (left) and COPD (right) according to severity of underlying disease. Notice the consistent relationship between diseases of the changes in Rrs and Xrs with increasing severity. In both cases, as severity increases, Rrs rises and becomes more frequency dependent, especially at lower frequencies (< ~16 Hz), and Xrs falls to more negative values, with an increase in the resonant frequency (point at which Xrs crosses zero). (Left = From Cavalcanti 2006, with permission from Elsevier. Right = From DiMango 2006, with permission from Elsevier)

f_{res} is dominated by inertance of the airway gas. Xrs becomes more negative with severity of obstructive disease. As a result, the area under Xrs(*f*) below f_{res}, denoted A_X, also increases and thus serves as a robust, empirical measure of overall respiratory system elastance.

Unlike Raw measured by body plethysmography, Rrs(*f*) measured by the FOT represents total respiratory system resistance and thus contains contributions from both the lung and chest wall. At low frequencies (i.e., <5Hz), Rrs(*f*) is very comparable to Raw but slightly higher due to contributions from the chest wall. At higher frequencies, Rrs(*f*) tends to underestimate Raw, likely due to shunting of flow into the upper airways (i.e., cheeks, floor of mouth). There is no direct comparison that can be made between either Rrs(*f*) or Raw and FEV1 since these quantities reflect different physical phenomena. Nevertheless, both Rrs(*f*) and *Raw* have an important advantage over FEV1 in that they do not involve the subject taking a deep breath, which can reverse any bronchoconstriction that is induced by standard challenge test with a bronchial agonist. Because of this, Rrs(*f*) is highly sensitive to changes in bronchial tone, but it is not particularly specific for asthma or other unique disease states.

7.7 Clinical Utility of FOT

The FOT has become popular because of its ease of administration. It requires minimal subject cooperation and is thus suitable for use in children and any patient who cannot cooperate or manage spirometry (e.g., ventilated patients, paralyzed patients, elderly). The FOT has been used in many applications, including differentiating healthy from obstructed patients in COPD and asthma; detecting bronchoconstriction, which occurs at lower doses of methacholine for Rrs(*f*) than for FEV1; measuring the severity of obstruction in asthma and COPD (Fig. 7.10); detecting early smoking-related changes in lung mechanics in smokers with normal spirometry; and assessing respiratory mechanics in patient with obesity. Methacholine-induced dyspnea is significantly associated with changes in Rrs(5) and Xrs(5), sometimes referred to as R5 and X5, respectively, but not with changes in FEV1, suggesting that these FOT measures are more sensitive to symptoms. However, the most sensitive measurement method varies between healthy and asthmatic subjects and with the degree of severity in asthma.

Since the FOT requires no patient cooperation or technique, it can be applied widely in many clinical settings. For example, only FOT bronchodilator responses, and not responses measured by FEV1, were able to distinguish 4-year-old children at risk for persistent asthma participating in the Childhood Asthma Prevention Study. A similar finding was seen in a cohort of children from Belgium. The FOT has yielded insight into the mechanism of wheezing in infants. It also has unique application in studies of sleep and patients on mechanical ventilation, where the oscillatory signal can be applied on top of tidal breathing. The use of FOT in ventilated and critically ill patients has provided insight into lung derecruitment, parenchymal overdistention, and expiratory flow limitation and has the potential to optimize ventilator settings.

Recent studies are tending to focus more on Xrs(*f*), as opposed to Rrs(*f*), since Xrs(*f*) yields information specifically related to the elastic properties of the lung, and these properties often change dramatically in lung disease. In particular, the magnitude of Xrs(*f*) increases in proportion to the amount of lung volume that is lost via atelectasis or closure of small airways. Indeed, in patients with moderate to severe COPD, the fall in FEV1 with methacholine was more closely related to Xrs(*f*) becoming more negative rather than Rrs(*f*) increasing. This occurred in association with a decrease in inspiratory capacity, suggesting that airway closure was the main response to methacholine. Asthmatics had a smaller change in lung volume and a larger change in Rrs(*f*), suggesting they had more of an airway response. In other cases, increases in the magnitude of Xrs(*f*) are thought to be a consequence of the shunting of forced flow into the more central airways that can occur with a sufficient degree of peripheral airway constriction. Xrs(*f*) has been noted to signal mild airflow obstruction before changes in Rrs(*f*) occur and may detect flow limitation in patients with COPD. Also in COPD, there are strong associations between Xrs(5) and resonant frequency and FEV1 and Xrs(5) and f_{res} and sGaw. A recent study in pediatric asthma has shown that only A_X continues to improve after the initial 12 weeks of therapy with inhaled fluticasone during a 48-week total study, perhaps reflecting ongoing improvement in small airway function. Two studies from Japan note that Xrs(*f*) relates more closely with quality of life measures than FEV1 in patients with both asthma and COPD.

One of the benefits of the FOT is that one can separately measure inspiratory from expiratory parameters. While whole-breath FOT may not differentiate patients with asthma and COPD, patients with COPD may have a higher mean expiratory Xrs(5) than patients with asthma, which may be due to enhanced dynamic airway narrowing on expiration in these patients. In comparing FOT in patients with asthma and COPD, only patients with COPD show a significant difference in Xrs(*f*) between inspiration and expiration, which again may relate to dynamic airway narrowing on expiration due to loss of recoil in COPD.

The European Respiratory Society published guidelines on FOT methodology in 2003, and new guidelines are currently being developed. In general, the repeatability of the technique is similar to Raw from body plethysmography and Rint from the interrupter technique (see below). The correlation with spirometry is highly variable, in part because of the deep breath involved in spirometry and also due to the differing mechanics assessed by the two techniques. The FOT is subject to strong influence by upper airway shunting, and this must be carefully controlled. Many regression equations are now available, but they each come from different populations and use different devices and techniques, so their applicability is limited. Recently, normative reference values and bronchodilator responses have been published from healthy people using five different devices.

The FOT is used commonly in research, from clinical studies in human subjects to basic studies of lung mechanics in experimental animal models. For example, severe asthma is associated with increasing frequency dependence of elastance, thought to be due to more severe peripheral airway resistance causing shunting of flow back into central airways. The FOT applied through the wedged bronchoscope has allowed demonstration of airway hyperresponsiveness of the lung periphery in asthmatics. It must be remembered, however, that the interpretation of Zrs(*f*) depends on mathematical models of the lung, so the physiological information it yields depends on the particular model that is invoked.

7.8 Measurement of Airway Resistance by the Interrupter Technique

A third method to noninvasively measure airway resistance, used primarily in children, is the interrupter technique. The concept here is similar to that used in body plethysmography in the sense that alveolar pressure is estimated from mouth pressure during transient occlusion of the airway opening during which flow, and thus the resistive pressure drop along the airways, is zero. The interrupter technique also shares a formal similarity with the FOT in the sense that it involves an analysis between pressure-flow relationships recorded at the mouth while mouth flow is manipulated by the measuring system; small-amplitude oscillations are forced into the lungs in the case of the FOT, while with the interrupter technique, mouth flow is forced to go from some finite value to zero in a very short period of time by a shutter that closes within a few milliseconds.

Interrupter resistance (Rint) is determined by measuring the difference in mouth pressure immediately after (Ppost) relative to immediately before (Ppre) a rapid interruption of flow at the mouth and then dividing this pressure difference by the flow ($\dot{\text{V}}\text{pre}$) measured immediately prior to the interruption. That is,

$$\text{Rint} = \frac{\text{Post} - \text{Ppre}}{\dot{\text{V}}\text{pre}} \tag{7.8}$$

It is important that the flow be interrupted extremely abruptly, within a few milliseconds, or Rint may be significantly underestimated due to passage of flow past the interrupter value while it is closing. Also, immediately upon occlusion, mouth pressure invariably exhibits rapid damped oscillations due to inertive effects in the respiratory system followed by a slow pressure transient due to tissue viscoelasticity plus any ventilation heterogeneities that might be present (Fig. 7.11). The oscillations obscure Ppost, and by the time the oscillations have decayed away, the subsequent pressure transient is at a different level, so Ppost is estimated by back-extrapolating the transient through the oscillations to the point in time when the occlusion took place (different systems have different algorithms for exactly how this is done, depending on how fast their interruption shutters close). Accordingly, the value of Rint one obtains depends on a variety of technical matters, including whether a facemask or mouthpiece is used. Typically, several repeat measurements are made and the mean or median is reported.

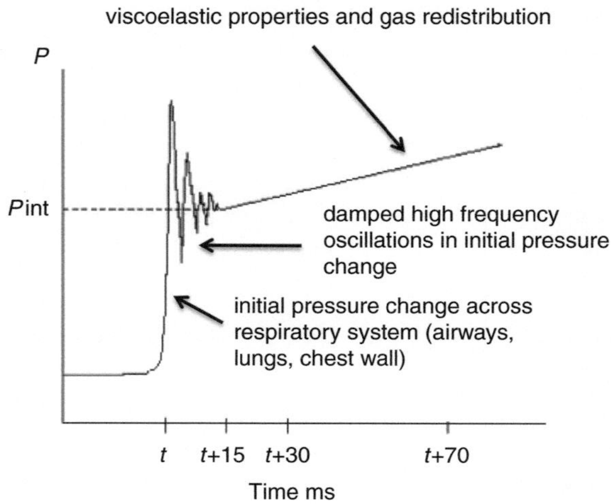

Fig. 7.11 Pressure vs. time during an interrupter maneuver during expiration. At $t = 0$, the airway is transiently occluded, resulting in an abrupt spike in pressure reflecting the initial pressure change across the respiratory system. The pressure then oscillates briefly before slowly climbing as pressure rises from viscoelastic properties and gas redistribution in the lung. By convention, a common method to calculate interrupter resistance (Rint) is to take the pressure at $t + 15$ ms determined by back extrapolation from $t + 30$ and $t + 70$ ms and divide this pressure by the flow immediately before the occlusion. (Adapted from Kooi 2006, with permission from Elsevier)

Animal studies have shown that Rint provides a measure of the flow resistance of the pulmonary airways when the chest is open but includes a contribution from the chest wall in the intact respiratory system, but this applies only when the lung is normal and functionally quite homogeneous. In obstructive pulmonary disease, as with body plethysmography, the assumption of rapid equilibration between mouth and alveolar pressures at zero mouth flow may not hold up very well, which can lead to difficulties in determining the value of Ppost. Nevertheless, because it is noninvasive and performed during normal breathing, the interrupter technique is especially suitable for use in young children and has been demonstrated feasible in children as young as 2 years old. The intrasubject coefficient of variation is similar to that of FOT (5–15%). There is a small group of reference equations that derives from pediatric studies.

7.9 Clinical Utility of Rint

Clinically, Rint has been used in discriminating between different phenotypes of wheezy children and between healthy children and children with asthma. In children with asthma, a correlation coefficient of 0.73 was found for baseline values of spirometry and Rint. Rint has also been used in conjunction with other measures to evaluate bronchodilator response in asthmatic children. In order of discriminating capacity, Raw, R5, Rint, and X5 were found to be useful with positive predictive values of 84%, 74%, 82%, and 76% respectively. The interrupter technique has also been used to assess the response to cold air inhalation, inhaled fluticasone, and oral montelukast therapy. An important issue with the interrupter technique has been deciding on the best cutoff for a bronchoconstrictor response. In adults, a 20% change in FEV1 following methacholine corresponds to different levels of change of Gaw (the reciprocal of Rint) determined by the interrupter technique, depending on the underlying degree of bronchial responsiveness.

7.10 Comparing sRaw, Rrs(*f*), and Rint

The limited studies directly comparing sRaw, Rrs(*f*), and Rint appear mainly in children. Even though these three measures of resistance are based on somewhat differing mechanical principles, all show consistent changes in relation to disease state or response to bronchodilator or bronchoconstrictor. Furthermore, these measures tend to be more sensitive to bronchodilation and bronchoconstriction than FEV1, with one study demonstrating that Raw was more sensitive than Rrs(*f*) and Rint in detecting bronchoconstriction in normal subjects. Technical factors are critical in achieving valid results, with special attention given to reducing thermal artifact in sRaw, and upper airway shunting in Rrs(*f*) and Rint. All three measures have shown higher values in children with asthma, but there is no clear agreement on cutoffs for abnormal values. This is especially important because even healthy children demonstrate reduced resistance in response to bronchodilators when using these highly sensitive measures. All three measures are commonly abnormal in young children with asthma, but none appear to associate with clinical outcomes assessed 3 years later. sGaw, Rrs(*f*), and Rint allow differentiation of inspiratory and expiratory resistance, and the dynamic looping of resistance and flow with use of sRaw and Rrs(*f*) may yield important information about laryngeal narrowing, a common occurrence during testing. Rrs(*f*) also provides information about frequency dependence, which yields additional insight into peripheral airway mechanics and inhomogeneities. In addition, the FOT and the interrupter technique provide information about the elastic properties of the respiratory system. A summary of the specific measurement properties of FEV1 in comparison with sRaw, sGaw, Rrs(*f*), and Rint is shown in Table 7.1.

7.11 Conclusions

Spirometry remains the gold standard pulmonary function test for determining the presence and severity of airflow limitation. However, spirometry has some key limitations: it is effort dependent and requires patient cooperation and skill, it involves a deep breath that can alter underlying airway resistance, and it provides limited insight into the link between lung structure and function. For subjects who cannot perform spirometry, measuring airway resistance by plethysmography, the FOT, and the interrupter technique remain important options. Measuring sRaw by body plethysmography involves bulky equipment that does not allow portable

Table 7.1 Characteristics of different lung function tests related to airway resistance

	Spiro (FEV1)	Pleth (sRaw, sGaw)	Rint	FOT (Rrs)
Requires patient cooperation/effort	+++	+++	+	+
Involves deep inhalation	+++	–	–	–
Adjusts for lung volume	–	++	–	–
Intrasubject variability (CV)	3–5%	8–13%	5–15%	5–15%
Sensitivity to airway location				
Central	+	++	+++	+++
Peripheral	++	+	+	+++
Cutoff for bronchodilator/ bronchoconstrictor responses	12/20%	25/40%	35%/3SDw	40/50%
Provides insight into respiratory system mechanics	+ Global, non-specific	+ sRaw: Raw, TGV sGaw: Raw	+ Lung + chest wall	+++ Lung + chest wall
Standardized methodology available	+++	++	+	++
Reference equations available	+++	++	++ (peds)	++

Abbreviations: *Spiro* spirometry, *FEV1* forced expiratory volume in 1 s, *Pleth* plethysmography, *sRaw* specific airway resistance, *sGaw* specific airway conductance, *Rint* interrupter resistance, *FOT* forced oscillation technique, *Rrs* respiratory system resistance, *SDw* within subject standard deviation, *TGV* thoracic gas volume, *Peds* pediatrics
"+" to "+++" = Yes, with increasing strength or prevalence of feature
"–" = No

measurement, and it provides an index that reflects both airway resistance and lung volume. In adults, sGaw is typically used to provide a sensitive measure of airway caliber. However, due to high sensitivity, sGaw has poor specificity for asthma or other unique disease states. The FOT is easy to perform with newly available commercial devices, but the method is very sensitive to upper airway shunting. Nevertheless, the FOT provides unique information related to lung mechanics that is not available by other noninvasive techniques. Measuring Rint also presents important technical issues including the upper airway shunt problem but is well-tolerated by very young children. There are no data comparing the clinical utility of these various measures head to head with each other and with spirometry, but measures of airway resistance may provide important physiological information that contributes to the care of the patient.

Appendix A

More Detailed Analysis of Raw by Body Plethysmography

To measure Raw by body plethysmography, one first needs to measure thoracic gas volume (TGV). During panting against an occluded mouthpiece ("closed-shutter panting"), a pressure transducer in the mouthpiece measures the changes in airway opening pressure (ΔPao) that occur with each breathing effort. As Dubois realized, because there is no airflow along the airways during this maneuver, ΔPao must equal the change in alveolar pressure that results in small changes in V_{TG} due to gas compression. At the same time, another pressure transducer measures the pressure changes within the plethysmograph (ΔPpleth). The changes in Ppleth occur because the air around the subject in the plethysmograph becomes cyclically compressed and decompressed as the subject decompresses and compresses, respectively, the air in their lungs as they try to breathe. In fact, the amounts by which V_{TG} and the gas in the plethysmograph change are always equal and opposite, so by knowing the compressibility of the air around the subject (which can be accurately estimated from the geometry of the plethysmograph and the weight of the subject), one can estimate from ΔPpleth what this volume change, ΔV, is. Boyle's law then states that

$$\frac{\mathrm{Atm}}{V_{\mathrm{TG}-\Delta V}} = \frac{\mathrm{Atm} + \Delta Pao}{V_{\mathrm{TG}}} \tag{7.9}$$

where Atm is atmospheric pressure. The only quantity in Eq. 7.6 that is not known is V_{TG}, so it can be solved for explicitly.

With V_{TG} in hand, one proceeds to measure Raw by having the subject breathe freely from the plethysmograph through a pneumotachograph so that mouth flow, $\dot{V}$, is recorded. The subject wears a nose clip and supports the cheeks and floor of the mouth with their hands in order to minimize any pressure losses in the soft tissues of the mouth and throat (so-called upper airway shunting). This ensures that any pressure changes measured are due to flow of air along the lower airways and into the lungs. This flow is caused by a pressure difference between mouth pressure (Pao), which is also recorded, and alveolar pressure (P_{A}). P_{A} itself causes the gas in the lungs to be compressed, or decompressed, according to Boyle's law, so this is reflected in changes in Ppleth as described above for the measurement of V_{TG}, and thus yields the amount of gas compression, ΔV, in the lungs. However, since V_{TG} is now known, P_{A} (relative to Atm) can be solved for through another statement of Boyle's law, namely,

$$\frac{\mathrm{Atm}}{V_{\mathrm{TG}} \mp \Delta V} = \frac{\mathrm{Atm} \pm P_{\mathrm{A}}}{V_{\mathrm{TG}}} \tag{7.10}$$

in which P_{A} is the only unknown quantity.

Finally, Raw is calculated from the defining equation for resistance,

$$\text{Raw} = \frac{\text{Pao} - P_A}{\dot{V}} \tag{7.11}$$

The difference between Ppleth and P_A during this measurement tends to be rather small, so it is necessary to have the subject breathe at a sufficient rate to make this difference measurable.

The closed-shutter panting maneuver used to measure V_{TG} is typically performed immediately after the open-shutter panting maneuver used to measure Raw, a so-called linked maneuver (Fig. 7.3). During the open-shutter panting maneuver, inspiratory and expiratory flows are plotted against Ppleth (often called *box pressure*, as in Fig. 7.4) and the slope of the relationship, S_{open}, determined. During the linked closed-shutter maneuver to measure V_{TG} (see chapter on lung volumes), inspiratory and expiratory mouth pressure is plotted against box pressure and the slope of the relationship, S_{closed}, determined. Dividing S_{open} by S_{closed} has the effect of combining Eqs. 7.9, 7.10, and 7.11 to provide Raw (Fig. 7.5).

More Detailed Interpretation of Impedance by the Forced Oscillation Technique (FOT)

Interpreting the physiological meaning of Rrs(f) and Xrs(f) must be done on the basis of some model idealization of the respiratory system. At the simplest level, one can think of the system as an elastic balloon on a flow-resistive airway, as was done above in deriving Eq. 7.1. In this case, Zrs(f) is a constant equal to R, while Xrs(f) is equal to $2\pi fI - E/2\pi f$, with E = elastance and I = inertance, as defined previously for the equation of motion of the lung. Importantly, Xrs(f) becomes zero at the so-called resonant frequency, f_{res}, when $2\pi fI - E/2\pi f$, which means that $f_{res} = \left(\sqrt{E/I}\right)/2\pi$. This model is far too simple to represent a real lung, of course, so one invariably finds that Rrs(f) and Xrs(f) exhibit dependencies on f that can only be reasonably interpreted in terms of more complex models.

Selected References

Bates JH, Ludwig MS, Sly PD, Brown K, Martin JG, Fredberg JJ. Interrupter resstance elucidated by alveolar pressure measurement in open-chest normal dogs. J Appl Physiol. 1988;65:408–14.

Bates JHT, Suki B. Assessment of peripheral lung mechanics. Respir Physiol Neurobiol. 2008;163:54.

Bisgaaard H, Nielsen K. Plethysmographic measurements of specific airway resistance in young children. Chest. 2005;128:355–62.

Black J, Baxter-Jones A, Gordon J, Findlay A, Helms P. Assessment of airway function in young children with asthma: comparison of spirometry, interrupter technique, and tidal flow by inductance plethysmography. Pediatr Pulmonol. 2004;37:548–53.

Blonshine S, Goldman M. Optimizing performance of respiratory airflow resistance measurements. Chest. 2008;134:1304–9.

Bosse Y, Riesenfeld E, Pare P, Irvin C. It's not all smooth muscle: non-smooth muscle elements in control of resistance to airflow. Annu Rev Physiol. 2010;72:437–62.

Cavalcanti J, Lopes A, Jansen J, Melo P. Detection of changes in respiratory mechanics due to increasing degrees of airway obstruction in asthma by the forced oscillation technique. Respir Med. 2006;100:2207–19.

Child F. The measurement of airways resistance using the interrupter technique (Rint). Paediatr Respir Rev. 2005;6:273–7.

Clement J, Landser F, Van de Woestijne K. Total resistance and reactance in patients with respiratory complaints with and without airways obstruction. Chest. 1983;83:215–20.

Criee C, Sorichter S, Smith H, Kardos P, Merget R, Heise D, Berdel D, et al. Body plethysmography – its principles and clinical use. Respir Med. 2011;105:959;xx1–13.

De Haut P, Rachiele A, Martin R, Malo J. Histamine dose-response curves in asthma: reproducibility and sensitivity of different indices to assess response. Thorax. 1983;38:516–22.

Dellaca R, Santus P, Aliverti A, Stevenson N, Centanni S, Macklem P, Pedotti A, et al. Detection of expiratory flow limitation in COPD using the forced oscillation technique. Eur Respir J. 2004;23:232–40.

Di Mango A, Lopes A, Jansen J, Melo P. Changes in respiratory mechanics with increasing degrees of airway obstruction in COPD: detection by forced oscillation technique. Respir Med. 2006;100:399–410.

Dubois A, Botelho S, Bedell G, Marshall R, Comroe J. A new method for measuring airway resistance in man using a body plethysmograph; values in normal subjects and in patients with respiratory disease. J Clin Invest. 1956a;35:327–35.

Dubois A, Brody A, Lewis D, Burgess B. Oscillation mechanics of lungs and chest in man. J Appl Physiol. 1956b;8:587–94.

Dubois A. Airway resistance. Am J Respir Crit Care Med. 2000;162:345–6.

Fish J, Peterman V, Cugell D. Effect of deep inspiration on airway conductance in subjects with allergic rhinitis and allergic asthma. J Allergy Clin Immunol. 1977;60:41–6.

Goldman M. Clinical application of forced oscillation. Pulm Pharm Therap. 2001;14:341–50.

Hellinckx J, Cauberghs M, De Boeck K, Demedts M. Evaluation of impulse oscillation system: comparison with forced oscillation technique and body plethysmography. Eur Respir J. 2001;18:564–70.

Kaminsky DA. What does airway resistance tell us about lung function? Respir Care. 2012;57:85–99.

Khalid I, Morris Z, DiGiovine B. Specific conductance criteria for a positive methacholine challenge test: are the American Thoracic Society guidelines rather generous? Respir Care. 2009a;54:1168–74.

Khalid I, Obeid I, DiGiovine B, Khalid U, Morris Z. Predictive value of sGaw, FEF 25-75, and FEV1 for development of asthma after a negative methacholine challenge test. J Asthma. 2009b;46:284–90.

Klug B, Bisgaaard H. Measurement of the specific airway resistance by plethysmography in young children accompanied by an adult. Eur Respir J. 1997;10:1599–605.

Kooi E, Schokker S, van der Moken T, Duiverman E. Airway resistance measurements in pre-school children with asthmatic symptoms: the interrupter technique. Respir Med. 2006;100:955–64.

Marchal F, Schweitzer C, Thuy L. Forced oscillations, interrupter technique and body plethysmography in the preschool child. Paediatr Respir Rev. 2005;6:278–84.

Merkus P, Mijnsbergen J, Hop W, de Jongste J. Interrupter resistance in preschool children. Measurement characteristics and reference values. Am J Respir Crit Care Med. 2001;163:1350–5.

Nielsen K. Plethysmographic specific airway resistance. Paediatr Respir Rev. 2006;7S:S17–9.

Oostveen E, Dom S, Desager K, Hagendorens M, De Backer W, Weyler J. Lung function and bronchodilator response in 4 year old children with different wheezing phenotypes. Eur Respir J. 2010;35:865–72.

Oostveen E, MacLeod D, Lorino H, Farre R, Hantos Z, Desager K, Marchal F. The forced oscillation technique in clinical practice: methodology, recommendations and future developments. Eur Respir J. 2003;22:1026–41.

Paredi P, Goldman M, Alamen A, Ausin P, Usmani O, Pride N, Barnes P. Comparison of inspiratory and expiratory resistance and reactance in patients with asthma and chronic obstructive pulmonary disease. Thorax. 2009;65:263–7.

Parker A, McCool F. Pulmonary function characteristics in patients with different patterns of methacholine airway hyperresponsiveness. Chest. 2002;121:1818–23.

Phagoo S, Watson R, Silverman M, Pride N. Comparison of four methods of assessing airflow resistance before and after induced airway narrowing in normal subjects. J Appl Physiol. 1995;79:518–25.

Pride N. Forced oscillaiton techniques for measuring mechanical properties of the respiratory system. Thorax. 1992;47:317–20.

Sly P, Lombardi E. Measurement of lung function in preschool children using the interrupter technique. Thorax. 2003;58:742–4.

Smith H, Irvin C, Cherniack R. The utility of spirometry in the diagnosis of reversible airways obstruction. Chest. 1992;101:1577–81.

Stocks J, Godfrey S, Beardsmore C, Bar-Yishay E, Castile R. Plethysmographic measurements of lung volume and airway resistance. Eur Respir J. 2001;17:302–12.

Sundblad B-M, Malmberg P, Larsson K. Comparison of airway conductance and FEV1 as measures of airway responsiveness to methacholine. Clin Physiol. 2001;21:673–81.

Yaegashi M, Yalamanchili V, Kaza V, Weedon J, Heurich A, Akerman M. The utility of the forced oscillation technique in assessing bronchodilator responsiveness in patients with asthma. Respir Med. 2007;101:995–1000.

Chapter 8
Initiating the Breath: The Drive to Breathe, Muscle Pump

Jeremy Richards, Matthew J. Fogarty, Gary C. Sieck, and Richard M. Schwartzstein

8.1 Introduction

Ten to 16 times a minute of every minute of every day, whether awake or asleep, we take a breath. Why? The typical answer is teleological: we need to get oxygen into the blood and remove carbon dioxide from the body. While we have central and peripheral chemoreceptors that can sense changes in partial pressure of gases and related pH changes in the blood, these do not appear to be the source of the signal that initiates resting breathing. So, what initiates the breath and how is the signal transformed to movement of the chest wall and the creation of a negative intrathoracic pressure?

When asleep, we are all dependent on the activity of inspiratory neurons in the brainstem to maintain normal ventilation. These neurons, to which we often refer as the "central pattern generator," are located in the medulla and have an independent firing frequency that ultimately is transformed into a breathing rate and tidal volume. Our central drive to breathe, however, can be influenced by a range of sensory inputs including the chemoreceptors, vascular receptors (heart and pulmonary circulation), and lung fibers sensitive to stretch and inflammation.

Breathing while awake, however, does not seem to be completely dependent on these inspiratory centers. Individuals with congenital central hypoventilation syn-

J. Richards · R. M. Schwartzstein (✉)
Division of Pulmonary, Critical Care, and Sleep Medicine, Beth Israel Deaconess Medical Center, Harvard Medical School, Boston, MA, USA
e-mail: rschwart@bidmc.harvard.edu

M. J. Fogarty
Department of Physiology and Biomedical Engineering, Mayo Clinic, Rochester, MN, USA

School of Biomedical Sciences, The University of Queensland, Brisbane, Australia

G. C. Sieck (✉)
Department of Physiology and Biomedical Engineering, Mayo Clinic, Rochester, MN, USA
e-mail: sieck.gary@mayo.edu

D. A. Kaminsky, C. G. Irvin (eds.), *Pulmonary Function Testing*, Respiratory Medicine, https://doi.org/10.1007/978-3-319-94159-2_8

drome (CCHS), for example, appear to lack a functioning respiratory center in the medulla, yet breathe relatively normally when awake. Wakefulness and the reticular activating system are presumed to have contributions to breathing that are independent of the medullary pattern generator.

There are many physiological functions that are essential for life and occur "in the background;" they do not require conscious thought. Breathing, contraction of the heart, and digestion of food all ensue in the absence of voluntary "commands." The control of ventilation, however, is different in that one can volitionally alter the automatic control mechanisms; we can all hold our breath or suddenly double our tidal volume or respiratory frequency on command, but have no similar control over cardiovascular or gastrointestinal function. Furthermore, emotional factors, such as anxiety, may lead to changes in one's breathing pattern independently of gas exchange considerations.

Once a neurological signal is generated in the brain, it must travel to the inspiratory muscles, which contract, move the chest wall, generate a negative intrathoracic pressure, and consequently produce a flow of gas into the lungs. The ventilatory pump, comprising the peripheral nervous system, bones and muscles of the chest wall, pleura, and airways, must all be functioning properly to create an inspiratory tidal volume. Thus, breathing requires a functional nervous system and pump.

Since the initiation of a breath must begin with a neurological impulse, assessment of the process ideally would include a measurement of the neural signal. In clinical settings, however, it is not feasible to access the activity of the inspiratory control centers in the brainstem. Downstream signals in the peripheral nervous system, primarily the phrenic nerve, are more accessible, but direct recordings are fraught with technical difficulties. Assessment of muscle activity with electromyography is feasible and commonly employed in experimental situations; clinical use of this technique, however, is less common. Often we are left with more global assessment of the controller by examining ventilation, particularly in response to stimuli such as acute hypoxemia or hypercapnia. In patient populations, however, the ventilatory pump may be compromised due to muscle weakness, hyperinflation of the lungs, changes in compliance of the chest wall or lungs, and airways disease. In the end, the initiation of the breath is an integrated function dependent upon both neurological and mechanical outputs.

In this chapter we will review the physiology underlying the control of breathing and the transformation of the neurological signals from respiratory centers into muscle contraction. We will also examine the role of peripheral sensory receptors in the control of breathing and the types of testing of the output of the ventilatory pump that enable us to begin separating out the assessment of neurological and pump function in the respiratory system.

8.2 Muscle Function and the Ventilatory Pump

Respiratory muscles can be broadly categorized as muscles that serve as a pump to move air into and out of our lungs (ventilation) and muscles responsible for maintaining the patency of the upper (the larynx and above) and lower (below the cricoid cartilage) airways. Ventilatory pump muscles provide movement of air from the mouth to alveoli allowing for gas exchange that supplies O_2 to arterial blood and eventually to metabolically active tissues in the body, while removing CO_2, the byproduct of tissue metabolism, from the blood.

The pump muscles are all skeletal (or striated). Similarly, respiratory muscles that control upper airway caliber are also skeletal muscles, whereas those comprising the lower airways are smooth muscles. Upper airway muscles fall into two categories, (1) muscles that control patency of nasal, oral, and pharyngeal conductive pathway for air and (2) muscles that control opening (abductors) or closing (adductor) of the laryngeal inlet for airflow to the trachea. Smooth muscles line lower airways from the trachea and bronchi down to alveoli. Contraction and relaxation of airway smooth muscles control airway resistance to airflow.

Ventilatory Pump Muscles The pump muscles are categorized as inspiratory or expiratory based on their mechanical action on the chest and abdominal walls and the functional translation to a decrease (inspiratory) or increase (expiratory) in thoracic pressure. Inspiration is an active process requiring contraction of chest wall inspiratory muscles. By contrast, expiration is generally passive due to elastic recoil of the lung and chest wall; the latter recoils inward only at higher lung volumes when it is above its resting position. Consequently, this chapter will focus primarily on inspiratory pump muscles.

Diaphragm muscle The major inspiratory muscle is the diaphragm, which is unique to mammals. The diaphragm separates the thoracic (pleural) and abdominal (peritoneal) compartments. With contraction, the diaphragm moves caudally, creating a negative intrathoracic pleural pressure (P_{pl}) and inspiratory airflow. This downward motion of the diaphragm produces positive abdominal pressure (P_{ab}). The resulting transdiaphragmatic pressure ($P_{di} = P_{pl} - P_{ab}$) reflects force generation by the diaphragm muscle.

Based on muscle fiber origins, the diaphragm is typically separated into three major regions: (1) sternal region in which muscle fibers originate from the posterior portion of xyphoid process and xiphisternal junction and insert into the central tendon, (2) costal region in which fibers originate from the broad expanse of the lower rib cage (ribs 7–12 and their costal cartilage) and insert into the central tendon, and (3) the crural region in which fibers originate from and insert into the central tendon. During normal breathing, the fibers of the diaphragm are longest at end exhalation, which facilitates generation of tension in the muscle.

The diaphragm muscle comprises right and left sides, which are generally symmetrical (some differences present based on structures that pass through the diaphragm). The orientation of fibers in the two sternal regions of the diaphragm is parallel, whereas radiating orientation of fibers in the costal regions is in series. In addition, fiber orientation in the costal regions of the diaphragm is curved into a dome shape. Contraction of muscle fibers in the costal regions causes this curvature to flatten downward, thereby pushing on the abdominal cavity and increasing abdominal pressure.

The orientation of fibers in the right and left crural regions of the diaphragm is more complex. The right side is larger and longer compared to the left side. The medial margins of the right and left cural regions encompass the esophagus and act as a sphincter during inspiratory contractions, decreasing the risk of gastric reflux. The descending aorta passes dorsal behind the right crural diaphragm, whereas the inferior vena cava passes through the central tendon such that blood blow in both structures is unimpaired by diaphragm contractions. Indeed, the negative transdiaphragmatic pressure generated during inspiration promotes an increase in venous return to the right atrium.

The diaphragm is innervated by the phrenic nerve, which originates from the lower cervical spinal cord (C3 to C6, depending on species). There is a somatotopic pattern in the innervation of the diaphragm muscle, with rostral segments of the phrenic motor neuron pool innervating the sternal region and more ventral portions of the costal and crural regions.

Intercostal muscles In addition to the diaphragm muscle, some intercostal muscles also serve as an inspiratory pump by directly affecting chest wall expansion. There are three layers of intercostal muscles: external, internal, and innermost portions. Inspiratory pump action occurs only with contraction of the external intercostal muscles and depends on the origin, insertion, and orientation of these muscle fibers. The ribs on each side curve downward and anteriorly and comprise a bony (lateral) and cartilaginous (medial) portion. Particularly in the lower ribs, the shapes of the downward curving portions appear as bucket handles that can be lifted by contraction of the external intercostal muscles that project obliquely downward and forward to insert on the ribs below.

The internal intercostal muscles originate inferiorly from the 2nd through 12th ribs and project obliquely upward and medially to insert on ribs above. Therefore, contraction of internal intercostal muscle fibers causes depression of the ribs above, compression of the chest wall, and an expiratory effect. In contrast, ventral internal intercostal muscle fibers that originate from medial cartilaginous portion of the ribs near the sternum cause these ribs to lift upward with contraction, expanding the thoracic cavity resulting in an inspiratory effect similar to that of external intercostal muscles. These ventral internal intercostal muscle fibers are often characterized as a separate group, called the parasternal intercostal muscles.

The innermost or deepest layer of the intercostal muscles is separated from the internal intercostal muscles by the neurovascular bundle. These muscle fibers form a thin musculo-tendinous layer that is continuous with fibers of the transversus abdominis muscle. Contraction of innermost intercostal muscle fibers exerts relatively minor mechanical effects on the chest wall, but may aid when expiratory efforts are forceful, together with the transversus abdominis muscle. The intercostal nerves innervate intercostal muscles segmentally with motor neurons located in the T1 through T11 spinal cord.

In addition to intercostal muscles, other muscles insert on ribcage may be involved in our inspiratory efforts. For example, the scalene muscles originate from transverse processes of the lower five cervical vertebrae and insert on the upper surfaces of the first two ribs. Contraction of scalene muscle fibers causes elevation of these upper ribs and can contribute to inspiration.

Classification of motor unit and muscle fiber types In the diaphragm, as in other skeletal muscles, the final output of neural control is the motor unit (Fig. 8.1), comprising a phrenic motor neuron located in the cervical spinal cord, and the group of

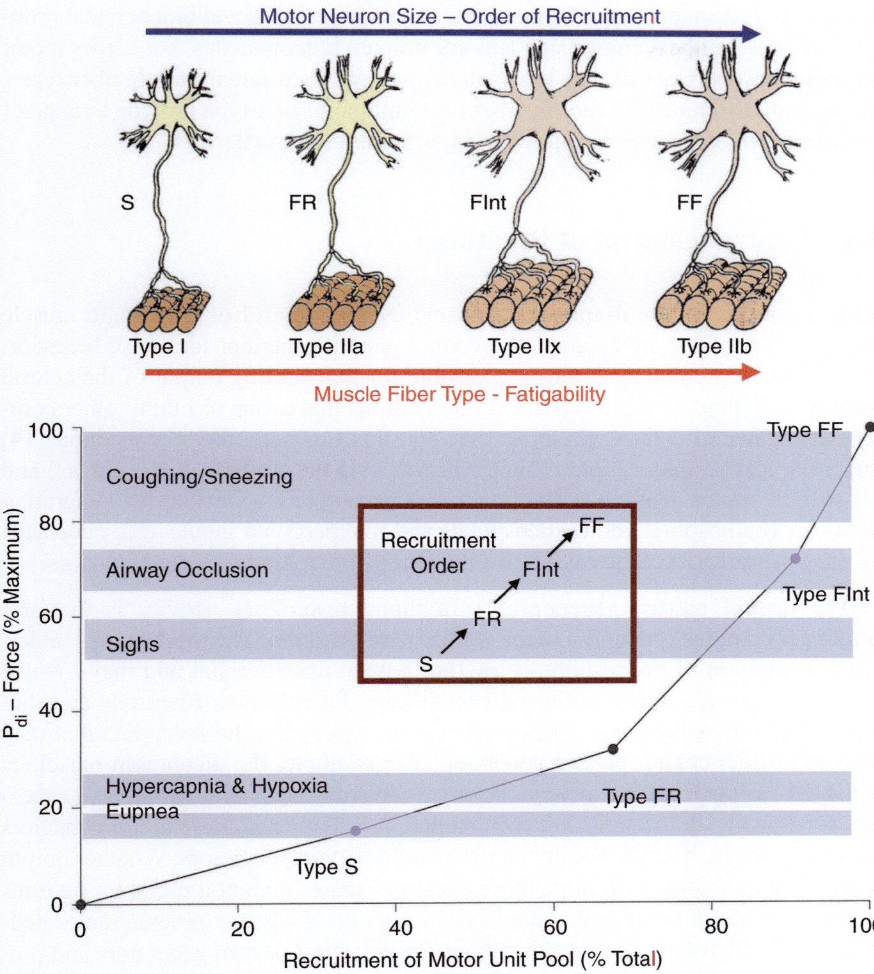

Fig. 8.1 Diaphragm motor units comprise phrenic motor neurons (PhMNs) and the diaphragm muscle fibers they innervate. Four motor units can be classified: (1) type S motor units, which have smaller PhMNs and innervate type I fibers that exhibit slower contraction time and velocity of shortening, produce lower specific force, and are resistant to fatigue during repetitive activation; (2) type FR motor units, which also have smaller PhMNs and innervate type IIa fibers that exhibit faster contraction time and velocity of shortening, produce greater specific force, and are fatigue resistant; (3) type FInt motor units, which have larger PhMNs and innervate type IIx fibers that exhibit faster contraction time and velocity of shortening, produce greater specific force, but are more susceptible to fatigue during repetitive activation; and (4) type FF motor units, which have larger PhMNs that innervate type IIx/IIb fibers that exhibit the fastest contraction time and velocity of shortening, produce the greatest specific force, but are highly fatigable. Different diaphragm motor unit types are recruited based on PhMN size to accomplish a range of motor behaviors. Ventilation (eupnea, hypercapnia, and hypoxia) is accomplished by recruitment of only smaller PhMNs comprising type S and FR motor units, whereas higher force, airway clearance behaviors require recruitment of larger PhMNs comprising more fatigable motor units

muscle fibers it innervates. The mechanical, fatigue-related, and biochemical properties of muscle fibers comprising a motor unit are homogeneous, but across motor units these properties can vary substantially and define different muscle fiber types. The overall differences in muscle fiber type and motor unit type provide a range of neural control of force generation during different motor behaviors.

8.3 Central Control of Breathing

Neural control of the diaphragm muscle Neural control of diaphragm muscle involves five main components: (1) a central pattern generator for motor behavior; (2) medullary premotor neurons responsible for transmitting output of the central pattern to phrenic motor neurons; (3) interneurons that excite or inhibit other components of neural control via direct synaptic input or neuromodulatory input; (4) direct cortical premotor input to motor neurons via the corticospinal pathway; and (5) phrenic motor neurons as the final common output responsible for integrating premotor (bulbospinal and corticospinal) and interneuronal inputs and, once activated, generating forces necessary for the range of diaphragm motor behaviors.

The central pattern generator for rhythmic respiratory activity is the pre-Bötzinger complex (preBötC) in the ventrolateral medulla. The mechanisms underlying generation of the respiratory rhythm remain controversial and may involve neuronal networks and/or neuronal pacemakers. Phrenic motor neurons and diaphragm muscle activation are involved in other types of motor behaviors that may involve distinct central pattern generators. For example, the diaphragm muscle is activated during expulsive airway clearance behaviors such as coughing and sneezing, swallowing, defecation, and vocalization. It is likely that these motor behaviors are controlled by discrete but interactive central pattern generators. Whether output from these individual central pattern generators shares common premotor neurons is unclear. Thus, a fundamental unresolved question is whether phrenic motor neurons receive distributed or selective inputs from central pattern generators and premotor neurons that are specific to different motor behaviors or whether components of these neural circuits are shared across different motor behaviors.

For rhythmic ventilatory behaviors, phrenic motor neurons receive premotor input primarily from the rostral ventral respiratory group in the ventrolateral medulla and to a lesser extent for the dorsal respiratory group in the dorsomedial medulla. This premotor output is bilateral, but primarily ipsilateral, and conveyed via bulbospinal pathways in the ventrolateral and dorsomedial funiculi of the spinal cord. This excitatory premotor input to phrenic motor neurons for ventilatory behaviors is mediated through glutamatergic (Glu) neurotransmission.

Premotor neurons are also a major site of integration of sensory and other neuromodulatory effects on respiration, particularly neural drive. Examples of such neuromodulation of the respiratory pattern generator and premotor output include effects of afferent inputs from mechanoreceptors and irritant receptors in the lung, peripheral chemoreceptors, central chemoreception, and serotonergic projections emanating from the raphe and catecholamine sources that mediate sleep-wake state and emotional state modulation. Lung mechanoreceptors respond to transient or sustained lung inflation, and are thus sensitive to mechanical loading of breathing, and prevent airway overinflation by peaking in afferent activity at the end of inspiration. These afferents, which travel via the vagus nerve to the nucleus tractus solitarius (NTS), exert their effect on the central pattern generator for ventilatory behaviors with early termination of inspiratory efforts. Laryngeal mechanoreceptors also exert an indirect effect on phrenic motor neurons, decreasing inspiratory drive during upper airway collapse. Peripheral chemoreceptors, primarily located in the carotid bodies, respond to hypoxia and/or hypercapnia, and their output travels via the carotid sinus nerve to the NTS. Stimulation of the peripheral chemoreceptors affects the respiratory pattern generator and premotor out to increase ventilation via an effect on both respiratory rate and tidal volume. Central chemoreceptors are found in many brainstem areas and are exquisitely sensitive to an increase in CO_2 and decrease in pH, resulting in an increase in ventilation. Serotonergic neurons within the caudal raphe within the medulla project to brainstem respiratory regions and the phrenic motor pool and have effects on both medullary and brainstem output and phrenic motor neuron excitation. Catecholamine modulation of respiration also occurs via an activation of $\alpha 1$ or $\alpha 2$ adrenoreceptors, respectively, enhancing or inhibiting respiratory rhythm central pattern generation.

In contrast to locomotor motor neurons, the diaphragm muscle has very few muscle spindles; thus, there is very little contribution of direct proprioceptive feedback to phrenic motor neurons. However, muscle spindles located in intercostal muscles exert inhibitory effects on phrenic motor neurons. In addition, local inhibition of phrenic motor neurons from other interneurons within the spinal cord has been characterized.

In humans, direct corticospinal inputs onto phrenic motor neurons allow for voluntary breathing control and the interplay between ventilation and behaviors such as speech. Phrenic motor neuron integration of rhythmic pattern inputs, modulatory inputs, and cortical inputs is illustrated in the difference in drive to breathe during the waking state, whereby the awake state provides a resilience to apnea in hypocapnic conditions. By contrast, sleep predisposes to episodes of apnea in the hypocapnic condition, yet it remains unknown how influential cortical arousal states are in the maintenance of eupnea.

Although much is still to be defined with regard to phrenic motor neuron inputs and the central pattern generation of respiratory behavior, the individual phrenic motor neuron is the final integrator of these signals. The phrenic motor unit remains the final executor of neuromotor control and produces respiratory motor force output across a multitude of ventilatory and non-ventilatory behaviors. Whether different types of motor units receive differing premotor inputs, or if intrinsic properties of motor units provide the nuances of control, remains to be elucidated. Regardless, different diaphragm neuromotor behaviors require differing levels of force generation, a property intrinsically dependent upon motor units.

8.4 Peripheral Inputs that Affect Central Control

While the brain is ultimately the source of neurological impulses to the ventilatory muscles, there are multiple sensory and mechanoreceptors located in the upper airway, lung parenchyma, pulmonary vasculature, and chest wall that contribute to the control of breathing. While individuals have different degrees of responses to signals provided by these receptors, their general effects on increasing awareness of respiratory sensations and on increasing the drive to breathe are reproducible across subjects. In the end, the stimulus to breathe and the resulting mechanical output of the respiratory system is a complicated integrative process that accounts for more than merely ensuring adequate levels of oxygen and carbon dioxide in the blood.

Voluntary/behavioral effects Neurologic signals from brainstem respiratory center (during normal breathing) and from the frontal voluntary respiratory centers (during volitional, conscious breathing) to the motor cortex activate the muscles of ventilation. Simultaneously, the motor cortex sends output to the sensory cortex, a central signaling pathway referred to as "corollary discharge," which is believed to produce a sense of "effort" of breathing. The sensory cortex also receives and processes signals from peripheral mechano- and chemoreceptors of the respiratory system (referred to as "reafferent signals"). Reafferent signals are produced by afferent receptors in response to efferent neurologic output from the motor cortex. For example, when one takes a voluntary deep breath, efferent signals from the motor cortex to muscles of ventilation result in muscle activation and contraction, respiratory system expansion, and inspiratory airflow. The mechanical motion and resulting flow of gas through the airways, changes in position of the chest wall, and generation of force by muscle contraction and shortening of the muscles result in peripheral mechanoreceptor activation, and reafferent information from these receptors is transmitted to the sensory cortex.

When one makes a voluntary effort to take a deep inspiratory breath, the motor cortex produces a large efferent signal to the muscles of ventilation (and a concomitant large corollary discharge to the sensory cortex). In disease states, a disparity may exist between the magnitude of efferent signaling and respiratory system movement and expansion. For example, if a patient's respiratory muscles are weak or at a mechanical disadvantage (e.g., due to hyperinflation or due to airways obstruction), the chest wall and lung expansion produced by motor cortex efferent signaling may be discordant, i.e., less volume is generated than would otherwise be expected for the neural discharge. This discordance is referred to as efferent-reafferent dissociation (or neuromechanical dissociation), and the neurologic perception of efferent-reafferent dissociation is a sensation of breathlessness or dyspnea, and this unpleasant sensation affects the control of breathing leading to an increase in respiratory drive.

8.5 Lung/Airway/Vascular/Chest Wall Receptors

Flow receptors Receptors on the face, oropharynx, and nasopharynx and airways respond to changes of airflow; these "flow" receptors are actually responding to change in temperature consequent to flow. Blowing cool air on one's face can activate trigeminal nerve sensory receptors and decrease symptoms of breathlessness. In addition, naso- and oropharyngeal receptors can modulate the drive to breathe, as evidenced by increased severity of dyspnea when oropharyngeal receptor signaling was decreased by breathing through a mouthpiece, applying topical lidocaine to the oropharynx, and breathing warm humidified air, and ventilation is reduced when compressed air is blown into the nasopharynx.

Upper airway receptor stimulation may affect control of breathing and the drive to breathe by decreasing central respiratory drive. In experimentally induced hypercapnia, blowing cool air through the nasopharynx decreased the expected amplification of minute ventilation from elevated $PaCO_2$. Furthermore, stimulating upper airway receptors reduces respiratory drive and increases exercise tolerance in patients with COPD. The mechanism by which upper airway receptors affect the drive to breathe is likely through modulation of efferent-reafferent dissociation, as greater stimulation of upper airway receptors is perceived as an appropriate mechanical respiratory system response to efferent messages from the motor cortex. This central processing effect reduces efferent-reafferent dissociation and reduces centrally mediated drive to breathe.

Irritant receptors C-fibers (or irritant receptors) are airway epithelial receptors that are activated by mechanical and chemical stimuli such as bronchoconstriction and inhalational irritants. Airway receptors stimulated by bronchoconstriction of airways can precipitate a sensation of breathlessness and affect respiratory drive and control of breathing.

Juxtapulmonary or J receptors are a type of C-fibers. The role of J receptors and pulmonary vascular receptors in respiratory signaling and the control of breathing are not well elucidated. J receptors are thought to be activated by fluid (e.g., interstitial liquid associated with pulmonary edema) or stretch signals in the pulmonary parenchyma and can generate signals that augment the drive to breathe and efferent output from the motor cortex.

Stretch receptors in the lung (inflation and deflation reflexes) Pulmonary stretch receptors affect the control of breathing by modulating efferent-reafferent dissociation. The role of stretch receptors on respiratory drive has been demonstrated in descriptive studies of subjects with high cervical spinal injuries who were ventilator-dependent. Under experimental conditions of acute hypercapnia, dyspnea and the drive to breathe were decreased by providing higher tidal volumes via the ventilator. The decreased drive to breathe could not be attributed to peripheral chest wall receptors given the high level of subjects' cervical spinal injury. Rather, increased signaling via intrapulmonary stretch receptors through the vagus nerve was postulated to be the mechanism for decreased dyspnea and drive to breathe.

Atelectasis causes increased respiratory drive through signaling from intrapulmonary stretch receptors (likely related to the Hering-Breuer deflation reflex). The tachypnea and increased drive to breathe associated with large pleural effusions may, in part, be due to compressive atelectasis of the underlying lung. Signaling via upper airway and intrapulmonary stretch receptors may be one of the mechanisms by which positive pressure modulates efferent-reafferent dissociation and the drive to breathe.

Muscle spindles (chest wall vibration) Receptors located in the joints, tendons, and muscles of the chest wall communicate with the central nervous system and affect control of breathing and the drive to breathe. Experimental assessments of the role of chest wall receptors using externally applied vibration to normal subjects and subjects with COPD have demonstrated decreased dyspnea and ventilation attributable to vibration and chest receptor stimulation. This indicates that stimulation of chest wall receptors, similar to C-fibers and pulmonary stretch receptors, results in decreased respiratory drive, likely by decreasing efferent-reafferent dissociation (the vibration may simulate greater movement of the chest wall).

Chemoreceptors Peripheral chemoreceptors, located in the carotid and aortic bodies, produce afferent responses to changes in $PaCO_2$, PaO_2, and pH (arterial hydrogen ion levels.) The carotid body is more sensitive to increases in $PaCO_2$, decreases in PaO_2, or decreases in pH, whereas the aortic body is less sensitive to $PaCO_2$ and PaO_2 and does not appear to monitor pH directly. In humans, aortic chemoreceptors appear to have a minimal role in control of ventilation.

Central chemoreceptors located in the medulla respond to changes in $PaCO_2$ and arterial pH. In addition, skeletal muscle is also thought to have metaboreceptors, which are not typically described as chemoreceptors, but appear to be capable of detecting local changes in metabolites produced by anaerobic metabolism at the tissue level. Metaboreceptors are likely important in conditions such as strenuous exercise or heart failure, when tissue oxygen demand may exceed oxygen delivery.

Case Example 1

A patient with interstitial lung disease and dyspnea with minimal activity insists that his breathing is more comfortable with supplemental oxygen via nasal cannula despite the fact that his oxygen saturation remains above 90% breathing ambient air. How do you explain this finding?

Answer: You assess his total ventilation and $P_{0.1}$ (see description of this technique below), to determine if there is a change in his drive to breathe under three conditions: (1) no nasal cannula, (2) supplemental oxygen at 3 L/min via nasal cannula, and (3) compressed air at 3 L/min via nasal cannula. Total ventilation and $P_{0.1}$ are reduced to the same degree with compressed air and supplemental oxygen compared to no nasal flow. While an argument can be made that this result is the consequence of placebo effect, experimental studies are consistent with a direct effect of stimulation of upper airway receptors on ventilatory drive.

8.6 Measurements

Hypoxic ventilatory response Acute hypoxemia is a less important modulator of control of breathing as compared to acute hypercapnia. From an evolutionary biology perspective, hyperventilation does not increase O_2 saturation significantly due to the sigmoid shape of the oxygen-hemoglobin saturation curve; thus, there is little physiologic benefit to a robust ventilatory response to hypoxemia. In contrast, hyperventilation makes a substantial difference for $PaCO_2$ due to the relatively linear relationship of CO_2-hemoglobin binding; given the importance of maintaining pH of the blood in a narrow range, a robust ventilatory response to hypercapnia and acidemia is advantageous. In clinical practice, patients with chronic cardiopulmonary disease often have mild to moderate hypoxemia without breathlessness. In experimental settings, however, during heavy exercise at a constant workload, drive to breathe is significantly increased when subjects inspired hypoxic gas mixtures compared with ambient air. Furthermore, subjects were also less breathless with decreased drive to breathe when exercising and breathing 100% oxygen as compared to air.

Functionally, the hypoxic ventilatory response is characterized as ($\Delta Ve/\Delta SpO_2$). Hypoxic ventilatory response can be assessed using a closed rebreathing system, in which a subject breathes through facemask or mouthpiece connected to tubes that allow for control of inspired gases. SpO_2, end tidal CO_2 ($EtCO_2$), respiratory rate, and tidal volume are measured throughout the assessment of hypoxic ventilatory response. To precipitate hypoxia, a poikilocapnic study (i.e., $PaCO_2$ is allowed to vary naturally) is performed in which a subject rebreathes exhaled air from which CO_2 is filtered (to avoid precipitating hypercapnia); alternatively, the patient may be given a gas mixture with 10% O_2, and CO_2 is added to the inspired gas to maintain isocapnia as ventilation increases. Changes in respiratory rate and tidal volume are tracked as PaO_2 falls, and tests are stopped if significant symptoms occur, significant vital signs changes manifest, or when the SpO_2 reaches 75% or lower. The change in minute ventilation for a given change in PaO_2 or oxygen saturation ($\Delta Ve/\Delta SpO_2$) is reported as the hypoxic ventilatory response. The normal value for the hypoxic ventilatory response is 0.2–5 L/min/%SpO_2, with a wide degree of variability and a hyperbolic increase in Ve below a PaO_2 of 60 mmHg.

Hypercapnic ventilatory response Acute hypercapnia is a major driver of increased ventilatory response, as small increases in $PaCO_2$ result in significant augmentation of minute ventilation. The central nervous system mediator of the hypercapnic ventilatory response is likely the retrotrapezoid nucleus in the ventral medulla, which augments efferent signaling when stimulated.

Increasing levels of inhaled carbon dioxide in patients with quadriplegia and in normal subjects under conditions of total neuromuscular blockade in experimental settings in which the minute ventilation is held constant result in increased $PaCO_2$ and $EtCO_2$. Under these conditions, subjects describe severe "air hunger." These studies demonstrate that acute hypercapnia (independent of ventilatory muscle function and efferent-reafferent dissociation) causes stimulation of chemoreceptors, producing increased drive to breathe and sensations described by subjects such as "air hunger," "urge to breathe," and "need to breathe." Chronic elevations in $PaCO_2$ do not cause as severe drive to breathe as compared to acute elevations in $PaCO_2$. Renal compensation resulting in less severe acidemia in chronic respiratory acidosis likely modulates the effects of $PaCO_2$ on the drive to breathe.

The hypercapnic ventilatory response is expressed as the change in minute ventilation (Ve in liters) per change in $EtCO_2$ in mmHg ($\Delta Ve/\Delta EtCO_2$); the $EtCO_2$ provides a rough estimate of arterial PCO_2, assuming equilibration of gas between the alveolus and pulmonary capillary. The hypercapnic ventilatory response is measured in a manner similar to the procedure for evaluating the hypoxic ventilatory response, with a facemask or mouthpiece connected to a circuit that is linked to a reservoir bag with 5–7 l of gas containing a fixed proportion of CO_2 (usually 7–10%), O_2 (40%), and nitrogen (remainder). The reservoir bag is connected to the circuit with a one-way value that allows inhalation only, such that the concentration of inhaled CO_2 and O_2 is controlled by the relative amounts of gases in the reservoir and not by rebreathing effects. SpO_2, EtO_2, respiratory rate, and tidal volume are measured during testing, and the test is terminated when symptoms occur, when vital sign changes are noted, or when the $EtCO_2$ reaches a preset threshold (typically 7–8%). $\Delta Ve/\Delta EtCO_2$ is reported as the output of the hypercapnic ventilatory response maneuver. A normal value for the hypercapnic ventilatory response is 2–5 L/min/mmHg; there is some evidence that genetic factors may influence one's ventilatory response.

$P_{0.1}$ The $P_{0.1}$, also termed the tension time index, the pressure time index, and the P_{100}, is a measure of the mechanical work being done by the ventilatory muscles during inspiratory efforts against a closed airway. As the mechanical manifestation of the neural signal to the muscles, one infers information about the drive to breathe from the force of muscular contraction.

The $P_{0.1}$ is performed during normal tidal volume breathing. To perform the $P_{0.1}$ maneuver, the tube through which a subject is breathing is transiently occluded for 0.1 s (100 ms) at the beginning of inspiration. The occlusion is released as quickly as possible thereafter. It is believed that conscious perception of occluding the tube does not occur during the first 0.1 s of occlusion; thus, the $P_{0.1}$ maneuver is believed to reflect the patient's intrinsic, unconscious, inspiratory respiratory drive at that moment, unaffected by the reflexive response to "breathe harder" that occurs when one notices an obstructed airway. The negative airway pressures generated by the subject during the 0.1 s occlusion are representative of normal, unconscious ventilatory work during inhalation. $P_{0.1}$ is typically measured at the airway opening (P_{mouth} or P_m), but for patients with obstructive airway disease and inhomogeneous and slow equilibration of pressure throughout the respiratory system during the ventilatory cycle, $P_{0.1}$ may be more accurately measured by an esophageal balloon ($P_{esophagus}$ or P_e), which provides an approximation of pleural pressure.

Measuring $P_{0.1}$ is well-tolerated by subjects and is considered to be a relatively accurate assessment of ventilatory muscle strength and inspiratory effort during normal tidal volume breathing. Again, the $P_{0.1}$ represents the initial inspiratory force generated by muscles of inspiration and is considered to be independent of airway resistance (there is no flow during the obstruction; this is a quasi-static maneuver), input from peripheral mechanoreceptors, or conscious voluntary modulation. To date, the $P_{0.1}$ has been used primarily in research settings, but can be measured clinically and may provide useful data in specific clinical scenarios. The normal range of $P_{0.1}$ is 1.5–5 cm H_2O.

To assess the function of the central respiratory controller in a standardized manner, $P_{0.1}$ is often assessed during stimulation with hypercapnia. When $P_{0.1}$ is plotted against $PetCO_2$ in normal subjects, the resultant graph is curvilinear with $P_{0.1}$ increasing more rapidly at higher $PaCO_2$ levels, with an average normal value of 0.5–0.6 cm H_2O increase per unit increase mm $PaCO_2$. As $P_{0.1}$ is a reliable and accurate indicator of respiratory systemic output, patients with impaired central respiratory controller function, such as those with congenital central hypoventilation syndrome (CCHS) or brainstem damage, will have blunted $P_{0.1}$ versus $PaCO_2$ relationships as compared to normal subjects. A major limitation of the $P_{0.1}$ measurement is that it is dependent on muscle function; thus, in a patient with weakened muscles (e.g., myopathy) or shortened inspiratory muscles (e.g., with elevated functional residual capacity [FRC] as seen in patients with severe emphysema), pressure generation is compromised.

Case Example 2

A patient with very severe COPD (FEV1 21% predicted) and chronic hypercapnia (baseline $PaCO_2$ 50–55 mmHg) undergoes pulmonary function testing to determine if her hypercapnia is due to central hypoventilation (respiratory controller pathology) or due to obstructive ventilatory disease (ventilatory pump pathology.) The patient's FRC is measured before $P_{0.1}$ testing, and the FRC is normal. $P_{0.1}$ is measured at different PCO_2 levels to endeavor to differentiate between controller and ventilatory pump pathology. The patient's average $P_{0.1}$ over multiple measurements as a function of PCO_2 levels is graphed below (Fig. 8.2).

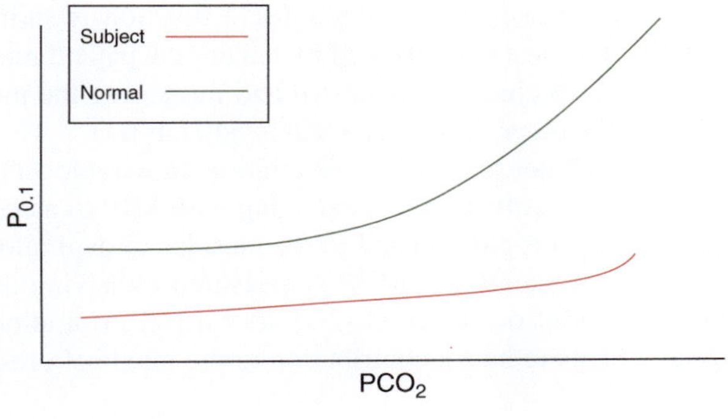

Fig. 8.2 Plot of $P_{0.1}$ as a function of PCO_2 during a progressive hypercapnic stimulus

Based on these results, how do you interpret this patient's hypercapnia?

Answer: The abnormal response of the $P_{0.1}$ is consistent with an alteration in ventilatory control. If ventilatory control were intact, the $P_{0.1}$ would be expected to increase in a manner similar to the "normal" graph, with the inflection point of $P_{0.1}$ occurring above the patient's baseline $PaCO_2$ levels. That the $P_{0.1}$ is essentially unchanged with increased $PaCO_2$ indicates that there is a central nervous system issue with processing and interpreting elevated systemic CO_2. The normal FRC argues against hyperinflation as a cause of the reduced $P_{0.1}$ measurement.

Maximal Inspiratory Pressure (MIP) The maximum inspiratory pressure (MIP) and maximal expiratory pressure (MEP) are the primary measurements of the force generated by respiratory muscles when stimulated by conscious command. By extension, the MIP and MEP provide information about subjects' nervous system function and respiratory muscle strength and function, which may help in determining whether low ventilation is due to problems with respiratory drive or the function of the neuromuscular ventilatory pump.

MIP and MEP are particularly useful measurements in assessing patients with possible congenital or acquired neuromuscular processes. MIP is measured starting from maximal expiration as the patient is instructed to inspire forcefully against an occluded airway for 1–2 s. Usually a small leak is present in the system between the occlusion and the patient's mouth in order to minimize glottis closure. Normal measured values for MIP are less than (more negative than) −50 cm H_2O in women and − 75 cm H_2O in men. Low MIPs may be due to submaximal effort by the subject during the procedure, elevated FRC with hyperinflation, and/or neuromuscular pathology. Performing the MIP maneuver can be uncomfortable for a subject, and early termination of inspiratory effort before generating a true maximal inspiratory effort is common, affecting the accuracy and reliability of the MIP measurement. Typically, one must ask the subject to perform the MIP maneuver three times to ensure a maximal effort is attained.

A low MIP may indicate issues with central ventilatory control, neuromuscular pathology (e.g., spinal cord injury, phrenic nerve injury, Guillain-Barre syndrome, myasthenia gravis), or primary muscle pathology. Potential causes of a low MIP may be further assessed by electroneurogram (ENG) and/or electromyogram (EMG.)

Another test of inspiratory muscle function is sniff nasal inspiratory pressure (SNIP). This test is performed by having the patient maximally inspire from RV or FRC while occluding one nostril and measuring the maximal inspiratory pressure through the other. A normal SNIP is >40 cm H_2O.

Although not reflective of inspiration, measurement of maximal expiratory pressure (MEP) is often performed along with MIP to assess overall breathing muscle strength, in this case related to the muscles of expiration, including the abdominal and accessory muscles. MEP is measured by having the patient forcefully exhale against a brief occlusion (1–2 s) after a full inspiration. Here a small leak in the system helps reduce a contribution to the maximal pressure by the cheek muscles.

The normal range for MEP is >80 cm H_2O in women and > 100 cm H_2O in men. While a low MEP often indicates expiratory muscle weakness, it is also entirely dependent on effort and may also be reduced by hyperinflation such as seen in COPD.

Case Example 3

A 67-year-old man with severe COPD (FEV1 40% predicted) undergoes pulmonary function testing for evaluation of progressive dyspnea on exertion over the past several weeks. He undergoes spirometry, lung volume measurements (via helium dilution), and MIP measurements.

Parameter	Measured value	Predicted value	Percent predicted
FEV1	1.3 L	3.7 L	41%
FVC	2.5 L	5.0 L	50%
FEV1/FVC	0.52		
TLC	3.8 L	5.5 L	69%
FRC	2.1 L	2.3 L	91%
RV	1.3 L	0.8 L	160%
MIP	24 cm H_2O	92 cm H_2O	26%

How do you use these tests to understand the etiology of the patient's dyspnea?

Answer: Although the patient demonstrates evidence of increased expiratory airway resistance, the markedly reduced MIP, the elevated RV, and the low TLC are consistent with either neurologic disease and/or inspiratory muscle weakness. The patient's inability to inhale to a predicted TLC and to exhale to a predict RV imply neuromuscular pathology, and the markedly reduced MIP is further confirmation of a neurologic and/or muscular process contributing to dyspnea and pulmonary function abnormalities. The normal FRC further indicates that the ventilatory pump is implicated in the patient's symptoms, as opposed to a controller or primary pulmonary process.

8.7 Exercise

As with resting conditions, respiratory control during exercise is complex, and the mechanisms by which ventilation increases during exercise are not fully understood. Nevertheless, the characterization of the normal ventilatory response to exercise is well established. Healthy subjects with normal cardiopulmonary function do not become hypercapnic, hypoxemic, or acidemic during mild to moderate exercise. Increases in ventilation are likely linked to inputs from peripheral muscles (metaboreceptors, muscle spindles), joints, and behavioral factors. With severe exercise beyond the anaerobic threshold, chemoreceptors may also contribute to control of ventilation during exercise.

Ventilatory Phases of Exercise: Neural Phase, Metabolic Phase, and Compensatory Phase Exercise influences ventilation in three distinct phases: the neurologic phase, the metabolic phase, and the compensatory phase. The neurologic phase occurs early in exercise and is characterized by an increase in Ve that is out of proportion to the body's metabolic needs. The increase in ventilatory effort and Ve is beyond hypoxic or hypercapnic demands and may reflect a central anticipatory component of exertion (e.g., augmenting ventilation in anticipation of increased systemic metabolic requirements). Experimental work with animals, in which passive motion of the limbs was associated with increased ventilation, suggests that input from joint and muscle receptors may also play a role in this phase of ventilation.

The metabolic phase of the ventilatory response to exercise occurs after the neurologic phase, during aerobic metabolism. Ve matches oxygen needs (oxygen consumption or VO_2) and increased systemic production of metabolic waste byproducts, such as CO_2 (CO_2 production or VCO_2). During the metabolic phase, increases in VO_2 and/or VCO_2 result in linear increases in ventilation. The precise mechanism(s) by which ventilation and metabolic demands are sensed during the metabolic phase of exercise are not precisely known, but peripheral metaboreceptors may play a role.

The compensatory phase of the ventilatory response to exercise occurs after the body reaches the anaerobic threshold, which is when cellular metabolism has reached the point that aerobic processes are not sufficient to meet cellular energy needs. At the anaerobic threshold, cellular anaerobic metabolism increases, and lactic acid, produced as a metabolic byproduct, accumulates in the blood. This results in an increase in systemic CO_2 levels, as lactic acid and increased systemic H^+ production are buffered by bicarbonate to create CO_2. Increased CO_2 production and lowered pH are direct stimuli to control of breathing, and Ve increases at an accelerated rate during the compensatory phase as compared to the metabolic phase. In the compensatory phase of ventilation, systemic CO_2 production is now the combination of CO_2 produced by cellular metabolism and CO_2 produced by the buffering of lactic acid by bicarbonate. When graphing Ve as a function of VO_2, the slope of the curve increases at anaerobic threshold (see section on VE/VCO_2 curve below). Mechanistically, peripheral chemoreceptors are the primary mediators of increased Ve during the compensatory phase.

Functionally, the anaerobic threshold correlates to cardiopulmonary fitness and exercise performance. Specifically, a higher (i.e., occurring at a greater VO_2) anaerobic threshold has been correlated with performance time and running efficiency in 5 km races, 10 km races, and marathons. These considerations emphasize how the timing of and the degree of exertion at which the anaerobic threshold occurs during exercise has implications for exercise performance and control of breathing during exertion.

VE/VO_2 curve and the anaerobic threshold One can detect the anaerobic threshold and the transition from the metabolic to compensatory phase of the ventilatory response to exercise, by plotting the change in Ve as a function of changes in VO_2

and VCO_2 to generate Ve/VO_2 and Ve/VCO_2 curves. The anaerobic threshold is defined by the point at which the slope of the Ve/VO_2 curve increases and marks the end of the metabolic phase of exercise ventilation. As compared to measuring and comparing the VO_2 and VCO_2 curves independently of Ve (and determining when VCO_2 changes disproportionately to VO_2), measuring and plotting the Ve/VO_2 provides a more accurate assessment of the anaerobic threshold in experimental and clinical conditions (see Fig. 8.3).

Case Example 4

As part of an evaluation of progressive dyspnea on exertion over the past several weeks, a patient with moderate pulmonary arterial hypertension (PASP 51 mmHg on right heart catheterization) undergoes a cardiopulmonary exercise test (CPET); see Fig. 8.3. The patient's performance on the CPET is graphed below (panel A). Identify the neural phase, metabolic phase, and compensatory phase of the patient's ventilatory response to exercise, and identify the anaerobic threshold. Interpret the patient's CPET performance as compared to expected performance for the patient's age, sex, and height (panel B).

Answer: 1 = neurological phase, 2 = metabolic phase, 3 = compensatory phase; the anaerobic threshold occurs at the break point in slope between phases 2 and 3 (Fig. 8.4).

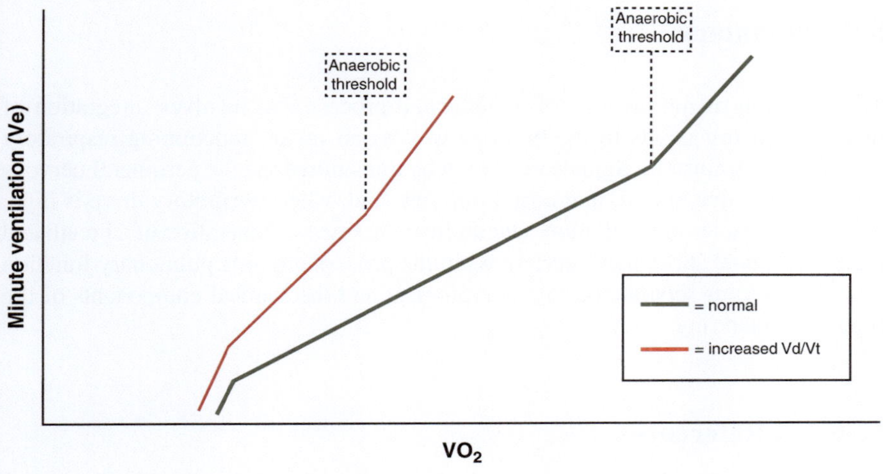

Fig. 8.3 The green bar indicates a healthy individual; note the three phases of increased ventilation during exercise. In a patient with increased *Vd/Vt*, greater ventilation is required for any degree of oxygen consumption. In addition, due to the chronic lung disease, the level of aerobic fitness is less, resulting in a lower anaerobic threshold (which is indicated by the onset of the compensatory phase of ventilation at a lower VO_2 than in the healthy individual)

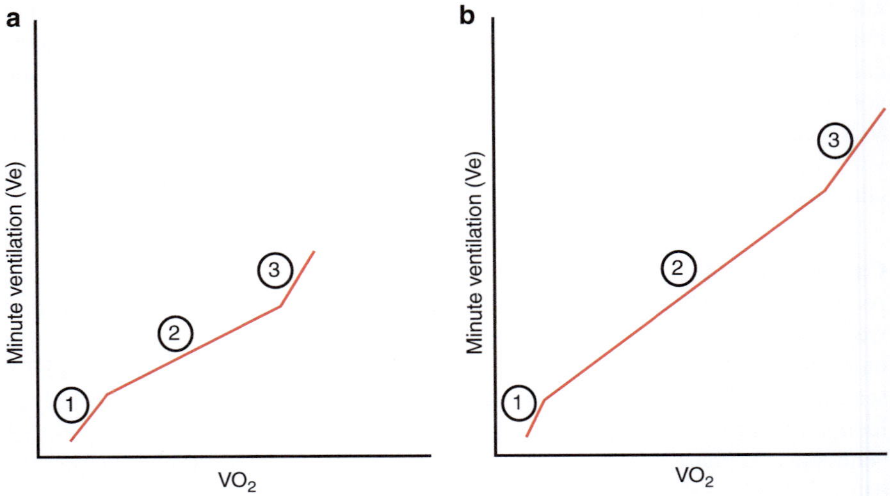

Fig. 8.4 Minute ventilation as a function of oxygen consumption during an exercise test. Panel A reflects the patient. Panel B reflects a healthy individual

The anaerobic threshold is reduced (lower VO_2) in the patient compared to the healthy individual suggesting a lower degree of cardiovascular fitness and earlier development of lactic acidosis.

8.8 Summary

The initiation of the breath is a complicated process that involves integration of multiple sensory inputs to the brain as well as an intact, functioning respiratory center in the brainstem. Signals must then be transmitted via the peripheral nervous system to the diaphragm, intercostal muscles, and, when respiratory drive is high, accessory muscles of ventilation. Our ability to assess the generation of a breath and the pathological states that interfere with this process requires pulmonary function tests that help us separate out the neurological and mechanical components of the process of inspiring.

Selected References

Banzett RB, Lansing RW, Brown R, et al. "Air hunger" from increased P_{CO2} persists after complete neuromuscular block in humans. Respir Physiol. 1990;81(1):18.

Banzett RB, Lansing RW, Reid MB, Adams L, Brown R. "Air hunger" arising from increased P_{CO2} in mechanically ventilated quadriplegics. Respir Physiol. 1989;76:53–68.

Brusasco V, Crapo R, Viegi G, American Thoracic Society, European Respiratory Society. Coming together: the ATS/ERS consensus on clinical pulmonary function testing. Eur Respir J. 2005;26:1–2.

Burgess KR, Whitelaw WA. Reducing ventilatory response to carbon dioxide by breathing cold air. Am Rev Respir Dis. 1984;129:687–90.

Burke RE. Motor units: anatomy, physiology and functional organization. In: Brookhart JM, Mountcastle VB, editors. Handbook of physiology, Sec. 1, Vol. III, Part 1, The nervous system. Bethesda: American Physiological Society; 1981. p. 345–422.

Chronos N, Adams L, Guz A. Effect of hyperoxia and hypoxia on exercise-induced breathlessness in normal subjects. Clin Sci. 1988;74:531–7.

Datta AK, Shea SA, Horner RL, Guz A. The influence of induced hypocapnia and sleep on the endogenous respiratory rhythm in humans. J Physiol. 1991;440:17–33.

Dick TE, Kong FJ, Berger AJ. Correlation of recruitment order with axonal conduction velocity for supraspinally driven motor units. J Neurophysiol. 1987;57:245–59.

Edström L, Kugelberg E. Histochemical composition, distribution of fibers and fatiguability of single motor units. J Neurol Neurosurg Psychiatry. 1968;31:424–33.

Enad JG, Fournier M, Sieck GC. Oxidative capacity and capillary density of diaphragm motor units. J Appl Physiol. 1989;67:620–7.

Fournier M, Sieck GC. Mechanical properties of muscle units in the cat diaphragm. J Neurophysiol. 1988;59:1055–66.

Gandevia SC, Rothwell JC. Activation of the human diaphragm from the motor cortex. J Physiol. 1987;384:109–18.

Geiger PC, Cody MJ, Macken RL, Sieck GC. Maximum specific force depends on myosin heavy chain content in rat diaphragm muscle fibers. J Appl Physiol. 2000;89:695–703.

Geiger PC, Cody MJ, Sieck GC. Force-calcium relationship depends on myosin heavy chain and troponin isoforms in rat diaphragm muscle fibers. J Appl Physiol. 1999;87:1894–900.

Henneman E. Relation between size of neurons and their susceptibility to discharge. Science. 1957;126:1345–6.

Liddell EGT, Sherrington CS. Recruitment and some other factors of reflex inhibition. Proc R Soc Lond (Biol). 1925;97:488–518.

Liss HP, Grant BJB. The effect of nasal flow on breathlessness in patients with chronic obstructive pulmonary disease. Am Rev Respir Dis. 1988;137:1285–8.

Lois JH, Rice CD, Yates BJ. Neural circuits controlling diaphragm function in the cat revealed by transneuronal tracing. J Appl Physiol (1985). 2009;106:138–52.

Manning HL, Basner R, Ringler J, et al. Effect of chest wall vibration on breathlessness in normal subjects. J Appl Physiol. 1991;71:175–81.

Manning HL, Shea SA, Schwartzstein RM, Lansing RW, Brown R, Banzett RB. Reduced tidal volume increases 'air hunger' at fixed P_{CO2} in ventilated quadriplegics. Respir Physiol. 1992;90:19–30.

Marazzini L, Cavestri R, Gori D, Gatti L, Longhini E. Difference between mouth and esophageal occlusion pressure during CO2 rebreathing in chronic obstructive pulmonary disease. Am Rev Respir Dis. 1978;118:1027–33.

Matthews AW, Howell JB. The rate of isometric inspiratory pressure development as a measure of responsiveness to carbon dioxide in man. Clin Sci Mol Med. 1975;49:57–68.

McCloskey DI, Gandevia S, Potter EK, Colebatch JG. Muscle sense and effort; motor commands and judgments about muscular contractions. In: Desmedt JE, editor. Motor control mechanisms in health and disease. New York: Raven Press; 1983.

Miller MR, Crapo R, Hankinson J, et al; ATS/ERS Task Force. General considerations for lung function testing. Eur Respir J 2005;26:153–61.

Nattie E, Li A. Central chemoreception is a complex system function that involves multiple brain stem sites. J Appl Physiol (1985). 2009;106:1464–6.

O'Donnell DE, Sanii R, Anthonisen NR, Younes M. Effect of dynamic airway compression on breathing pattern and respiratory sensation in severe chronic obstructive pulmonary disease. Am Rev Respir Dis. 1987;135:912–8.

Rebuck AS, Campbell EJM. A clinical method for assessing the ventilatory response to hypoxia. Am Rev Respir Dis. 1974;109:345–54.
Schwartzstein RM, Lahive K, Pope A, Weinberger SE, Weiss JW. Cold facial stimulation reduces breathlessness induced in normal subjects. Am Rev Respir Dis. 1987;136:58–61.
Schwartzstein RM, Manning HL, Weiss JW, Weinberger SE. Dyspnea: a sensory experience. Lung. 1990;169:185–99.
Seven YB, Mantilla CB, Sieck GC. Recruitment of rat diaphragm motor units across motor behaviors with different levels of diaphragm activation. J Appl Physiol. 2014;117:1308–16.
Shea SA, Andres LP, Guz A, Banzett RB. Respiratory sensations in subjects who lack a ventilatory response to CO2. Respir Physiol. 1993;93(2):203–19.
Sieck GC, Han YS, Prakash YS, Jones KA. Cross-bridge cycling kinetics, actomyosin ATPase activity and myosin heavy chain isoforms in skeletal and smooth respiratory muscles. Comp Biochem Physiol. 1998;119:435–50.
Sieck GC. Neural control of the inspiratory pump. NIPS. 1991;6:260–4.
Sieck GC, Fournier M. Diaphragm motor unit recruitment during ventilatory and nonventilatory behaviors. J Appl Physiol. 1989;66:2539–45.
Smith JC, Ellenberger HH, Ballanyi K, Richter DW, Feldman JL. Pre-Botzinger complex: a brainstem region that may generate respiratory rhythm in mammals. Science. 1991;254:726–9.
Spence DPS, Graham DR, Ahmed J, Rees K, Pearson MG, Calverley PMA. Does cold air affect exercise capacity and dyspnea in stable chronic obstructive pulmonary disease? Chest. 1993;103:693–6.
Whitelaw WA, Derenne JP, Milic-Emili J. Occlusion pressure as a measure of respiratory center output in conscious man. Respir Physiol. 1975;23:181–99.

Chapter 9
Measurement of Airway Responsiveness

Teal S. Hallstrand, John D. Brannan, Krystelle Godbout, and Louis-Philippe Boulet

9.1 Introduction

Airway hyperresponsiveness (AHR) refers to the increased propensity of the airways to narrow when challenged with a stimulus that induces airway narrowing. This tendency of airways to respond too much and too easily to various stimuli that induce airway narrowing is assessed with bronchoprovocation tests. The majority of subjects with symptomatic asthma have AHR as a key manifestation of airway dysfunction. As a corollary, a negative bronchoprovocation test in an asymptomatic period does not exclude the presence of asthma as the feature of AHR is not constant. The measurement of AHR provides an objective measure of the variability of airway obstruction, supporting the diagnosis of asthma, particularly in subjects with normal baseline spirometry.

Some forms of AHR can also be observed in many other conditions that affect airway and lung structure such as chronic obstructive pulmonary disease (COPD) and in some subjects who are at increased risk of asthma such as those with allergic rhinitis, although the prevalence of AHR is lower in these populations. Individuals with asthma have an increased response to a variety of specific agents

T. S. Hallstrand (✉)
Department of Medicine, Division of Pulmonary, Critical Care and Sleep Medicine, University of Washington, Seattle, WA, USA

Center for Lung Biology, University of Washington, Seattle, WA, USA
e-mail: tealh@uw.edu

J. D. Brannan
Department of Respiratory and Sleep Medicine, John Hunter Hospital, Newcastle, NSW, Australia

K. Godbout · L.-P. Boulet
Institut universitaire de cardiologie et de pneumologie de Québec, Québec, Canada

D. A. Kaminsky, C. G. Irvin (eds.), *Pulmonary Function Testing*, Respiratory Medicine, https://doi.org/10.1007/978-3-319-94159-2_9

including cholinergic agonists (e.g., methacholine), histamine, the cysteinyl leukotrienes (CysLT, LTs C_4, D_4, and E_4) LTC_4 and LTD_4, prostaglandins (PG) PGD_2 and $PGF_2\alpha$, and adenosine, in addition to physiological stimuli including hyperpnea induced by exercise, particularly in cold and dry air, and hypertonic or hypotonic solutions.

The prevalence of AHR in the general population varies from about 4% to 35% according to the specific population studied, the type of AHR assessed, and the criteria for a positive test. AHR is more commonly observed in atopic individuals than in the non-atopic general population. The distribution of AHR in the general population follows a continuous or unimodal distribution with asthmatic individuals representing the more hyperresponsive segment of the AHR distribution curve. In the general population, asymptomatic AHR can be identified infrequently with a prevalence of less than 15%. Among individuals with known AHR, symptoms may be absent in approximately 30–50% of those tested for AHR. Some individuals with asymptomatic AHR may evolve into symptomatic asthma, particularly if regularly exposed to sensitizing agents.

There is generally a correlation between the severity of AHR and clinical features of asthma such as the severity of the disease, expiratory airflow variability, bronchodilator response, and the amount of anti-inflammatory therapy needed to achieve disease control. The presence of AHR has also been associated with an accelerated decline in lung function, even in asymptomatic subjects. The severity or even presence of AHR can change over time, either spontaneously, or in response to exposure to relevant sensitizers that increase AHR, or with anti-inflammatory medications that can decrease AHR. Thus, AHR can be stable or show episodic changes. Because of this variability in AHR, the repeatability observed with measurements of AHR over time is moderate.

Direct or indirect bronchoprovocation tests can be used to evaluate the presence of AHR. Direct tests include methacholine and histamine bronchoprovocation tests that act directly on muscarinic receptors or H1 receptors, respectively, while indirect tests act through the endogenous release of mediators by inflammatory or neuronal cells that are present in the airways (Fig. 9.1).

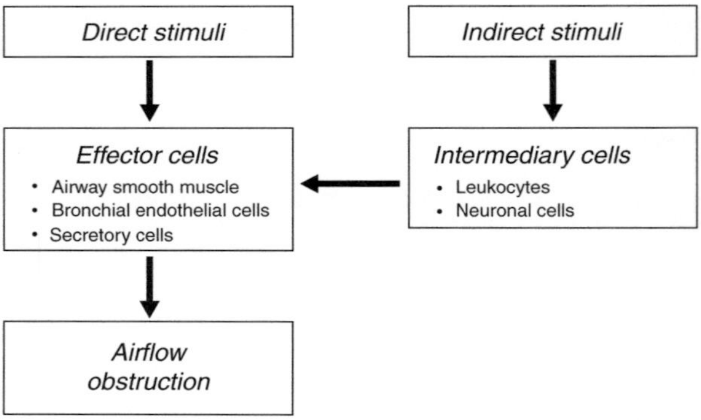

Fig. 9.1 Conceptual framework for the difference between direct and indirect challenge tests. Indirect challenge tests act indirectly through the activation of leukocytes and/or neuronal cells that lead to the subsequent development of airflow obstruction. (Adapted from Van Schoor et al. Eur Respir J 2000;16(3):514–33 with permission)

9.2 Components of Airway Hyperresponsiveness

There are three basic components of AHR. First, "airway sensitivity," or "responsiveness," represents the position of the dose-response curve relative to the dose of the agonist used to provoke bronchoconstriction, with a lower dose representing greater airway sensitivity. Such measurements of airway sensitivity are typically based on the reduction in forced expiratory volume in the first second (FEV_1) and are used most commonly in clinical practice. Second, "airway reactivity" is measured by the slope of the dose-response curve with a steeper slope representing increased airway reactivity. Finally, "maximal bronchoconstrictor response" is demonstrated by the plateau that can be observed where further increases in the bronchoconstrictor does not causes further airway narrowing; this plateau is present in healthy controls, but is lost in subjects with asthma (Fig. 9.2).

For clinical purposes, the sensitivity or responsiveness is considered the most relevant measurement. It is usually quantified as the provocative dose or concentration of an agonist (e.g., methacholine) inducing a 20% fall in FEV_1 (PD_{20} or PC_{20}). The most recent guideline from the Bronchoprovocation Task Force of the American Thoracic Society (ATS) and the European Respiratory Society (ERS) recommends using the PD_{20} so that the results are consistent across a variety of delivery devices. Measurement of the slope of the dose-response curve can allow assessment of airway function even in subjects not reaching a 20% fall in FEV_1 although the clinical relevance of this outcome is less well established than for responsiveness. The loss of the plateau response is not typically assessed in clinical testing as this feature of AHR could allow life-threatening bronchoconstriction in extreme cases. Incremental dose-response tests facilitate the early identification

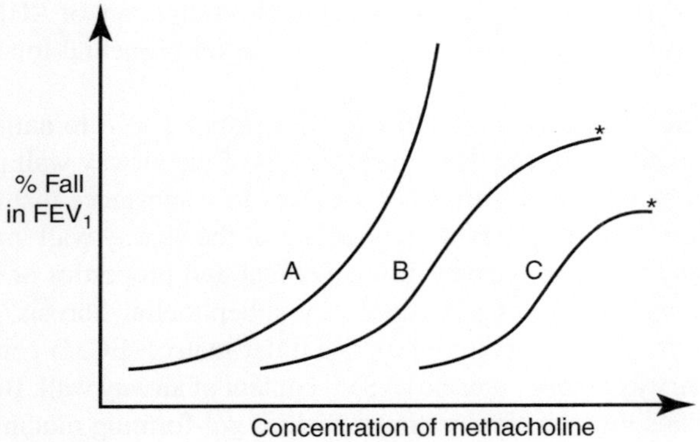

Fig. 9.2 Differences in the response to a direct-acting stimulus for bronchoconstriction in individuals with asthma. Individuals with asthma respond to a lower dose or concentration of agonists to initiate bronchoconstriction, have a steeper dose-response curve, and show an increased maximal bronchoconstrictor response (loss of plateau) to bronchoconstrictors, particularly when asthma is severe. (A) Moderate asthma. (B) Mild asthma. (C) Normal subject (*plateau effect observed). (Adapted from Woolcock et al. Am Rev Respir Dis 1984;130(1):71–75 with permission)

of severe AHR and generally avoid severe bronchoconstriction. In contrast, the hyperpnea challenge tests use a single strong stimulus for bronchoconstriction that can lead to severe bronchoconstriction in some individuals and should be used with caution in individuals with poorly controlled asthma or low baseline lung function.

9.3 Factors that Modulate Airway Hyperresponsiveness

Although AHR can be transient, there is typically a persistent component to AHR. The exposure to relevant allergens or sensitizing agents can increase AHR in susceptible individuals, either at home or work or following natural exposure, after respiratory irritant exposure such as ozone, and following repeated training in high-level athletes. For example, AHR typically increases following specific allergen challenge, in association with an increase in features of airway inflammation including the influx of T-cells and eosinophils to the airways. Following a single allergen challenge, levels of AHR return to baseline after approximately 1 week. During periods of natural allergen exposure, the severity of AHR can also be reduced by environmental control measures and anti-inflammatory medications, such as inhaled corticosteroids. It is generally accepted that some components of AHR are related to alterations in airway and lung structure and remain persistent over time, while there is a reversible component of AHR that is related to airway inflammation, although the precise components of airway inflammation that are critical to the development of AHR are not fully understood. Indirect tests of AHR have a stronger association with airway inflammation, reflecting their dependence on the release of endogenous mediators that caused bronchoconstriction. Airway neural pathways and both local axonal effects and those modulated by the autonomic nervous system are involved in the variable component of AHR as increased parasympathetic tone can have a modulatory role on bronchial tone and increase AHR.

The persistent component of AHR does not respond well to anti-inflammatory treatments because such changes in the structure of the airway wall predispose the airways to narrowing and closure when exposed to a substance that causes airway narrowing. These factors related to remodeling of the airway wall include thickening of the airway wall and changes in the content and properties of structural elements. Airway wall thickening is caused by subepithelial fibrosis, angiogenesis, glandular hypertrophy, deposition of extracellular matrix (ECM) components, and an increase in airway smooth muscle (ASM) content of airway wall. Both the release of airway sections into the airway lumen such as gel-forming mucins and changes in ASM contractile properties are involved in the increased AHR. Changes in ECM components are key features of airway remodeling, and it has been suggested that an increased content of ECM elements between smooth muscle fibers could increase their contractility. Furthermore, an increase in basal ASM tone may be involved in increasing airway responsiveness.

9.4 Etiology of Airway Hyperresponsiveness

AHR is multifactorial in origin, reflecting the properties of ASM, airway geometry and physical properties, and characteristics of the type and intensity of airway inflammation. The key factors involved are the airway geometry, airway wall thickness, ASM mass and function, and the activation of these systems through infiltration of the airway wall with leukocytes. How these various mechanisms interact to cause AHR may vary from one individual to another. The basis for AHR involves both genetic susceptibility and environmental exposures as well as the interaction between these two factors. The "inheritability" of AHR has been estimated to be about 30%. Genome-wide association studies based on direct AHR have revealed associations between a number of gene variants and the susceptibility to AHR and asthma. Environmental exposures are also clearly important as allergen-specific challenge in individuals sensitized to aeroallergens leads to an increase in both direct and indirect AHR. Allergen exposure in non-asthmatic allergically sensitized subjects with rhinitis alone can lead to an increase in AHR.

9.4.1 Reduction in Airway Caliber

The reduction in expiratory flows observed during spirometry is the result of changes in the elastic recoil force of the lung and a component of airway resistance that reflects airway narrowing mediated in part by airway wall thickening, which leads to greater airway narrowing as the volume of the lung decreases during expiration. A reduction in airway caliber and the thickening of the airway wall increase direct AHR because these changes lead to a more rapid reduction in the radius of the airway when constricted with an agonist, causing an exponential rise in the resistance which is proportionate to the radius cubed according to the Hagen-Poiseuille equation (Fig. 9.3). Such changes in airway geometry play a major role in direct AHR in COPD. In asthma, baseline airway narrowing and thickening, as well as losses in lung elastic recoil, contribute to AHR; however, changes in airway caliber alone do not always correlate with improvements in AHR.

9.4.2 Altered ASM "Plasticity" and the Effect of Deep Inspiration

Another mechanism that increases airway responsiveness in asthma is the loss of the bronchoprotective effect of a deep inspiration. A rapid deep inspiration protects against methacholine-induced bronchoconstriction in healthy individuals, but it is less effective in individuals with asthma. When a deep inspiration is taken after inhalation of a direct bronchoconstrictor agent, it reverses the induced

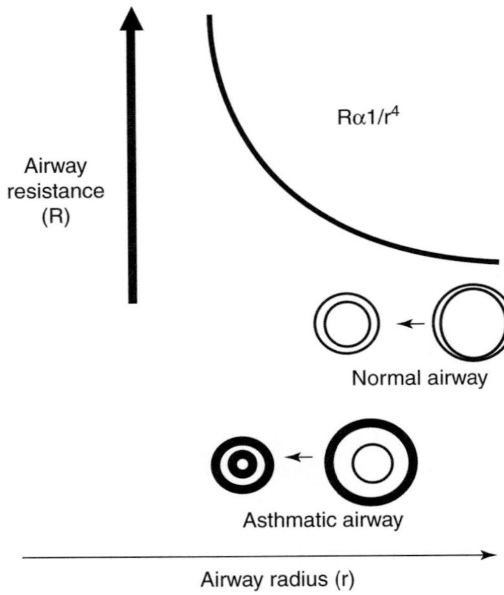

Fig. 9.3 Schematic of the effect of baseline airway narrowing and airway wall thickness on the radius of the lumen and airway resistance. As the lumen of the airway narrows under the influence of a direct-acting agonist of bronchoconstriction such as methacholine, the resistance climbs exponentially as described by the Hagen-Poiseuille equation. In asthma, thickening of the airway wall, enhanced airway tone, luminal obstruction with mucus, and loss of lung elastic recoil can each contribute to the propensity of the airways to narrow when challenged with an agonist of bronchoconstriction (Adapted from O'Byrne et al. Clin Exp Allergy 2009; 39(2): 181-92 with permission)

bronchoconstriction, while a deep inspiration before administration partially prevents the development of bronchoconstriction (i.e., bronchoprotection). In asthma, this bronchodilatory response to deep inspiration is reduced, and there is less bronchoprotection, suggesting that the loss of deep-inspiration-induced bronchoprotection could be a major determinant of AHR. Such inability of a deep breath to reverse or prevent airway narrowing in asthma may reflect a change in mechanisms leading to relaxation of contracted ASM when subjected to stretch, although other mechanisms are possible.

Some aspects of airway remodeling associated with airway thickening may also play a protective role in preventing further airway narrowing as an inverse relationship between airway reactivity and airway wall thickness has been reported. This relationship may be mediated by increased airway stiffness that can counteract the tendency of the airways to narrow in the face of ASM constriction. Thickening of the reticular basement membrane can make the airways stiffer, with a reduction in its distensibility. Such increased airway stiffness increases the load on airway smooth muscle to reduce bronchoconstriction, although the increased load on the ASM could also promote AHR if intrinsic properties of ASM change.

9.4.3 Changes in ASM Mass or Contractility

During induced bronchoconstriction, airway narrowing is mainly due to airway smooth muscle contraction, in association with contributing factors such as airway wall edema and mucus secretion. In cross-sectional bronchoscopy studies, an increase in ASM mass has been described in asthma, particularly ASM hypertrophy in subjects with severe asthma and ASM hyperplasia in mild asthma. An autopsy series evaluating ASM in different regions of the lung found hypertrophy of ASM cells occurs in the large airways in both nonfatal and fatal cases of asthma, while hyperplasia of ASM cells was only observed only in the large and small airways of subjects with fatal asthma. These changes in the amount and size of the ASM are accompanied by peribronchial edema and an increase in the ECM components, which may promote airway narrowing by "uncoupling" the airway from lung parenchyma and enhancing bronchoconstriction by reducing the load against ASM.

Some studies have found that ASM from subjects with asthma have an intrinsic hypercontractile phenotype in vitro, while others have not confirmed these findings, suggesting that the local environment in the airways influences the contractile state of the ASM. Additionally, an increase in the "basal tone" of the ASM in asthma is associated with the responsiveness of the small airways to methacholine and loss of the bronchodilatory effect of deep inspiration.

9.4.4 Regional Heterogeneity of Bronchoconstriction and Airway Closure

Recent studies using detailed images of regional ventilation demonstrate that airway narrowing in asthma is heterogeneous suggesting that some areas of the airways are more prone to narrowing than others. An important revelation from these studies in both humans and in murine models is that airway closure is an important mechanism leading to reduced expiratory airflow following challenge. The regional pattern and extent of airway closure measured by three-dimensional ventilation imaging is associated with the severity of AHR, particularly in the component of ventilation in the periphery of the lung.

9.5 Direct Challenge Tests

Direct bronchoprovocation challenge refers to tests using agents that directly cause bronchoconstriction predominantly through direct stimulation of specific receptors on the ASM. These tests are highly sensitive measures of the propensity of the airways to constrict and consequently work best to exclude asthma in the appropriate setting. Although methacholine is the agent most commonly used in clinical

Table 9.1 Agents that directly induce bronchoconstriction

Agent	Class	Characteristics
Methacholine	Cholinergic agonist	Possesses a third of the affinity of acetylcholine for true cholinesterase and totally resistant to pseudocholinesterase
Histamine	Inflammatory mediator	More flushing and systemic side effects than methacholine
Acetylcholine	Cholinergic agonist	Very short half-life
Carbachol	Cholinergic agonist	Resistant to true cholinesterase and pseudocholinesterase and not fully antagonized by atropine
Prostaglandin D_2	Inflammatory mediator	Higher potency than methacholine (about 30 times)
Leukotriene D_4	Inflammatory mediator	Highly potent endogenous bronchoconstrictor (100–1000 times more potent than methacholine or histamine)

Adapted from Van Schoor et al. Eur Respir J 2000;16(3):514–33.
However, only methacholine is commercially available.

practice, other direct-acting agents have been described. The properties of direct-acting stimuli leading to airway narrowing are shown in Table 9.1.

The ASM is innervated by parasympathetic neurons that modulate airway tone through acetylcholine released from nerve endings acting primarily through M3 muscarinic receptors to contract the ASM. Patients with asthma and AHR have airway narrowing that is greater and occurs at a lower dose of acetylcholine stimulation. Because of the short half-life of acetylcholine, it is impractical to use this agent in bronchoprovocation testing. Methacholine chloride is a synthetic derivative of acetylcholine that has a longer duration of action and favorable side effect profile, making it the preferred agent for direct bronchoprovocation testing. Other direct-acting agents are typically reserved for research purposes and have not been standardized in population-based studies. Thus, we focus on the detailed methods for the methacholine challenge test (MCT).

9.6 Indications and Contraindications for Direct Challenge Tests

Tests of direct AHR are predominantly used clinically to either exclude or alternatively increase the probability of asthma. A diagnosis of asthma is often established based on the appropriate history, as well as confirmatory tests including the demonstration of reversible airflow obstruction either following a bronchodilator or resolution of an exacerbation. If the diagnosis of asthma is uncertain, a direct bronchoprovocation test can increase or decrease the probability of asthma and should be interpreted within the appropriate clinical context. Because of the high sensitivity of a direct bronchoprovocation test such as the MCT, the test is especially useful to exclude the diagnosis of asthma in an individual with ongoing symptoms of asthma. Direct bronchoprovocation tests are also useful as an outcome

Table 9.2 Contraindications for methacholine challenge testing

Airflow limitation
FEV_1 < 60% predicted or 1.5 L
Spirometry quality
Inability to perform acceptable-quality spirometry
Medical conditions
Cardiovascular conditions
Recent eye surgery
Intracranial pressure elevation risk
Contraindication to methacholine chloride
Pregnancy
Nursing mothers
Use of cholinesterase inhibitor medication (e.g., for myasthenia gravis)

Adapted from Coates et al. Eur Respir J 2017;49(5): pii: 1601526.

measurement in clinical research and genetic and epidemiological studies of asthma. A MCT is also used to support a diagnosis of occupational asthma when performed before and after the exposure to a specific agent.

Direct bronchoprovocation tests are contraindicated in the presence of conditions that compromise the quality of the test or expose the patient to significant risks (Table 9.2). Although the MCT is a graded challenge designed to induce a modest increase in airway narrowing at each dose step, the drug methacholine still has the potential to provoke severe bronchoconstriction in susceptible individuals. Because the increase in airflow obstruction can be more severe in presence of significant airflow limitation, a pre-bronchodilator FEV_1 of >60% predicted or 1.5 L is the generally accepted threshold above which the MCT is deemed safe. As the change in FEV_1 is usually the primary endpoint measured during bronchoprovocation testing, any factor that reduces the quality or reproducibility of spirometry affects the ability to interpret the test. If an individual is not able to perform reliable, acceptable-quality spirometry, it is possible to choose an endpoint that is less dependent on patient effort such as airway resistance to circumvent this limitation in the appropriate setting (see below).

Medical conditions other than airway disorders also need to be considered in performing direct challenge tests safely. In particular, several cardiovascular conditions, recent eye surgery, and other disorders where elevated intracranial pressure would be harmful are contraindications for the test. In the case of cardiovascular conditions, individuals with a recent myocardial infarction or stroke (<3 months), uncontrolled hypertension (systolic >200 mmHg and diastolic >100 mmHg), or a known aortic aneurysm should not undergo bronchoprovocation testing. In these conditions, extra care is advised as the bronchoconstriction provoked during the procedure adds to the sole cardiovascular stress of spirometry.

The drug methacholine chloride is a pregnancy category C drug (unknown effects on the fetus), and its excretion in breastmilk is unknown. Thus, pregnancy and nursing are considered relative contraindications to the MCT. Cholinesterase inhibitors (e.g., for myasthenia gravis) block the degradation of methacholine and can increase the effects of the drug. A MCT should be performed with caution in patients taking cholinesterase inhibitors.

9.7 Methods for Conducting the Methacholine Challenge Test

The MCT is conducted with a series of increasing amounts of methacholine delivered to the lower airways, with an assessment of the amount of airway narrowing at each step. Thus, the MCT is a graded challenge test that is designed to assess direct AHR without inducing severe bronchoconstriction. The accuracy of the MCT can be affected by medications and other substances consumed by individuals taking the test and by several critically important technical factors that affect the delivery of methacholine to the lower airways. Recent work comparing modern nebulizers to the delivery devices that were initially described in the 1999 guideline has validated an approach that standardizes the methacholine challenge across a variety of delivery devices through the assessment of the dose delivered to the lower airways.

9.7.1 Withholding Times

As for other lung function tests, patients should refrain from drinking alcohol and smoking respectively 4 h and 1 h before the test. Medications causing bronchodilation decrease airway responsiveness when administered prior to the test and should be withheld according to their duration of action (Table 9.3). Anti-inflammatory medications like inhaled corticosteroids and leukotriene modifiers have little acute effect on direct AHR measured by methacholine and do not need to be routinely withheld. If a reduction in the anti-inflammatory effect of a medication is desired, a withhold time of 4–8 weeks is reasonable. Although earlier guidelines recommended withholding antihistamines, it is not necessary to withhold these drugs as they do not affect methacholine response and can be continued.

Table 9.3 Withholding times for medications prior to direct challenge testing

Medication		Minimum withholding time (h)
β-Agonist	Short-acting	6
	Long-acting (e.g., salmeterol)	36
	Ultra-long-acting (e.g., vilanterol)	48
Antimuscarinic	Short-acting	12
	Long-acting	168
Oral theophylline		12–24

Adapted from Coates et al. Eur Respir J 2017;49(5): pii: 1601526.

9.7.2 *Delivery of Methacholine for Challenge Testing*

The amount of airway narrowing induced in any individual is directly related to the dose of methacholine delivered to the lower airways. The dose of methacholine delivered varies according to the concentration of the solution, the output rate of the nebulization device, the inhalation time, and the portion of the nebulized particles that are of a size that reach the lower airways called the respirable fraction. Thus, the same concentration of solution delivers a different dose of methacholine, depending on the nebulizer used.

To enable the use of modern nebulizers and better standardization of the test, the recent European Respiratory Society (ERS) guideline that was also endorsed by the American Thoracic Society (ATS) adopted the delivered dose causing a 20% fall in FEV_1 (PD_{20}) instead of the PC_{20}. This new guideline also removed the use of the traditional dosimeter method, although a dosimeter can be used with tidal breathing rather than a deep inspiration. This strategy allows for a more consistent evaluation, removing the variability introduced by the use of different methods of inhalation and nebulizers, and makes comparisons across different laboratories possible. To implement the new guideline, the specific inhalation time and methacholine concentration at each step needs to be calculated according to the characteristics of the nebulizer used to deliver the desired dose.

When using the PD_{20}, any nebulizer can be employed provided the manufacturer provides sufficient information about the output of the device and particle size so that a schedule of methacholine concentrations and the delivered dose of methacholine to the lower airways can be calculated. The characteristics of the nebulizer need to be specified by the manufacture, as gravimetrically measuring output should not be used to calculate the delivered dose of methacholine since most of the weight loss is from evaporation. Methods of aerosol delivery involving deep breaths, including the five-breath dosimeter method, are no longer recommended because of the bronchodilating and bronchoprotective effect of deep inhalation to TLC, which reduces the sensitivity of the test. Methacholine should be inhaled through calm tidal breathing.

9.8 Methacholine Challenge Protocol

The MCT involves the inhalation of progressively increasing doses of nebulized methacholine chloride until a drop of 20% in FEV_1 is provoked or the patient reaches the highest dose or concentration in the protocol (usually 16 mg/ml or 400 μg).

Methacholine chloride is available as a dry crystalline powder and available under United States (US) Food and Drug Administration (FDA) approval in the USA and increasingly available elsewhere under the name Provocholine®. Methacholine solutions used during MCT are prepared beforehand using sterile normal saline with or without 0.4% phenol (to reduce bacterial contamination) and stored in a refrigerator for up to 2 weeks. Buffered solutions are less stable and should be avoided as diluent.

Nebulization time is computed from the output of the nebulizer, the breathing pattern, respirable fraction, and concentration used to deliver the desired dose. The starting dose for MCT is usually 1–3 μg with doubling or quadrupling in the delivered doses at each subsequent step until reaching ≥400 μg. The increase in methacholine dose during the MCT is achieved through increases in methacholine concentrations, while the inhalation time is kept constant. Because the new guideline recommends a breathing time of at least 1 min of tidal breathing to reduce the variability in delivered dose, many nebulizers will need further dilution of the methacholine concentrations to achieve the desired dose.

An optional diluent step is frequently used before the first dose of methacholine, mainly to familiarize the patient with the nebulizer and spirometry maneuvers. The diluent step is not needed for safety as the first concentration of methacholine delivered has been chosen to provoke significant bronchoconstriction in only the patients with the most severe AHR.

9.9 Interpretation of the Methacholine Challenge Test

The primary outcome measure for the MCT is the FEV_1 measured by spirometry. As forced vital capacity (FVC) measures are not required, spirometry is frequently shortened to 2 s of forced exhalation during the test. Spirometry should be performed at least twice after each dose of methacholine at 30 s and 90 s to insure repeatability. Only acceptable-quality FEV_1 maneuvers are kept, but no more than three or four maneuvers should be done after each dose, within a 3-min timeframe.

PD_{20} and PC_{20} are calculated by interpolation from the doses (D_1 and D_2) or concentrations delivered between the two final steps and the percent reduction in FEV_1 at those two time points (R_1 and R_2) without consideration of any cumulative effect of methacholine (Eq. 9.1). The time interval between doses should be kept constant at 5 min so that any effect of cumulative dose is similar between different laboratories. The short-term within-subject repeatability in PD_{20} and PC_{20} is usually within 1.5 doubling doses.

$$PD_{20} = 10^{\left[\log D_2 + \frac{(\log D_2 - \log D_1)(20 - R_1)}{R_1 - R_2}\right]} \tag{9.1}$$

As an alternative to measuring expiratory airflow changes measured by spirometry, changes in airway resistance (Raw), usually expressed as specific conductance (sGaw), have also been described as an outcome for direct bronchoprovocation testing. Body plethysmography or forced oscillation can be used to measure changes in Raw, but this outcome measurement has not been fully standardized. Because of the increased variability of the test and greater change in conductance corresponding to a 20% change in FEV_1, a larger percent decrease is usually required for a positive test (35–45% in sGaw), but the optimal cutoff to differentiate individuals with asthma from individuals without asthma has not been clearly established. Airway resistance measures are not routinely used, but may have some value in children and individuals unable to perform acceptable-quality spirometry.

Methacholine can elicit paradoxical vocal cord motion in susceptible individuals. If suspected or if stridor is observed during the exam, full inspiratory and expiratory flow-volume loops can be conducted at baseline and throughout the test. Abnormalities in the inspiratory part of the curve such as a plateau, a sawtooth pattern, or irregularities suggest the diagnosis of inducible laryngeal obstruction.

9.9.1 Interpretation and Clinical Relevance

The interpretation of a methacholine challenge test is based on the PC_{20} or PD_{20} and the pretest probability of disease using a Bayesian analysis with a series of receiver operating characteristic (ROC) curves that represent different PC_{20} or PD_{20} categories. In this interpretive scheme, 8 mg/ml or 200 ug was chosen as the cutoff point that neither increases nor decreases the posttest probability of asthma; there are a significant portion of healthy young adults that will have a PD_{20} in this range. As the PD_{20} decreases, the likelihood of asthma increases, and results inferior to 1 mg/ml (25 µg) are considered highly specific for asthma. In the 1999 guideline, the cutoff point was expanded to include *a* ± 1 doubling dose. The resulting interval (4–16 mg/ml or 100–400 µg) signifies borderline AHR. Abnormal response is further categorized as mild AHR (1–4 mg/ml or 25–100 µg), moderate AHR (0.25–1 mg/ml or 6–25 µg), and marked AHR (<0.25 mg/ml or < 6 µg).

Direct bronchoprovocation tests are highly sensitive and consequently most useful to exclude asthma in the appropriate setting. A negative MCT result ($PD_{20} > 400$ µg or $PC_{20} > 16$ mg/ml) in the presence of symptoms in the last 2 weeks makes the diagnosis of asthma unlikely.

A positive test supports the diagnosis, but is not specific for asthma as direct AHR occurs in other airway disorders and can occur transiently in certain populations. In one series, 21% of patients without asthma or rhinitis had a PC_{20} less than 16 mg/ml. Several chronic conditions have been associated with a positive MCT including allergic rhinitis, COPD, bronchiectasis, cystic fibrosis, and heart failure. Allergic rhinitis is the condition apart from asthma most associated with a positive MCT, with prevalence rates as high as 50%. Respiratory infection, especially those caused by viruses or mycoplasma, also causes a temporary increase in AHR that lasts for weeks. The underlying mechanism is thought to be direct damage to the airway epithelium. Environmental exposures to allergens (seasonal asthma), chemical irritants leading to reactive airway dysfunction syndrome (RADS), or occupational sensitizers (occupational asthma) can lead to a persistent increase in direct AHR.

False-negative MCT are less frequent because of the high sensitivity but can occur in individuals that predominantly have indirect AHR. Several studies focusing on elite athletes have identified individuals with indirect AHR to hyperpnea challenge who have a negative MCT. Inhaled corticosteroids have also been found to slightly decrease sensitivity to direct bronchoprovocation tests with a magnitude of effect of around 1.2 doubling dose. Conflicting data exist on whether these relations are dependent on the dose of inhaled corticosteroid. Four to 8 weeks of withholding time is necessary to remove this effect, but this is less relevant if the patient still experience symptoms.

9.10 Indirect Challenge Tests

In contrast to direct challenge tests, indirect challenge tests rely on physical or pharmacological stimuli that lead to the activation of endogenous pathways that cause airway narrowing through the activation of inflammatory or neuronal cells (Fig. 9.4). Because indirect challenge tests act through mediators and mechanisms that are involved in asthma pathogenesis, these tests tend to be specific for asthma, but less sensitive as a general test to detect asthma. Direct challenge tests such as methacholine challenge are sensitive to detect asthma, but are not specific for asthma as direct AHR occurs in other airway disorders. The indirect challenge tests are useful to understand the underlying immunopathology of asthma and can be useful to guide therapy for specific manifestations of asthma. The classic manifestation of indirect AHR is a syndrome that is called exercise-induced bronchoconstriction (EIB) in which bronchoconstriction develops in response to the hyperpnea that occurs during exercise. Most patients with EIB have direct AHR to methacholine, but many

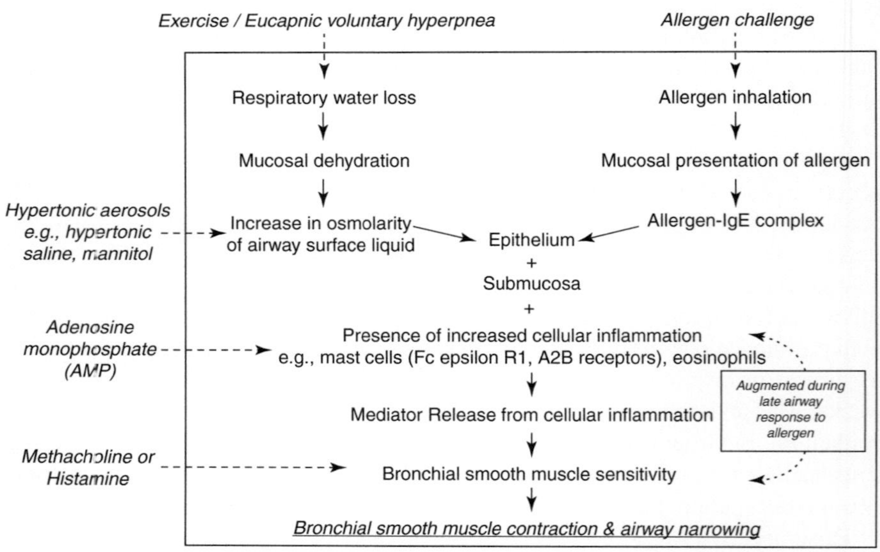

Fig. 9.4 Mechanisms of action of indirect challenge tests used in the clinical and research setting. In contrast to the indirect mechanisms of indirect AHR, methacholine and histamine are examples of direct challenge test that cause airway narrowing directly through airway smooth muscle contraction. (Adapted from Woolcock et al. Am Rev Respir Dis 1984; 130(1): 71-75 with permission)

patients with a positive methacholine challenge do not have EIB. Thus, a positive methacholine challenge test does not rule in EIB. Further, a negative methacholine challenge does not entirely exclude EIB, as some athletes have been described with EIB in the absence of a positive methacholine challenge, as well as some who have early clinical signs of asthma and EIB.

There are two general categories of tests used to detect indirect AHR. Hyperpnea challenge tests such as exercise challenge and eucapnic voluntary hyperpnea (EVH) provide a single strong stimulus for bronchoconstriction, while incremental challenge tests are conducted with a series of increasing doses of a stimulus such as inhaled mannitol, much in the same manner to the "dose-response" protocols using methacholine. Because the hyperpnea challenge tests use a single strong stimulus to induced bronchoconstriction, caution is warranted as severe bronchoconstriction can be triggered. Specific allergen challenge, which also assesses an allergen-specific form of indirect AHR, is conducted predominantly in the research setting, should be used with caution and is not covered in this chapter, but has been reviewed recently. We will discuss the pathophysiological rational for indirect challenge tests, and the specific methods of hyperpnea challenge tests and incremental challenge tests.

9.11 Pathophysiological Basis and Rationale

The susceptibility to develop airway narrowing in response to an indirect stimulus varies markedly among the general population and among subjects with asthma. Although some have contended that nearly all subjects with asthma will respond to indirect stimuli, cross-sectional studies identify EIB in about 30–60% of patients with asthma. In some individuals with asthma, the lack of EIB is due to the regular use of inhaled corticosteroids or leukotriene inhibitors that reduce the severity of EIB. There is also evidence from cross-sectional studies in the general population that between 10% and 20% of children and young adults have features of EIB and that this represents a risk for development of other features of asthma. Several studies reported an association between atopy in the form of allergic rhinitis or atopic dermatitis with exercise-related symptoms and EIB and that susceptibility to EIB increases in the allergy season.

Indirect AHR is associated with specific features of airway inflammation in asthma. Patients with EIB tend to have higher levels of exhaled nitric oxide (FENO), especially in the presence of atopy. Consistent with elevated levels of FENO, a relationship between the percentage of sputum eosinophils and the severity of EIB has also been identified. There is a remarkably clear relationship between infiltration of the airway epithelium with mast cells and the susceptibility to EIB identified in a detailed quantitative immunopathology study. As leukocytes such as eosinophils and mast cells are major sources of CysLTs, it is not surprising that these mediators are elevated in the airways of subjects with EIB as are nonenzymatic products of lipid peroxidation such as 8-isoprostanes. Airway injury has been implicated in EIB as elite athletes without a prior history of asthma, who train in environments in which they inspire large volumes of cold dry air, have a high prevalence of asthma and EIB.

A common pathway leading to airway narrowing and mucus release through the activation of sensory nerve pathways has been clearly demonstrated in animal models and is further supported by findings in humans. Although inflammatory pathways are activated in response to indirect challenge tests, there is no clear evidence of a cellular influx into the airways or an increase in direct AHR following exercise challenge.

9.12 Hyperpnea Challenge Tests

During periods of increased ventilation, large volumes of inspired air are rapidly equilibrated to the humidified conditions of the lower airways, leading to transfer of water with resulting osmotic stress as well as cooling of the airways that results from evaporation of water. The role of cooling per se remains controversial since very cold temperatures are required to accentuate airway narrowing, cold air is not required for bronchoconstriction, and EIB occurs following inspiration of warm dry air. The severity of bronchoconstriction induced on any one occasion is strongly related to the amount of ventilation achieved, up to a maximal level, and is directly related to the amount of water transferred out of the airways. As such, the water content and temperature of the inspired air can modulate the intensity of the stimulus during periods of increased ventilation.

Because exercise, EVH, and cold air hyperpnea challenge tests build rapidly to a strong stimulus for bronchoconstriction, it is imperative that the laboratory has appropriate equipment to manage severe bronchoconstriction. A physician and cardiopulmonary resuscitation equipment should be present or immediately available during the study, and oxygen saturation, heart rhythm, and blood pressure should be monitored. With exercise challenge, it is important to monitor subjects with cardiovascular risk factors using a 12 lead EKG and to confirm the rise in systolic blood pressure throughout exercise. It is recommended that the FEV_1 before challenge should be ≥75% predicted and pulse oximetry saturation should be above 94%. Additional absolute and relative contraindications are the same as those outlined for direct challenge tests (Table 9.1), including pregnancy as an absolute contraindication due to the potential hypoxia risk to the fetus.

Subjects should consume no more than a light meal before testing, and both short- and long-term medications that are known to inhibit EIB should be withheld for the recommended times before testing to prevent the possibility of a false-negative test (Table 9.4). Notation of all medications is important as regular use of bronchodilators increases the severity of EIB, and some studies have found short-term preventative effects of inhaled steroids, although most studies support a longer period of use for efficacy. Dietary factors including a low salt diet, supplemental omega-3 fatty acids, and antioxidants and the acute consumption of high doses of caffeine may also influence the severity of EIB. Regardless of the type of challenge, vigorous exercise should be avoided for at least 4 h before testing, as exercise may cause a period where the subject is refractory to further challenge. Diurnal variation has also been described with greater EIB severity in the afternoon relative to the morning.

It is critical to obtain reliable baseline spirometry prior to hyperpnea challenge since the results are based on the change in FEV_1 from baseline. It is ideal to obtain two baseline spirometry tests separated by 10–20 min before the challenge test to confirm the stability of spirometry.

9.13 Exercise Challenge Testing

Exercise testing in the laboratory can be accomplished using a motorized treadmill or a cycle ergometer. The rapid increase in ventilation during treadmill running makes it the preferable test; however, a cycle ergometer can be used effectively provided that the work rate is increased rapidly to reach the target ventilation or heart rate. Regardless of the mode of exercise test, the protocol should be designed to reach the target heart rate or minute ventilation over a short period of time, on the order of 2–3 min. The rapid rise in work rate is needed because a warm-up period or the more gradual ramp used in standard cardiopulmonary exercise testing may reduce the sensitivity for detection of EIB.

Following the rapid increase in work, the target level should be maintained for at least 4 min, but ideally for 6 min. If the equipment is available, it is preferable to achieve a ventilation target rather than a heart rate target to monitor the intensity of the challenge. The target ventilation is 60% of the predicted maximum voluntary ventilation (MVV, estimated as $FEV_1 \times 40$). An acceptable alternative is a target heart rate of >85% of the predicted maximum (calculated as 220 age in years); however, this approach may not achieve the target ventilation in all subjects.

The inspired air should be relatively dry and less than 25 °C. This can be accomplished by conducting the study in an air-conditioned room (with ambient temperature at 20–25 °C) with low relative humidity (50% or less). The temperature and relative humidity should be recorded. An ideal system delivers dry air through a mouthpiece and a two-way valve from a talc-free reservoir filled with medical grade compressed air. The use of compressed air is preferred because it is completely dry and will cause greater water loss from the airways, thus generally increasing the sensitivity of the test. During exercise, the patient should wear nose clips as nasal breathing decreases water loss from the airways.

On the treadmill, speed and grade are progressively advanced during the first 2–3 min of exercise until the target level is obtained. The degree of physical fitness and body weight will strongly influence the grade and speed necessary to obtain the desired ventilation or heart rate. A reasonable procedure is to quickly advance to a rapid but comfortable speed at a treadmill incline of 5.5% (3°) and then raise the slope until the desired heart rate or ventilation is obtained up to an incline of 10%.

The test ends when the patient has exercised at the target ventilation or heart rate for at least 4 min, but preferably 6 min. The treadmill challenge protocol has a high degree of reproducibility.

For cycle ergometer exercise, work rate is rapidly increased using the electromagnetic braking system to achieve the target ventilation. Direct measurement of ventilation is easier with the stable position on an ergometer and is the preferred target. The target heart rate or ventilation should be reached within 2–3 min. A valid test requires the target exercise intensity to be sustained for 6 min, although sustained exercise of at least 4 min may be acceptable if the subject fatigues. Although the reproducibility of the bicycle protocol has not received extensive study, the reproducibility in a limited number of individuals was excellent.

There are several tests to detect EIB outside of the laboratory setting, including a free run test followed by serial spirometry. Sport-specific tests in which the athlete performs the level of exercise that triggers their symptom have also been used in competitive athletes.

9.14 Eucapnic Voluntary Hyperpnea

EVH is an alternative to exercise challenge that utilizes medical dry air from a reservoir with an admixture of 4.9% CO_2 that enables the study subject to breathe at high ventilation without the adverse consequences of hypocapnia. The subject is instructed to perform voluntary hyperpnea for 6 min aiming at a target ventilation of 85% of MVV and with a minimum ventilation threshold of 60% of MVV. Like exercise challenge, the volume and water content of the inspired air are important determinants of the severity of bronchoconstriction following EVH, and the use of certain asthma medications before the challenge can alter the sensitivity and specificity of the test (Table 9.4). When standardized properly, the EVH test has a high degree of reproducibility. A consistent finding when comparing EVH to exercise challenge is a higher sensitivity for EVH than exercise challenge for the detection of bronchoconstriction.

9.15 Cold Air Hyperpnea Challenge

Cold air has a low water carrying capacity, resulting in greater heat and water transfer necessary to condition the inspired air at any minute ventilation. Cold air generators that produce dry air at below-freezing temperatures are commercially available and are in use in some laboratories; however, the additive effects of cold air depend on the intensity of the ventilation stimulus. When using a cold air generator, the device is either held by the patient or is supported in such a way as to deliver the air immediately before inspiration. The target range for inspired air temperature is -10 to -20 °C and should be recorded by the technologist during the challenge.

Table 9.4 Withholding times prior to indirect challenge testing

Medication/activity/food	Withholding time	Max duration[a]
SABA (albuterol, terbutaline)	8 h	<6 h
LABA (salmeterol, eformoterol)	24 h	12 h
LABA in combination with an ICS (salmeterol/fluticasone, formoterol/budesonide)	24 h	NA
Ultra-LABAs (indacaterol, olodaterol, vilanterol)	72 h	NA
ICS (budesonide, fluticasone propionate, beclomethasone)	6 h	NA
Long-acting ICS (fluticasone furoate)	24 h	NA
Leukotriene receptor antagonists (montelukast, zafirlukast)	4 d	24 h
Leukotriene synthesis inhibitors (zileuton/slow-release zileuton)	12 h/16 h	4 h
Antihistamines (loratadine, cetirizine, fexofenadine)	72 h	<2 h
Short-acting muscarinic acetylcholine antagonist (ipratropium bromide)	12 h	<0.5 h
Long-acting muscarinic acetylcholine antagonist (tiotropium bromide, aclidinium bromide, glycopyrronium)	72 h	NA
Cromones (sodium cromoglycate, nedocromil sodium)	4 h	2 h
Xanthines (theophylline)	24 h	NA
Caffeine	24 h	NA
Vigorous exercise	4 h	<4 h

Adapted from Weiler at al. J Allergy Clin Immunol 2016;138(5):1292–95.e36.
SABA short-acting beta-agonist, *LABA* long-acting beta-agonist, *ICS* inhaled corticosteroid.
[a]The maximum duration of protection refers to the potential effects of a single dose and may not apply to chronic dosing.

While some studies have found that adding cold air to a hyperpnea challenge enhances bronchoconstriction, others do not. These differences can be reconciled because of the plateau that occurs with exercise or EVH challenge where further increases in ventilation and water transfer do not increase bronchoconstriction. Thus, the inhalation of cold air, which increases ventilation and provides greater water transfer in certain conditions, may shorten the duration of the stimulus needed to achieve a positive test. Studies also indicate that the airway response to exercise in cold temperatures may be partially due to exposure of the face and body to cold temperatures.

9.16 Assessment and Interpretations of Hyperpnea Challenge Tests

Serial measurements of lung function by FEV_1 over the first 30 min after challenge are used to determine whether the test is positive and quantify the severity of bronchoconstriction. Many laboratories conduct the first lung function measurements immediately after challenge and then 3, 6, 10, 15, and 30 min after challenge. It is acceptable to initiate assessments 5 min after challenge; however, earlier assessments are useful to detect severe bronchoconstriction if present. At least two acceptable FEV_1 maneuvers within 0.150 L or 5% should be obtained at each testing interval, and the best FEV_1 at each interval reported to calculate % fall in FEV_1. As deep inspiration may inhibit bronchoconstriction, it is best to limit the number of spirometry maneuvers. It is also acceptable to shorten the duration of exhalation to 2–3 s if the technician monitors for the presence of technical factors such as reduced inspiratory effort and submaximal exhalation that can occur following exercise. The nadir in FEV_1 generally occurs within 5–10 min of the end of exercise but can occur as late as 30 min post exercise.

The presence of EIB is defined by plotting FEV_1 as a percent decline from the pre-exercise baseline FEV_1 at each postexercise interval. A decrease of $\geq$10% from baseline FEV_1 is considered abnormal relative to population normal values, but the specificity is higher with a criterion of 15% from baseline. The threshold for EVH testing is also typically set at a fall in FEV_1 of $\geq$10% below baseline based on the response in normal subjects. Exercise or EVH challenge tests that include the addition of cold air should be interpreted in the same manner as the test conducted without cold air. The threshold for a positive response also depends on the indication for the test, such that a more sensitive test (i.e., 10%) might be useful to understand the origin of symptoms in athletes, while a more specific test (i.e., 15%) may be needed for research studies. A method primarily used in the research setting to quantify the overall severity of EIB is to measure the area under the curve (AUC) for time multiplied by the percent fall in FEV_1.

If the patient experiences symptoms that are too severe, or there is concern that bronchoconstriction will progress to dangerous levels, or if FEV_1 has not recovered to within 10% of baseline, a short-acting β_2-agonist bronchodilator should be administered. It is also important to remain observant for other causes of exercise-related symptoms including cardiovascular disease and upper airway abnormalities including fixed upper airway obstruction (i.e., subglottic stenosis) and inducible laryngeal obstruction (iLO). Upper airway abnormalities may be apparent on the flow-volume loops obtained during spirometry, or other techniques such as direct laryngoscopy may be needed to establish a specific diagnosis.

9.17 Incremental Indirect Challenge Tests

Indirect bronchoprovocation tests where increasing doses of provoking stimuli are delivered incrementally have been validated for routine use for the assessment of AHR in asthma and also have an ongoing role in research investigating mechanisms of asthma. The osmotic challenge tests such as mannitol and hypertonic saline cause changes in the osmolarity of the airway surface, leading to the release of endogenous mediators from airway inflammatory cells (e.g., mast cells, eosinophils). Adenosine 5′-monophosphate (AMP) is considered an indirect test as it is converted to adenosine and activates human airway mast cells via activation of the adenosine A2b receptor.

These incremental tests can identify the presence of EIB in an individual, and there is a relationship between the airway sensitivity to these tests and the percent fall in FEV_1 after exercise challenge. Further, the airway sensitivity to all these tests is related to the degree of airway inflammation such as eosinophils in sputum and mast cells in biopsy, as well as the nonspecific marker of inflammation such as eNO.

While AHR assessment with nebulized hypertonic saline using an ultrasonic nebulizer has clinical and research applications, the mannitol challenge test was developed to make an indirect test that is more clinically accessible and does not require specialized pulmonary function laboratory testing equipment. Nebulized hypertonic saline has several disadvantages including the variation in the delivered dose based on the characteristics of the nebulizer and the expiration of a wet nebulizer solution with potential exposure of the technical staff to infectious agents. Mannitol dry powder is produced using spray drying in order to provide a uniform particle size that was found to be stable and suitable for encapsulation. The preprepared package of mannitol provides a common operating standard for bronchoprovocation tests with potential to compare results in different laboratories. Incremental challenge tests have demonstrated adequate safety and do not cause large falls in FEV_1.

9.18 Mannitol Challenge Test

Following the establishment of reproducible baseline spirometry, the mannitol test requires the patient to inhale increasing doses of dry powder mannitol, with the FEV_1 measured in duplicate 60 s after each dose. The test protocol consists of 0 mg (empty capsule), 5 mg, 10 mg, 20 mg, 40 mg, 80 mg (2 × 40 mg capsules), and three doses of 160 mg (4 × 40 mg capsules) of mannitol. The maximum cumulative dose of mannitol that is administered is 635 mg. A positive test result is defined as either a fall in FEV_1 of 15% from baseline (i.e., post 0 mg capsule) or a 10% fall in FEV_1 between two consecutive doses. If a patient presenting with symptoms suggestive of EIB has a fall of greater than 10% but less than 15% following the maximum cumulative dose of 635 mg (i.e., only documenting a PD_{10}), then mild EIB should be considered.

The mannitol test should be performed in a timely manner so that the osmotic gradient is increased with each dose. The time to complete a positive test, as observed in a large Phase 3 trial, was 17 min for a positive test and 26 min for a negative test. A test taking more than 35 min may lead to a false-negative result. Recovery to baseline lung function following mannitol occurs with a standard dose of short-acting beta-agonist, and the rate of recovery is similar to that following methacholine bronchoprovocation test. Coughing during a mannitol challenge test is common; however, the severity of cough is typically mild, and only 1–2% of challenge tests were stopped prematurely due to excessive cough in Phase 3 studies. The severity of AHR to mannitol is characterized by the dose of mannitol administered to cause a 15% fall in FEV_1 (PD15). A PD15 < 35 mg is mild, between 35 and 155 mg is moderate, and > 155 mg and < 635 mg indicates mild bronchial hyperresponsiveness.

9.19 Summary

Assessments of AHR play key diagnostic roles in the diagnosis of airway disorders such as asthma. The basis of AHR includes alterations in airway inflammation, airway remodeling, and lung structure. Tests for AHR are useful as diagnostic tests for asthma and can reveal specific information about the underlying basis of airway dysfunction. Because an exogenous stimulus is used to induce airway narrowing in direct tests of AHR, such tests are sensitive to alterations in airway remodeling and lung structure that tend to be present in the majority of subjects with asthma and in individuals with other disorders affecting airway and lung structure such as COPD. As such, direct tests are sensitive tests to detect the presence of asthma, but are not specific for a diagnosis of asthma. In contrast, indirect challenge tests for AHR are dependent upon the endogenous release of mediators that causes airway narrowing and therefore predominantly reflect the degree of airway inflammation present prior to the challenge test. These indirect tests reveal significant information about the underlying biology of asthma and tend to be specific for the diagnosis of asthma and the type of inflammation that is present in asthma. Thus, direct challenge tests have the greatest value in the exclusion of asthma in the presence of symptoms that are suggestive of asthma, while indirect challenge tests are most useful to confirm a diagnosis of asthma and to understand the specific basis of symptoms suggestive of asthma. Both types of tests should be interpreted carefully along with clinical features of asthma and other respiratory disorders.

Selected References

An SS, Fredberg JJ. Biophysical basis for airway hyperresponsiveness. Can J Physiol Pharmacol. 2007;85(7):700–14.

Anderson SD. Indirect' challenges from science to clinical practice. Eur Clin Respir J. 2016;3:31096.

Anderson SD, Brannan JD. Methods for "indirect" challenge tests including exercise, eucapnic voluntary hyperpnea, and hypertonic aerosols. Clin Rev Allergy Immunol. 2003;24(1):27–54.

Anderson SD, Schoeffel RE, Follet R, Perry CP, Daviskas E, Kendall M. Sensitivity to heat and water loss at rest and during exercise in asthmatic patients. Eur J Respir Dis. 1982;63(5):459–71.

Argyros GJ, Roach JM, Hurwitz KM, Eliasson AH, Phillips YY. Eucapnic voluntary hyperventilation as a bronchoprovocation technique: development of a standardized dosing schedule in asthmatics. Chest. 1996;109(6):1520–4.

Black JL, Roth M, Lee J, Carlin S, Johnson PR. Mechanisms of airway remodeling. Airway smooth muscle. Am J Respir Crit Care Med. 2001;164(10 Pt 2):S63–S6.

Bougault V, Turmel J, St-Laurent J, Bertrand M, Boulet LP. Asthma, airway inflammation and epithelial damage in swimmers and cold-air athletes. Eur Respir J. 2009;33(4):740–6.

Boulet LP. Asymptomatic airway hyperresponsiveness: a curiosity or an opportunity to prevent asthma? Am J Respir Crit Care Med. 2003a;167(3):371–8.

Boulet LP. Physiopathology of airway hyperresponsiveness. Curr Allergy Asthma Rep. 2003b;3(2):166–71.

Brannan JD, Lougheed MD. Airway hyperresponsiveness in asthma: mechanisms, clinical significance, and treatment. Front Physiol. 2012;3:460.

Brannan JD, Anderson SD, Perry CP, Freed-Martens R, Lassig AR, Charlton B. The safety and efficacy of inhaled dry powder mannitol as a bronchial provocation test for airway hyperresponsiveness: a phase 3 comparison study with hypertonic (4.5%) saline. Respir Res. 2005;6:144.

Cabral AL, Conceicao GM, Fonseca-Guedes CH, Martins MA. Exercise-induced bronchospasm in children: effects of asthma severity. Am J Respir Crit Care Med. 1999;159(6):1819–23.

Chapman DG, Irvin CG. Mechanisms of airway hyper-responsiveness in asthma: the past, present and yet to come. Clin Exp Allergy. 2015;45(4):706–19.

Chapman DG, Berend N, King GG, Salome CM. Increased airway closure is a determinant of airway hyperresponsiveness. Eur Respir J. 2008;32(6):1563–9.

Coates AL, Dell SD, Cockcroft DW, Gauvreau GM. The PD20 but not the PC20 in a methacholine challenge test is device independent. Ann Allergy Asthma Immunol. 2017a;118(4):508–9.

Coates AL, Wanger J, Cockcroft DW, Culver BH, the Bronchoprovocation Testing Task Force, Kai-Hakon C, Diamant Z, et al. ERS technical standard on bronchial challenge testing: general considerations and performance of methacholine challenge tests. Eur Respir J. 2017; 49(5): pii: 1601526.

Cockcroft DW, Davis BE. The bronchoprotective effect of inhaling methacholine by using total lung capacity inspirations has a marked influence on the interpretation of the test result. J Allergy Clin Immunol. 2006;117(6):1244–8.

Crapo RO, Casaburi R, Coates AL, Enright PL, Hankinson JL, Irvin CG, et al. Guidelines for methacholine and exercise challenge testing-1999. This official statement of the American Thoracic Society was adopted by the ATS Board of Directors, July 1999. Am J Respir Crit Care Med. 2000;161(1):309–29.

Crimi E, Pellegrino R, Milanese M, Brusasco V. Deep breaths, methacholine, and airway narrowing in healthy and mild asthmatic subjects. J Appl Physiol (1985). 2002;93(4):1384–90.

De Fuccio MB, Nery LE, Malaguti C, Taguchi S, Dal Corso S, Neder JA. Clinical role of rapid-incremental tests in the evaluation of exercise-induced bronchoconstriction. Chest. 2005;128(4):2435–42.

Dell SD, Bola SS, Foty RG, Marshall LC, Nelligan KA, Coates AL. Provocative dose of methacholine causing a 20% drop in FEV1 should be used to interpret methacholine challenge tests with modern nebulizers. Ann Am Thorac Soc. 2015;12(3):357–63.

ElHalawani SM, Ly NT, Mahon RT, Amundson DE. Exhaled nitric oxide as a predictor of exercise-induced bronchoconstriction. Chest. 2003;124(2):639–43.

Clinical exercise testing with reference to lung diseases: indications, standardization and interpretation strategies. ERS Task Force on Standardization of Clinical Exercise Testing. European Respiratory Society. Eur Respir J. 1997;10(11):2662–89.

Gazzola M, Lortie K, Henry C, Mailhot-Larouche S, Chapman DG, Couture C, et al. Airway smooth muscle tone increases airway responsiveness in healthy young adults. Am J Physiol Lung Cell Mol Physiol. 2017;312(3):L348–L57.

Gibson PG, Saltos N, Borgas T. Airway mast cells and eosinophils correlate with clinical severity and airway hyperresponsiveness in corticosteroid-treated asthma. J Allergy Clin Immunol. 2000;105(4):752–9.

Hallstrand TS. Approach to the patient with exercise-induced bronchoconstriction. In: Franklin N, Adkinson J, Bochner BS, Wesley Burks A, Busse WW, Holgate ST, Lemanske Jr RF, O'Hehir RE, editors. Middleton's allergy principles and practice, vol. 1. Philadelphia: Elsevier; 2013. p. 938–50.

Hallstrand TS, Curtis JR, Koepsell TD, Martin DP, Schoene RB, Sullivan SD, et al. Effectiveness of screening examinations to detect unrecognized exercise-induced bronchoconstriction. J Pediatr. 2002;141(3):343–8.

Hallstrand TS, Moody MW, Aitken ML, Henderson WR Jr. Airway immunopathology of asthma with exercise-induced bronchoconstriction. J Allergy Clin Immunol. 2005a;116(3):586–93.

Hallstrand TS, Moody MW, Wurfel MM, Schwartz LB, Henderson WR Jr, Aitken ML. Inflammatory basis of exercise-induced bronchoconstriction. Am J Respir Crit Care Med. 2005b;172(6):679–86.

Hallstrand TS, Altemeier WA, Aitken ML, Henderson WR Jr. Role of cells and mediators in exercise-induced bronchoconstriction. Immunol Allergy Clin North Am. 2013;33(3):313–28. vii

Hayes RD, Beach JR, Rutherford DM, Sim MR. Stability of methacholine chloride solutions under different storage conditions over a 9 month period. Eur Respir J. 1998;11(4):946–8.

Hopp RJ, Townley RG, Biven RE, Bewtra AK, Nair NM. The presence of airway reactivity before the development of asthma. Am Rev Respir Dis. 1990;141(1):2–8.

James AL, Pare PD, Hogg JC. The mechanics of airway narrowing in asthma. Am Rev Respir Dis. 1989;139(1):242–6.

Jeffery PK, Wardlaw AJ, Nelson FC, Collins JV, Kay AB. Bronchial biopsies in asthma. An ultrastructural, quantitative study and correlation with hyperreactivity. Am Rev Respir Dis. 1989;140(6):1745–53.

Johansson H, Norlander K, Berglund L, Janson C, Malinovschi A, Nordvall L, et al. Prevalence of exercise-induced bronchoconstriction and exercise-induced laryngeal obstruction in a general adolescent population. Thorax. 2015;70(1):57–63.

Joos GF, O'Connor B, Anderson SD, Chung F, Cockcroft DW, Dahlen B, et al. Indirect airway challenges. Eur Respir J. 2003;21(6):1050–68.

Khalid I, Morris ZQ, Digiovine B. Specific conductance criteria for a positive methacholine challenge test: are the American Thoracic Society guidelines rather generous? Respir Care. 2009;54(9):1168–74.

Langdeau JB, Boulet LP. Is asthma over- or under-diagnosed in athletes? Respir Med. 2003;97(2):109–14.

Laprise C, Laviolette M, Boutet M, Boulet LP. Asymptomatic airway hyperresponsiveness: relationships with airway inflammation and remodelling. Eur Respir J. 1999;14(1):63–73.

Modrykamien AM, Gudavalli R, McCarthy K, Liu X, Stoller JK. Detection of upper airway obstruction with spirometry results and the flow-volume loop: a comparison of quantitative and visual inspection criteria. Respir Care. 2009;54(4):474–9.

Nair P, Martin JG, Cockcroft DC, Dolovich M, Lemiere C, Boulet LP, et al. Airway hyperresponsiveness in asthma: measurement and clinical relevance. J Allergy Clin Immunol Pract. 2017;5(3):649–59.e2.

O'Byrne PM, Gauvreau GM, Brannan JD. Provoked models of asthma: what have we learnt? Clin Exp Allergy. 2009;39(2):181–92.

Parsons JP, Kaeding C, Phillips G, Jarjoura D, Wadley G, Mastronarde JG. Prevalence of exercise-induced bronchospasm in a cohort of varsity college athletes. Med Sci Sports Exerc. 2007;39(9):1487–92.

Parsons JP, Hallstrand TS, Mastronarde JG, Kaminsky DA, Rundell KW, Hull JH, et al. An official American Thoracic Society clinical practice guideline: exercise-induced bronchoconstriction. Am J Respir Crit Care Med. 2013;187(9):1016–27.

Perkins PJ, Morris MJ. Vocal cord dysfunction induced by methacholine challenge testing. Chest. 2002;122(6):1988–93.

Petak F, Czovek D, Novak Z. Spirometry and forced oscillations in the detection of airway hyperreactivity in asthmatic children. Pediatr Pulmonol. 2012;47(10):956–65.

Postma DS, Kerstjens HA. Characteristics of airway hyperresponsiveness in asthma and chronic obstructive pulmonary disease. Am J Respir Crit Care Med. 1998;158(5 Pt 3):S187–92.

Pralong JA, Lemiere C, Rochat T, L'Archeveque J, Labrecque M, Cartier A. Predictive value of nonspecific bronchial responsiveness in occupational asthma. J Allergy Clin Immunol. 2016;137(2):412–6.

Prieto L, Ferrer A, Domenech J, Perez-Frances C. Effect of challenge method on sensitivity, reactivity, and maximal response to methacholine. Ann Allergy Asthma Immunol. 2006;97(2):175–81.

Scichilone N, Kapsali T, Permutt S, Togias A. Deep inspiration-induced bronchoprotection is stronger than bronchodilation. Am J Respir Crit Care Med. 2000;162(3 Pt 1):910–6.

Sterk PJ, Bel EH. Bronchial hyperresponsiveness: the need for a distinction between hypersensitivity and excessive airway narrowing. Eur Respir J. 1989;2(3):267–74.

Sumino K, Sugar EA, Irvin CG, Kaminsky DA, Shade D, Wei CY, et al. Variability of methacholine bronchoprovocation and the effect of inhaled corticosteroids in mild asthma. Ann Allergy Asthma Immunol. 2014;112(4):354–60 e1.

Thomson RJ, Schellenberg RR. Increased amount of airway smooth muscle does not account for excessive bronchoconstriction in asthma. Can Respir J. 1998;5(1):61–2.

Trankner D, Hahne N, Sugino K, Hoon MA, Zuker C. Population of sensory neurons essential for asthmatic hyperreactivity of inflamed airways. Proc Natl Acad Sci U S A. 2014;111(31):11515–20.

Van Schoor J, Joos GF, Pauwels RA. Indirect bronchial hyperresponsiveness in asthma: mechanisms, pharmacology and implications for clinical research. Eur Respir J. 2000;16(3):514–33.

Wanger JS, Ikle DN, Irvin CG. Airway responses to a diluent used in the methacholine challenge test. Ann Allergy Asthma Immunol. 2001;86(3):277–82.

Ward C, Pais M, Bish R, Reid D, Feltis B, Johns D, et al. Airway inflammation, basement membrane thickening and bronchial hyperresponsiveness in asthma. Thorax. 2002;57(4):309–16.

Weiler JM, Brannan JD, Randolph CC, Hallstrand TS, Parsons J, Silvers W, et al. Exercise-induced bronchoconstriction update-2016. J Allergy Clin Immunol. 2016;138(5):1292–5 e36.

Woolcock AJ, Salome CM, Yan K. The shape of the dose-response curve to histamine in asthmatic and normal subjects. Am Rev Respir Dis. 1984;130(1):71–5.

Wubbel C, Asmus MJ, Stevens G, Chesrown SE, Hendeles L. Methacholine challenge testing: comparison of the two American Thoracic Society-recommended methods. Chest. 2004;125(2):453–8.

Chapter 10
Field Exercise Testing: 6-Minute Walk and Shuttle Walk Tests

Annemarie L. Lee, Theresa Harvey-Dunstan, Sally Singh, and Anne E. Holland

10.1 Background to Field Exercise Testing

Assessment of exercise capacity is traditionally performed in a laboratory using cardiopulmonary exercise testing (CPET); however this method is time-consuming and requires expensive equipment and technical support, which may limit its application in some settings. As a result, the last three decades have seen the development of alternative approaches in the form of field-based walking tests. These are shown to be valid, reliable, and repeatable, are easy to perform for both the operator and the subject (although they do require initial training), and require little equipment. An added bonus of walking tests is that walking is a common and acceptable

A. L. Lee (✉)
Faculty of Medicine, Nursing and Health Sciences, Monash University, Frankston, VIC, Australia

Rehabilitation, Nutrition and Sport, La Trobe University, Bundoora, VIC, Australia

Institute for Breathing and Sleep, Austin Health, Heidelberg, VIC, Australia
e-mail: Annemarie.Lee@monash.edu

T. Harvey-Dunstan · S. Singh
Centre for Exercise and Rehabilitation Science, NIHR Leicester Biomedical Research Centre – Respiratory, Glenfield Hospital, Leicester, UK

Faculty of the College of Medicine, Biological Sciences and Psychology, University of Leicester, Leicester, UK
e-mail: sally.singh@uhl-tr.nhs.uk

A. E. Holland
Institute for Breathing and Sleep, Austin Health, Heidelberg, VIC, Australia

Alfred Health, Melbourne, VIC, Australia

Department of Rehabilitation, Nutrition and Sport, La Trobe University, Bundoora, VIC, Australia
e-mail: a.holland@alfred.org.au

D. A. Kaminsky, C. G. Irvin (eds.), *Pulmonary Function Testing*, Respiratory Medicine, https://doi.org/10.1007/978-3-319-94159-2_10

form of activity. This enables implementation across a variety of settings where people with chronic respiratory disease receive their care and is frequently used to guide exercise prescription for pulmonary rehabilitation programs.

The most commonly employed field walking tests are the 6-minute walk (6MWT) and the incremental shuttle walking tests (ISWT) and, its derivative, the endurance shuttle walking test (ESWT). The 6MWT is a self-paced test, while the ISWT is a maximal and incremental test that uses an audible prompt for progressive increases in walking speed. Within 3 min, the 6MWT achieves a plateau in VO_2 which is sustained for the remainder of the test. In contrast the ISWT demonstrates a gradual increase in VO_2 to the point of symptom limitation, matching closely the trajectory and peak values of the laboratory-based CPET.

The 6MWT and ISWT provide important information relevant to assessment of people with chronic respiratory disease, understanding treatment responses, and monitoring disease progress over time. In this chapter we will outline the rationale for each test, as well as their measurement properties, testing protocols, and interpretation. The testing procedures described in this chapter are consistent with those described in the European Respiratory Society/American Thoracic Society Technical Standard for field walking tests.

10.1.1 6-Minute Walk Test

10.1.1.1 Background

The 6MWT is a self-paced test of functional exercise capacity. The aim is to walk as far as possible in 6 min along a flat corridor. The main outcome is the 6-minute walk distance (6MWD), reported in meters or feet. Standardized instructions and encouragement are provided, to minimize variation in test performance. The 6MWT is widely used across many chronic respiratory diseases to assess functional capacity, estimate prognosis and disease progression, assess exertional desaturation, prescribe exercise for pulmonary rehabilitation, and assess response to treatments. It has been extensively studied, particularly in COPD, with good evidence for validity and reliability.

Validity

The validity of the 6MWT is well established in individuals with COPD, ILD, CF, and PAH and in individuals undergoing lung transplantation. There is a strong relationship between the 6MWD and other measures of exercise capacity, particularly peak oxygen uptake (VO_2 peak) from a CPET (correlation coefficients ranging from 0.40 to 0.80) and peak work (0.58–0.93). In patients with moderate to severe COPD, there is no difference in VO_2 peak between a CPET and a 6MWT, although the ventilatory requirements (peak carbon dioxide production, peak ventilation, and respiratory exchange ratio) during a 6MWT are lower. This may account for the excellent patient tolerance of the 6MWT across different chronic respiratory diseases. The high physiological load imposed by the 6MWT suggests it is not truly a submaximal test, particularly in individuals with more severe disease. There is a moderate to strong relationship between the 6MWD and measures of physical activity during daily life (walking time, daily energy expenditure, time spent in vigorous physical activity, number of steps) in a range of patient populations (COPD, ILD, CF, PAH), which supports the notion that the 6MWT is best conceptualized as a test of functional exercise capacity.

The relationship of 6MWD to measures of respiratory function is weaker than the relationship to exercise capacity and physical function. In COPD, correlation coefficients for FEV_1 ranged from 0.31 to 0.70, although a stronger relationship has been reported in those with more severe disease. In ILD, the relationship between FVC or DLCO and 6MWD ranged from $r = 0.06$ to 0.61, while in PAH, mean PAP and 6MWD are weakly to moderately related ($r = -0.2$ to -0.62). In lung cancer, a moderate relationship was evident with FEV_1 $r = 0.53$. In bronchiectasis, 6MWD has a moderate relationship with FVC ($r = 0.52$). For patient-reported outcomes, the strength of the relationship is similar, with weak to moderate relationships between 6MWD and symptoms of dyspnea, fatigue, or health-related quality of life (HRQOL) reported in all disease groups. The 6MWD should be considered as a global measure of functional capacity which is influenced by many important body systems including respiratory, cardiovascular, musculoskeletal, neurological, and psychological function.

Reliability and Learning

The 6MWD is a highly reliable measure of functional exercise capacity, with excellent intraclass correlation coefficients (ICCs ranging from 0.72 to 0.99) across COPD, CF, ILD, and PAH. Despite its reliability, there is consistent evidence of a learning effect for the 6MWD, with most patients walking further on a second test. In 1514 people with COPD, the average learning effect was 27 m, with 82% of patients improving their 6MWD on the second test. The size of the learning effect is sufficiently large to be of clinical significance. For this reason, if the 6MWD is being used to evaluate the effect of an intervention (e.g., pulmonary rehabilitation or medication prescription), either as clinical practice or as part of research, at least two tests should be completed in order to obtain an accurate measurement of functional exercise capacity, with the longest distance recorded.

When the 6MWD is applied to stage disease or assess morbidity, the presence and magnitude of the learning effect may be of lesser relevance, and one test may be sufficient. However, if the information obtained influences treatment decisions (e.g., decisions regarding transplantation or other surgical management), repeat testing should be considered. The learning effect may be moderated by test repetition and the duration between tests. For example, for people with COPD undertaking pulmonary rehabilitation, the learning effect is less if the test is repeated within a short period of time, such as the end of rehabilitation, but may reemerge by 3 months following rehabilitation. Clinicians should be mindful that learning effect may return after a longer duration of time between tests, and in these circumstances, two tests should be completed.

The reliability of other outcomes obtained during a 6MWT, including nadir oxyhemoglobin saturation and heart rate response, is more variable and may be influenced by the type of respiratory disease. For oxyhemoglobin saturation, excellent reliability is evident in COPD and CF, but in individuals with ILD, this measure may be influenced by the presence of underlying vascular disease, which can reduce oximetry signal quality and reduce reliability. For individual patients in whom detecting desaturation is the key indication for the 6MWT, this may influence further clinical decision-making. In COPD and CF, heart rate (HR) measures are more variable compared to oxyhemoglobin saturation, with differences between tests being from −4 bpm to +8 bpm. While this may be of little significance for some individual patients, those suspected of concurrent heart disease or a history of abnormal heart rate or rhythms, the degree of variability in this measure during the 6MWT may warrant additional measures to clarify HR response.

10.2 Relationship of 6MWT to Clinical Outcomes

The 6MWD has a strong relationship to important clinical outcomes in individuals with chronic respiratory disease, with a lower 6MWD consistently associated with increased mortality and morbidity. In COPD, the 6MWD threshold below which mortality is increased has varied across studies from 200 to 350 m, with similar values reported in IPF and PAH. The 6MWD is a component of the BODE index, a multidimensional disease rating for COPD which includes body mass index (BMI), degree of obstruction (FEV_1), functional exercise capacity (6MWT), and degree of dyspnea; in the BODE index, a 6MWD of less than 350 m predicts increased mortality. For individuals with COPD undergoing bilateral lung volume reduction survey, a reduced 6MWT distance (200 m or less) has been associated with a longer length of hospital stay (greater than 3 weeks) and increased likelihood of mortality within 6 months of surgery. Lower distances (<357 m) are also associated with an increased risk of exacerbation-related hospitalization. This metric is also associated with lung transplant waitlist mortality. For this reason, 6MWD is part of the lung allocation score and included as a standard component of pretransplant evaluation. In non-small cell lung carcinoma, the 6MWD offers a moderate prediction of post-operative outcomes and survival in those with advanced disease.

Monitoring of oxygen saturation during the 6MWT provides the opportunity to detect exercise-induced desaturation. The 6MWT is more sensitive for detecting exercise-induced desaturation compared to cardiopulmonary exercise testing, probably because it involves walking rather than cycling. Desaturation during a 6MWT is associated with greater disease severity and progression, more rapid decline in FEV_1, and worse prognosis. In addition, evidence of desaturation during a 6MWT can be used to establish the need for supplemental oxygen therapy, either during daily life or during pulmonary rehabilitation. The distance-saturation product (DSP) is defined as the product of the 6MWD and the nadir SpO_2 when the test is conducted on room air. A DSP $\leq$200 m% predicts mortality in individuals with IPF; the DSP is also an independent predictor of health-related quality of life (HRQOL) in people with sarcoidosis.

Although less commonly applied in clinical practice, HR monitoring during a 6MWT may provide additional information related to morbidity and mortality. The heart rate response (HRR) is the reduction in HR with rest following the exercise period. An abnormal HRR at 1 min (prolonged recovery, usually defined as ≤13–18 beats per min) is a predictor of clinical deterioration in people with idiopathic PAH and of mortality in people with IPF and is a significant predictor of an acute exacerbation of COPD.

10.3 Reference Equations for 6MWD

Reference equations describe the 6MWD for healthy individuals and allow results to be presented as a percentage of the predicted value. A large number of published reference equations are available for both children and adults. Factors influencing the 6MWD in healthy adults include age, height, weight, sex, grip strength, and percentage of maximum heart rate attained during walking. However the reference equations were generated using a wide range of different methods and in different populations. For instance, the walking tracks ranged from 20 to 50 m, and test repetition ranged from one to four 6MWTs. As a result, there is marked variability in the predicted 6MWD generated by different equations.

The impact of this variation in predicted 6MWD across reference equations is demonstrated in Fig. 10.1. A 74-year-old lady with COPD has FEV_1 48%, height

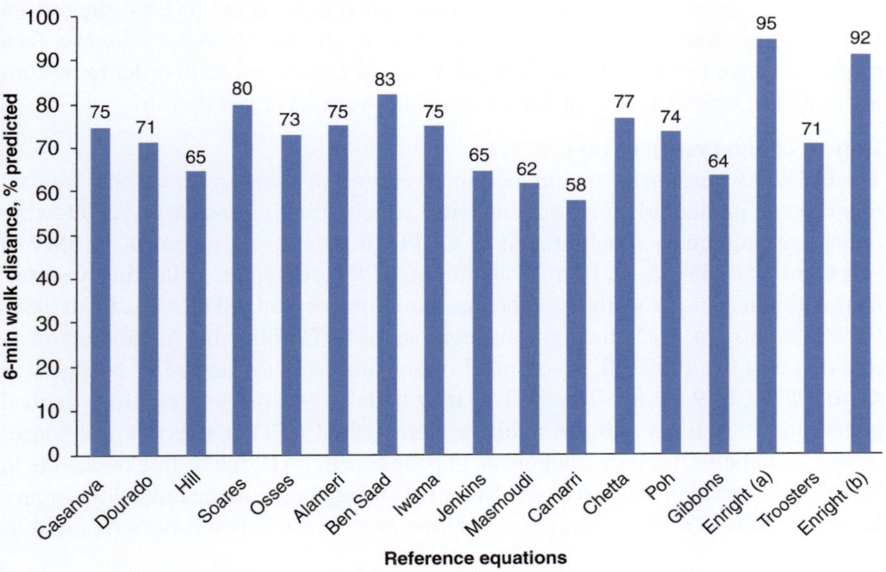

Fig. 10.1 Impact of different reference equations on the 6-minute walk percent predicted for a 74-year-old lady with COPD, FEV_1 48%, height 162 cm, weight 80 kg, 6MWD 365 m, 83% of predicted maximum HR

162 cm, and weight 80 kg. Her 6MWD is 365 m, and she reaches 83% of her predicted maximum HR. Her 6MWD ranges from 58% to 95% of the predicted maximum value, depending on the reference equation used. This could substantially affect interpretation. For this reason, it is recommended that if a reference equation is used, it should be one that was developed in a similar population that in whom it is being applied, using a similar 6MWT protocol. The name of the reference equation should also be provided.

10.4 Meaningful Change in 6MWD

Minimal Important Difference

The minimal important difference (MID) is the smallest difference in score in the outcome of interest that informed patients or informed proxies perceive as important and which would lead the patient or health professional to consider a change in the management. There have been a number of studies investigating the MID for 6MWD in adults with chronic lung disease, including over 5600 patients. Most are in COPD, with smaller numbers of trials in ILD and PAH, and most studies have been conducted in the context of a rehabilitation program. Recent studies report consistent estimates for the MID in the range 25–33 m, with a median value of 30 m. The MID estimates are consistent across patient groups and across study methods. At present there is no evidence that the MID varies according to disease severity or baseline 6MWD, although there are few studies examining these questions.

Current standards for the conduct and interpretation of the 6MWT suggest an MID of 30 m should be used in adult patients with chronic respiratory disease. As a result, a change in 6MWD of at least 30 m would need to occur in order to be confident that true clinical change had occurred between testing occasions.

Impact of Interventions on 6MWD

The 6MWD is responsive to common interventions in people with chronic respiratory disease, particularly for those involving exercise training and surgery. Following outpatient pulmonary rehabilitation in COPD, the mean improvement in 6MWD was 44 m (95% 33–55 m), from 38 studies of 1879 participants. Following hospitalization for an acute exacerbation, the mean improvement in 6MWD was 62 m (95% CI 38–86 m). In ILD, the improvement in 6MWD following rehabilitation is reported as 44 m (95% CI 26–63 m). In bronchiectasis, the degree of change was 41 m (95% CI 19–63 m). The 6MWD may be less responsive to pharmacological interventions. In trials of bronchodilator therapy for COPD or selective and nonselective endothelin receptor antagonists in people with PAH, the degree of change in 6MWD has varied between 6 m and 54 m. Following lung volume reduction surgery in people with COPD, the degree of improvement in 6MWD has been reported as high as 98 m.

10.5 Factors Affecting the 6-Minute Walk Distance

The 6MWD is highly sensitive to small changes in test methodology. The factors shown to influence 6MWD, and the magnitude of their effect on the measured distance, are presented in Table 10.1. Many of these effects exceed the MID. As a result of the substantial impact of variations in methodology, standardization of the testing procedure is very important.

Methodological factors requiring particular attention include:

- Use of standardized encouragement. Recommended phrases are provided below.
- Consistency in provision of supplemental oxygen within an individual, where 6MWD will be compared over time. This includes the method of transporting the supplemental oxygen, which can have a significant impact on 6MWD due to the added weight.
- Clear documentation regarding method for transporting supplemental oxygen (by patient or by tester) and use of gait aids.
- Treadmill testing is not recommended as 6MWD is substantially reduced.
- Track length and layout should be consistent between tests. To facilitate comparison across centers, a straight track, 30 m in length, has been recommended.

10.5.1 Performing the 6MWT

A 6MWT should be performed in a flat, straight corridor that is relatively free of pedestrian traffic. A course of 30 m is recommended, to be consistent with the courses on which most reference equations have been generated. The ends of the course should be marked such that they are clearly visible to the patient. Prior to the test, patients should take their usual medications at the usual times. Strenuous

Table 10.1 Factors affecting the 6-minute walk distance

Change to methodology	Average effect on 6-minute walk distance
Instructions (far vs fast)	↑ 53 m
Supplemental oxygen	↑ 35 m
Continuous track	↑ 34 m
Encouragement	↑ 30 m
Repeat testing	↑ 27 m
Rollator	↑ 14 m
Outdoors	No difference
Home (vs hospital)	↓ 27 m
Shorter track (10 m vs 30 m)	↓ 50 m
Treadmill	↓ 102 m

Data are from Holland et al. 2014

exercise should be discouraged on the day of the test. If respiratory function tests are to be performed on the same day, then these should be performed prior to the 6MWT due to the potential impact of exercise on respiratory function measures. Subsequent 6MWTs should ideally be performed at a similar time of day to the first test.

Contraindications and Precautions to the 6MWT
Because the 6MWT is a strenuous test which frequently elicits a VO_2 similar to CPET, it is recommended that the same contraindications and precautions are used. An extensive list has been published. Comorbidities and medication use should be recorded prior to the test.

Baseline Measurements
Patients should be seated in a chair close to the starting line. Measures to be taken at baseline, prior to test performance, are resting SpO_2 and HR from pulse oximetry; dyspnea and fatigue using a validated scale; and blood pressure, if this has not recently been documented.

Patient Instructions
Standardized instructions should be given before the test begins. These should be given every time the test is performed, regardless of whether the patient has previously performed the test. The ERS/ATS Technical Standard recommends specific, standardize wording be used.

Measurements Taken During the 6MWT
Continuous pulse oximetry should be performed during the 6MWT, in order to accurately determine the lowest SpO_2. This measure has important clinical implications for assessment of disease progression and need for oxygen therapy. The assessor should ensure that a quality signal is obtained. The assessor should not "pace" the patient during the test but should walk sufficiently behind the patient such that the pulse oximeter readings can be observed without influencing the patient's walking speed. This is usually achieved by placing the pulse oximeter in a pouch which is hung over the patient's torso.

Rests
The patient can rest at any time during the test, either in sitting or standing. However, the timer keeps going up until 6 min, to give the patient opportunity to resume walking when able, if SpO_2 is $\geq$85%. Record the start and end time of each stop.

Stopping the 6MWT
The Technical Standard suggests that the 6MWT is ceased if the SpO_2 falls to 80%, as this is associated with a very low rate of adverse events. The rate of adverse events if the SpO_2 is allowed to fall below 80% is not known. If the SpO_2 recovers to 85%, then the patient is asked to recommence walking. Other reasons the assessor may cease a test include chest pain, intolerable dyspnea, leg cramps, staggering or loss of balance, diaphoresis, or pale appearance. Emergency procedures should be instituted according to local protocols, including administration of oxygen as required.

Test Repetition
Due to the learning effect, two 6MWT are required in order to obtain a baseline value against which subsequent 6MWDs can be compared. The Technical Standard suggests an interval of 30 min between 6MWTs to allow physiological measures and symptoms (SpO_2, HR, blood pressure, dyspnea, and fatigue) to return to baseline.

Use of Oxygen During the 6MWT
If the patient has been prescribed oxygen therapy, then this should be used during the 6MWT. Ideally the flow rate should be kept constant for subsequent tests; if this is not possible due to a change in the patient's oxygen prescription, then this should be clearly documented, as direct comparison of 6MWD will not be possible. Oxygen should not be titrated during any 6MWT where 6MWD will be reported, as this is not reproducible and likely to have a highly significant effect on distance walked. For any test where oxygen is used, ensure that the flow rate, oxygen delivery device, and method by which it is transported (by patient or assessor, backpack or trolley, etc.) are recorded.

Recording Performance on the 6MWT
The primary outcome is the 6MWD, in meters or feet. During the tests the assessor should record the number of laps and the number of meters/feet walked in the final part-lap, so that a total distance walked can be reported. If the test is performed twice, then the best 6MWD should be reported, along with other variables recorded on the same test. The SpO_2 and HR at baseline and end test, the lowest SpO_2 recorded during the test, and the symptom scores obtained before and after the test should also be reported. It is also informative to ask the patient about what prevented them from walking further/faster during the test (dyspnea, leg fatigue, or others). If the patient stopped during the test, then the number of stops and the total time stopped are reported. This provides alternative metrics to describe disease progression and may assist with exercise prescription in pulmonary rehabilitation. An example of a recording form is available with the Technical Standard.

10.5.2 Safety Considerations for the 6MWT

The rate of adverse events during the 6MWT in people with chronic respiratory diseases is very low, particularly when the test has been conducted to an established protocol, which incorporates cessation of the test with oxygen desaturation less than 80%. With this protocol applied, one study documented complications on 6% of tests, with the most common complication being oxygen desaturation. Intolerable symptoms, including dyspnea, severe wheeze, lightheadedness, low back pain, chest pain, and tachycardia, were also noted. Predictors of desaturation during a 6MWT were a lower FEV_1 and lower pre-6MWT oxygen saturation.

The absence of documented long-term adverse sequelae related to oxygen desaturation may influence the differing approaches between clinical practices regarding permissible oxygen desaturation during a 6MWT. Some centers advocate for test termination before significant desaturation has the opportunity to occur, while others lend support an individual clinicians' judgment and experience regarding the safety level for cessation of a 6MWT for this metric. The safety of the 6MWT if severe desaturation (<80%) is permitted has not been documented.

10.6 Clinical Example Using the 6MWD

The following example illustrates the use of the 6MWT in clinical practice.

Mr. C is a 66-year-old gentleman who presents to a respiratory clinic with dyspnea and cough of 6-month duration. His respiratory function tests show a mild restrictive pattern with FVC 67% predicted and TLCO 60% predicted. Mr. C has no history of relevant exposures. High-resolution computed tomography shows a honeycombing pattern consistent with idiopathic pulmonary fibrosis (IPF).

The best of two 6MWDs at initial clinic visit is relatively well preserved at 520 m or 77% predicted using reference equations from Jenkins et al. The lowest SpO_2 during 6MWT is 92%, decreased from resting SpO_2 of 96%.

A diagnosis of IPF is confirmed after review by a multidisciplinary meeting. Mr. C is prescribed with pirfenidone, which he tolerates well. At repeat clinic visit 6 months later, his respiratory function tests are stable. His 6MWD shows a small increase (+22 m) which is not clinically significant, and his nadir oxygen saturation is unchanged at 91%.

Twelve months later Mr. C returns to clinic, reporting an increase in his dyspnea. There has been a small reduction in respiratory function (5% in FVC and TLCO). However, there has been a highly significant reduction in 6MWD, falling from 540 m to 480 m, with lowest SpO_2 of 86%. Mr. C's physician recommends that he remains on pirfenidone. He also refers Mr. C to pulmonary rehabilitation and to the oxygen clinical for consideration of ambulatory oxygen.

Key Points

- The 6MWT at baseline allows both assessment of Mr. C's functional capacity and exertional oxygen saturation.
- Regular monitoring of the 6MWD can alert clinicians to any significant changes, either improvement or decline. In this case the first follow-up 6MWD provided assurance that Mr. C's functional capacity remained stable. The second follow-up 6MWD showed a highly significant decline, indicating that more intensive treatment and monitoring may be required.
- The 6MWT provides sensitive information about exertional desaturation that can alert clinicians to change over time and suggests when initiation of oxygen therapy could be considered. It will also assist pulmonary rehabilitation practitioners to design a safe and effective training strategy for Mr. C.

10.6.1 *Incremental Shuttle Walk Test (ISWT)*

10.6.1.1 Background

The ISWT was developed as a way of performing an objective and standardized measure of functional capacity in patients with COPD. This test is performed around a 10-meter course, at speeds dictated by an external auditory cue. The speed of walking increases every minute and provokes a symptom-limited maximal performance. The primary outcome of the ISWT is distance which is recorded in meters to the last completed shuttle. Since initial development, it has been adopted for use in other respiratory and chronic conditions. The ISWT was developed and modified from earlier work where a test using a 20-m running track was used to measure the peak oxygen uptake ($\dot{V}O_2$Peak) in a sporting population. By adapting the incremental levels reported by Léger and Lambert, the ISWT was developed to include similar multistage speeds.

Validity
The ISWT distance related well to $\dot{V}O_2$Peak, the gold standard measure of cardiorespiratory fitness, during a CPET ($r = 0.88$). When comparing the distances walked between the ISWT to the previously established 6MWD, there was a good correlation ($r = 0.68$). From the initial validation data, Singh et al. established the following regression equation:

Estimated $\dot{V}O_2$Peak (ml.min^{-1}.kg^{-1}) = 4.19 (95% CI 1.12 to 7.17) + 0.025 (0.018 to 0.031) distance (m).

For patients with COPD, a moderate correlation has been observed between the ISWT and quadriceps strength ($r = 0.47$), symptom burden using the COPD assessment tool (CAT; $r = 0.50$), and physical activity ($r = 0.54$). Only weak correlations have been reported in COPD between ISWT distance and age or lung function, as might be expected. For patients with lung cancer, the ISWT correlates moderately to quadriceps and inspiratory muscle strength but only weakly to lung function. There is evidence that the ISWT is also a valid tool for use in bronchiectasis with moderate correlations observed for $\dot{V}O_2$Peak, steps per day, MRC, and peak workload.

For patients with asthma, the ISWT has been validated in those who do not demonstrate exercise-induced bronchodilation. When comparing the response between the ISWT and a constant work rate (CWR) treadmill-based CPET test, there were similar responses in ventilatory efficiency ($\dot{V}E/\dot{V}CO_2$ 32 ± 8 vs 19.7); however, the ISWT elicited a greater ventilatory demand than the CWR treadmill test (VE/MVV 0.5 ± 0.2 vs 0.4 ± 0.2). This may have been a relative effect of comparing an incremental test to a CWR test which was performed at 40% of an incremental alternative. The development of a modified ISWT (MST) has demonstrated a strong relationship in $\dot{V}O_2$Peak ($r = 0.95$, $p < 0.01$) for adult patients with cystic fibrosis. This relationship was expressed as $\dot{V}O_2$Peak = 6.83 [95% CI, 2.85–10.80] + 0.028 [0.019–0.024] × MST distance.

Reliability and Learning
The reliability of the ISWT for patients with COPD is strong when measured by intraclass correlation coefficients (ICC 0.88–0.93). While not measured with ICCs, initial data by Singh et al. reported an excellent correction between tests one and two ($r = 0.98$). This is also the case for patients with bronchiectasis and CF. The reliability of the ISWT has not been reported in either ILD or asthma.

Initial testing of the ISWT suggested a significant learning effect of 31 m between tests one and two, but this reduced to 2 m between tests two and three. A similar learning effect was also reported in a recent systematic review where a pooled mean difference of 20 m was reported in over 600 patients. For same-day repeatability, a learning effect of 20–40 m has been reported. For physiological variables, same-day repeatability of the ISWT has been described as −56 L/min for $\dot{V}O_2$Peak (coefficient of repeatability (CR) of 414 L/min), 56 L/min for $\dot{V}CO_2$Peak (CR of 329 L/min), 0.09 for RER (CR of 0.24), 4 bpm for end test HR (CR 13 bpm), and 0 for end test SpO_2 (CR of 4%). Expert opinion would suggest that two tests should be performed when establishing a baseline ISWT, with the best distance recorded. Recent audit data in the United Kingdom highlights that this is not routine practice for many clinical services. Many services may struggle with this repetition in terms of time and provision; however, its completion allows for accurate assessment of exercise performance and prescription required for optimal exercise training as recommended internationally.

Repeatability of the ISWT within other respiratory populations is unclear. In ILD the learning effect is suggested to be 29 m, while for bronchiectasis, this effect was absent between tests with only a 4-meter difference. In a population of adult patients with CF, there was no difference between the distance walked on two tests (mean 0, 95% CI −1–1). Repeatability of the ISWT has not been confirmed in adult patients with asthma.

10.7 ISWT as a Clinical Indicator

Performance of the ISWT has proven useful for predicting mortality in patients with COPD with a suggested distance threshold of <170 m indicating greater mortality and in predicting hospital readmission following an acute exacerbation of COPD. The test has also been incorporated into the multidimensional tool, the iBODE (body mass index, degree of airflow obstruction, dyspnea, and exercise capacity (by ISWT)), which has proven valuable as a composite measure for the categorization and prediction of outcome in patients with COPD. This has not been duplicated in other respiratory conditions.

10.8 Reference Equations

Numerous reference equations have been published for predicting $\dot{V}O_2$Peak from the ISWT. One of these studies was conducted in a South American population and was not age matched to a COPD population; however, another based in India grouped patients by three age ranges. A European-based study observed that age, body mass index (BMI), FEV_1, quadriceps strength, and physical activity explained 50% of the variation in the ISWT distance. No predictive equations have been reported within other respiratory populations.

10.9 Meaningful Change in the ISWT

Minimal Important Difference
The minimal important difference (MID) for the ISWT for patients with COPD and following pulmonary rehabilitation has been estimated at 48 m. This measure was calculated using a patient preference approach, rather than a statistical model. For patients with non-CF bronchiectasis, an MCID of 35 m has been identified.

Impact of Interventions on ISWT
The ISWT is sensitive in identifying exercise-induced desaturation in patients with COPD, and distance walked is sensitive for identifying improvements in oxygenation when ambulatory oxygen was administered. This study identified a significant increase of 33 m in ISW distance when patients received supplemental ambulatory oxygen when compared to air. Interestingly these authors also identified a significant reduction of 29 m in ISW distance in persons carrying an air cylinder when compared to an unencumbered control walk. This highlights the benefits of supplemental oxygen but also that the method of ambulation (i.e., carrying with a backpack or on a walker) should be documented, enabling standardization of the test on subsequent visits. The use of a walking aid has also demonstrated a useful tool worthy of prescription for increasing walking distance for patients with COPD.

The ISWT is sensitive to exercise-based interventions such as pulmonary rehabilitation for patients with COPD and a variety of respiratory and long-term chronic diseases (such as heart failure). Studies report a range of ISWT responses to pulmonary rehabilitation from 36 to 61 m. A pooled mean improvement of 40 m has been suggested in the latest Cochrane Review; however, only half of the studies achieved the suggested MID. An effect size of 0.65 has also been reported for the ISWT following pulmonary rehabilitation. For patients with ILD, significant improvements in ISWT distance have been reported following pulmonary rehabilitation; however, these gains were not observed for those patients prescribed with oxygen therapy. A recent systematic review in patients with non-CF bronchiectasis has suggested improvement of the ISWT following pulmonary rehabilitation with weighted mean difference of 67 m, coinciding with improvements in health status.

With relation to the sensitivity of the ISWT to detect changes following bronchodilation, significant improvements of 30 m have been reported following the administration of nebulized salbutamol and ipratropium. This was not however translated into any significant improvements in breathlessness scores. For patients with chronic asthma, the response of the ISWT has not been reported following either bronchodilation or exercise-based interventions.

10.9.1 Endurance Shuttle Walk Test (ESWT)

10.9.1.1 Background

The ESWT is an endurance or constant work rate derivative of the ISWT, using the same walking track and setup but with a different protocol. The primary outcome of the ESWT is time and should be reported in seconds or percent change following an intervention. For this test, after an initial warm-up period of 2 min, the speed of walking is kept constant. The speed of walking is derived from the results of the ISWT, and therefore the ESWT cannot be completed as a stand-alone test. The test was developed as a submaximal measure of function for the assessment of disability in patients with COPD as a companion to the ISWT. As such, an accurate prediction of 85% peak performance is dependent upon the patient completing an adequate ISWT prior to calculating the appropriate speed of the ESWT. An added benefit of performing an ESWT is that it allows a health-care provider to prescribe a level of exercise at a given threshold value, enabling accurate and optimal aerobic training. It also serves as a responsive outcome measure. At the present time, the majority of ESWT data has been reported within the COPD population; however there is growing use of this test within other respiratory populations.

Validity

There is limited evidence regarding the validity of the ESWT. However, during the developmental stages of the ESWT, the test was validated against a laboratory-based constant work rate treadmill test in patients with COPD. The ESWT and treadmill constant work rate test elicited similar physiological and metabolic responses for $\dot{V}O_2$Peak, $\dot{V}_E$Peak, breaths per minute, tidal volume, and heart rate per minute, when tests were performed at both 75 and 85% predicted $\dot{V}O_2$Peak (using the ISWT equation). This was not the case when patients performed near maximal testing (95% $\dot{V}O_2$Peak).

Reliability and Learning

For patients with COPD, the learning effect for the ESWT has been reported as 60 s between tests one and two, when the test is performed at 85% predicted $\dot{V}O_2$Peak obtained from the ISWT. While this was not statistically significant, there was a significant increase in distance between tests one and three by 74 s. The same authors who developed the ESWT also suggested a nonsignificant mean increase in ESWT duration of 12 s between tests one and two when measuring on the same day in 68 patients with COPD. This small difference in duration was confirmed by Bland and Altman (BA) plots where the coefficient of repeatability was ±100 s. Further studies have reported test-retest differences of −7 to −2 s. These data also identified some variability in ESWT performance associated with longer endurance time. This variation may be evident in patients who walk for longer as they are more sensitive to external influences such as motivation, mood, or boredom.

10.9.1.2 Meaningful Change in ESWT

Minimum Important Difference

Different values have been proposed for the MID of the ESWT, depending on the nature of the intervention. While Pepin et al. reported an MID of 45–85 s (or 60–115 m) following bronchodilation, the authors were unable to determine an MID for pulmonary rehabilitation using a preference-based approach. These authors did however report that a distribution-based analysis suggested an MID of 186–203 s. This was equivalent to 136% change in performance. Borel et al. (2014) more recently reported a similar MID range following a bronchodilation intervention of tiotropium plus additional fluticasone/salmeterol (fixed-dose combination), proposing that an improvement of 56–61 s, or distance of 70–82 m, was meaningful to patients. For patients with a diagnosis of respiratory failure, an MID in the range of 186–199 s or 154–164 m has been reported when anchored to health-related quality of life and exercise capacity.

Impact of Interventions

It is generally accepted that a constant work rate test is likely to be more sensitive to an intervention than a maximal exercise test, and this is observed when comparing the ISWT and ESWT. Given the increasing awareness of the responsive properties of the ESWT, there is a growing use of the test in clinical trials.

There is growing literature on ESWT response to bronchodilation. Pepin et al. have reported the response of the ESWT on two separate occasions found similar significant improvements (164 and 144 s, respectively) along with strong effect sizes (ES) of 0.93 and 0.66. Brouillard and colleagues reported similar responses with a significant improvement of 117 s and a moderate ES (0.56) following bronchodilation with salmeterol. A more recent study of tiotropium reported a difference of 117 s following 3 weeks of therapy. These improvements in exercise function were also translated into significant improvements in breathlessness at end test.

Response of ESWT to pulmonary rehabilitation has been reported as significant with improvement of 160 s from baseline and a strong ES of 2.90. Other trials have also reported significantly high responses with improvements ranging from 293 to 408 s. Unfortunately, the ESWT has not been included in any large Cochrane Reviews to date, and this may be a consequence of the small volume of literature available at the time of the review. However, a recent systematic review by Singh et al. reported the test responsiveness with standardized response means ranging from 0.52 to 1.27, with two of the six studies reported evaluating pulmonary rehabilitation.

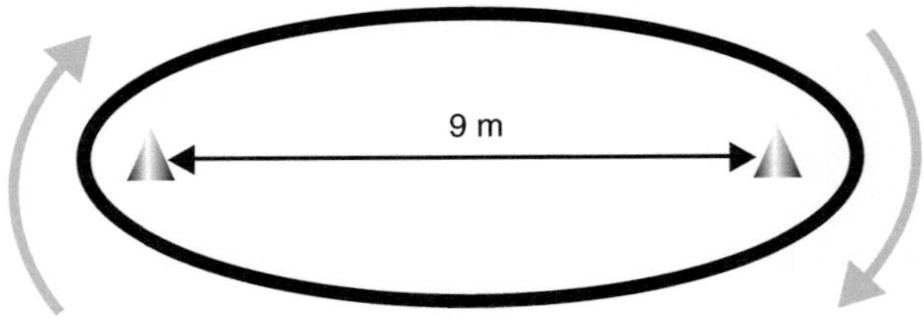

Fig. 10.2 Layout and conduct of the Shuttle Walk Test

10.10 Performing the ISWT and ESWT

Both incremental and endurance SWT utilize a 10-meter track marked with cones at either end Fig. 10.2. The remaining 1 m is accounted for in the turn required at either end of the track. The ISWT is a maximal and progressive symptom-limited test that is externally paced using an incremental speed which is indicated using an audio signal. The ESWT is a constant work rate test, which requires that an ISWT is performed first to establish the workload. The test should be conducted in a quiet corridor or dedicated exercise testing room. Standardized encouragement is required for both tests.

Contraindications and Precautions
As the ISWT is designed to elicit maximal exercise performance, the same contraindications and precautions as a CPET should be applied (TS).

Baseline Measurements
Before the test, physiological parameters should be collected including blood pressure, pulse rate, and oxygen saturation along with scales of perceived exertion and breathlessness.

Patient Instructions
Initial test instructions are given by the audio recording and are reproduced in the Technical Standard. An operator should pace the patient for the first minute/level of the test before stepping away, unless closer supervision is required for patient safety. Patients should not run during the ISWT. When running, $\dot{V}O_2$Peak increases in direct proportion to velocity and therefore is more efficient than walking. This change in metabolic demand would therefore render the predictive equation of the ISWT invalid.

Setting the Speed for the ESWT
The ESWT is calculated as a percentage of peak performance of the ISWT (e.g., 70–85% estimated $\dot{V}O_2$Peak) or a percentage of the peak speed achieved. The ESWT includes a warm-up period of 1.5 min, after which the patient should be paced for the first two shuttles. When choosing an appropriate speed, an operator should calculate the predicted $\dot{V}O_2$Peak (4.19 + (0.025 * ISWT distance)) followed by the percentage work the patient needs to work at (i.e., 70–85%). This percent-predicted $\dot{V}O_2$Peak can then be used to identify the appropriate walking speed for the ESWT.

Encouragement

For the ISWT, as the speed of walking increases every minute, indicated by a triple bleep, the patient should be advised:

"You now need to increase your speed of walking."

During both ISWT and ESWT, only one verbal cue can be used to encourage the patient to pick up their speed; if they are more than 0.5 m from the marker when the bleep sounds:

"You need to increase your speed to keep up with the test."

No other verbal cues should be given.

Measures Taken during the SWTs

The assessor counts the number of shuttles completed during the test. It is advisable to time the performance as an additional measure, to confirm manual recording of the number of shuttles completed.

Stopping the SWTs

The test is ceased if the patient is more than 0.5 of a meter from the marker when the auditory cue sounds for a second successive shuttle. The test is also ceased if the patent indicates symptom limitation (e.g., too breathless or tired to continue). It may also be terminated at the assessor's discretion should there be a drop of SpO_2 below 80%, an increase in cardiac frequency above 85% predicated heart rate maximum, or the patient feeling generally unwell. For an ESWT, the test should last between 180 and 480 s in duration, allowing for an optimal physiological response to the point of symptom limitation. If a patient exceeds this time, the test should be stopped and the patient allowed to rest. Once the patient has rested, a further test should be completed at one or two levels above the first. The operator's decision on prescribed speed should be guided by the patient's physiological and self-reported response to the first test.

Test Repetition

Due to the learning effect on the ISWT, two tests are recommended to obtain an accurate baseline. Repeat testing should occur following a 30-min rest or sufficient time to allow recovery of all physiological and symptom measures to baseline. Two tests do not appear to be required for an accurate baseline ESWT measurement. After an intervention the ESWT should be repeated at the same speed as at baseline, in order to accurately identify any treatment effects.

Use of Oxygen

In order to interpret change over time, the SWTs should be performed with oxygen delivered at the same flow rate and by the same method, where possible. The delivery system, flow rate, and method of carrying the oxygen (patient or assessor, backpack or trolley, etc.) should be documented on the testing form.

Recording Performance

The primary outcome of the ISWT is distance, reported as an accumulation of 10-m lengths. The minimum distance is 0 m if patients fail to complete the first shuttle, and the maximum is 1020 m. It can also be reported as percent predicted, noting the reference equation used. The ESWT is reported as time (minutes and seconds), although it can also be expressed as distance. The recording form should include

SpO_2, heart rate, dyspnea, and fatigue scores at the beginning and end of the test, as well as the lowest SpO_2 recorded during the test. The reason for test termination should be recorded. Examples of recording forms are available with the Technical Standard.

10.11 Safety of the Shuttle Walk Tests

Subjects with angina or a recent myocardial infarction (1 month) should be discussed with the referring physician and testing under physician supervision when clinically safe. Stable exertional angina is not an absolute contraindication for a field walking test, but subjects with these symptoms should perform the test after using their anti-angina medication, and rescue nitrate medication should be readily available. Indeed, the ISWT has been used as an outcome for cardiac rehabilitation and is therefore a safe test to perform on patients with cardiac disease.

10.12 Clinical Examples Using the ISWT and ESWT

The following examples illustrate the use of the ISWT and ESWT in clinical practice:

ISWT example: Patient with COPD referred for pulmonary rehabilitation. Mr. A, a 69-year-old gentleman, attended a pulmonary rehabilitation assessment clinic during the winter. He had a confirmed diagnosis of COPD with post-bronchodilator spirometry of FEV_1 54% predicted and FEV_1/FVC 52%. He had an MRC breathlessness score of four, regular sputum production, and cough. No cardiovascular symptoms on questioning. He had a symptom burden score (CAT score) of 30 and CRQ-dyspnea score of 2.2 indicating he was disabled with breathlessness. Comorbidities consisted of hypertension (managed with an ACE inhibitor and a diuretic) and previous DVT and PE for which he was on warfarin. Mr. A also had a BMI of 38.3 $kg.m^{-2}$. He was treated with a combination inhaler (steroid/long-acting β_2-agonist), along with long-acting muscarinic receptor antagonist (LAMA) and a short-acting $Beta_2$-agonist (SAMA) for acute relief. This gentleman's 85% heart rate maximum (HRmax) was estimated at 128.

At rest he had finger oximetry (SpO_2) of 93% on room air and a pulse rate (regular) of 92 with a blood pressure of 120/65. His Borg breathlessness score was one. No ankle swelling and JVP were unremarkable.

Mr. A performed 120 m in his first ISWT, and test termination was due to breathlessness and leg fatigue. At end test, his SpO_2 was 90% (nadir SpO_2 was 90%) on room air and a pulse rate (regular) at 133 with a blood pressure of 136/72. His perceived breathlessness score was five and rate of perceived exertion was 17. These values returned to baseline within minutes after a short period of rest. A second test was performed after 30 min. This second test measured 20 m less than the first (100 m) but with the same test termination (breathlessness and leg fatigue). At end test his SpO_2 was 92% on room air and a pulse rate (regular) at 103 with a blood pressure of 120/65. His perceived breathlessness score was five and rate of perceived exertion was 17.

Mr. A expressed that he was really happy with the distance that he had covered at the speed he had performed.

Key Notes

- Mr. A presents as a very symptomatic patient with moderate COPD (GOLD 2) with a very high CAT (30), an MRC of four, and an extreme breathlessness when measured using the CRQ dyspnea.
- The best test performed by Mr. A was test one despite both tests eliciting levels of severe breathlessness and leg fatigue. This is indicted by the first test provoking a good cardiovascular response to just above his predicted 85%HRmax. There was adequate rise in blood pressure within acceptable level for an exercise test.
- Mr. A displayed a decrease in his SpO_2 to 90%. While this would not constitute an additional prescription of oxygen, it would be clinically wise to monitor this during exercise training for any additional desaturation that may warrant further assessment.
- Given that Mr. A has a history of hypertension, the ISWT may identify excessive rises or even decompensation at end test if there was a drop in blood pressure below 10% of resting BP. It is therefore suggested that blood pressure is measured in all patients presenting in clinic for an ISWT. This allows a thorough interrogation of the systemic responses to exercise and hence optimizes the safety of patients entering pulmonary rehabilitation.
- ESWT example: calculation and performance of the ESWT.
- Using the example above, we can assume that Mr. A performed an accurate test (we know he performed a good maximal test due to his responses) and that his predicted $\dot{V}O_2$Peak, using the following predictive equation ($\dot{V}O_2$Peak (ml/min/kg) = 4.19 + (0.025 * ISWT distance)) was 7.19 (ml/min/kg).
- When choosing the speed for the ESWT, we calculate 85% of his predicated $\dot{V}O_2$Peak (7.19 * 0.85 = 6.11 (ml/min/kg). If we use the published equations, we find that in order for Mr. A to perform an endurance test at 60.11 (ml/min/kg) $\dot{V}O_2$Peak, the speed of choice was approximately 2.72 km/h (the closest level to the prediction).
- Using this calculation, Mr. A completed an ESWT at level four. The duration of his test was 240 s, exceeding the lower threshold of 3 min for conducting a good test. His end test responses were SpO_2 was 94% on room

air and a pulse rate (regular) at 118 with a blood pressure of 133/72. His perceived breathlessness score was five and rate of perceived exertion was 15. Reason for termination was breathlessness and leg fatigue.

- This endurance test elicited the suggested duration of a CWR test (180 s) and elicited a submaximal response at 85% of his predicted $\dot{V}O_2$Peak. When compared to his maximal test, these physiological responses are noted with less desaturation and less increase in cardiovascular outputs. While Mr. A reported severe breathlessness, his perceived leg fatigue was less than the ISWT.
- In terms of exercise prescription, level four would be an optimal training prescription for Mr. A with the aim to increase the duration of his walks over time. Clinically, and if Mr. A was finding training at level four too hard, the health-care professional could decrease to level three and be guided by the Borg breathlessness scale to gauge training efficiency.
- On completing pulmonary rehabilitation, the test should be repeated at the same level (level four in Mr. A's case). This enables the greatest changes to be assessed. If a new ESWT was calculated from a new ISWT, any treatment effect may be lost.

Selected References

American Thoracic S, American College of Chest P. ATS/ACCP statement on cardiopulmonary exercise testing. Am J Respir Crit Care Med. 2003;167(2):211–77.

Bolton CE, Bevan-Smith EF, Blakey JD, Crowe P, Elkin SL, Garrod R, Greening NJ, Heslop K, Hull JH, Man WD, Morgan MD, Proud D, Roberts CM, Sewell L, Singh SJ, Walker PP, Walmsley S. British Thoracic Society pulmonary rehabilitation guideline development G, British Thoracic Society standards of care C. British Thoracic Society guideline on pulmonary rehabilitation in adults. Thorax. 2013;68(Suppl 2):ii1–30.

Borel B, Pepin V, Mahler DA, Nadreau E, Maltais F. Prospective validation of the endurance shuttle walking test in the context of bronchodilation in COPD. Eur Respir J. 2014;44(5):1166–76. https://doi.org/10.1183/09031936.00024314.

Celli B, Cote C, Lareau S, Meek P. Predictors of survival in COPD: more than just the FEV1. Respir Med. 2008;102(Suppl 1):S27–35.

Chandra D, Wise R, Hrishikesh S, et al. Optimising the 6-min walk test as a measure of exercise capacity in COPD. Chest. 2012;142:1545–52.

Dyer CA, Singh SJ, Stockley RA, Sinclair AJ, Hill SL. The incremental shuttle walking test in elderly people with chronic airflow limitation. Thorax. 2002;57(1):34–8.

Eaton T, Young P, Milne D. Six-minute walk, maximal exercise tests: reproducibility in fibrotic interstitial pneumonia. Am J Respir Crit Care Med. 2005;171:1150–7.

Granger C, denehy L, Parry S, Martin J, Dimitriadis T, Sorohan M, Irving L. Which field walking test should be used to assess functional exercise capacity in lung cancer? An observational study. BMC Pulm Med. 2015;15:89.

Harrison SL, Greening NJ, Houchen-Wolloff L, Bankart J, Morgan MD, Steiner MC, Singh SJ. Age-specific normal values for the incremental shuttle walk test in a healthy British population. J Cardiopulm Rehabil Prev. 2013;33(5):309–13.

Hernandes N, Wouters E, Meijer K, et al. Reproducibility of 6-minute walking test in patients with COPD. Eur Respir J. 2011;38:261–7.

Hill K, Dolmage TE, Woon L, Coutts D, Goldstein R, Brooks D. Comparing peak and submaximal cardiorespiratory responses during field walking tests with incremental cycle ergometry in COPD. Respirology (Carlton, Vic). 2012;17(2):278–84.

Holland A, Spruit M, Singh S. How to carry out a field walking test in chronic respiratory disease. Breathe. 2015;11(2):129–39.

Holland A, Spruit M, Troosters T, Puhan M, Pepin V, Saey D, MCCormack M, Carlin B, Sciurba F, pitta F, Wanger J, MacIntyre N, Kaminsky D, Culver B, Revill S, Hernandres N, Andrianopoulos V, Camillo C, Mitchell K, Lee A, Hill C, Singh S. An official European Respiratory Society / American Thoracic Society technical standard: field walking tests in chronic respiratory disease. Eur Respir J. 2014;44(6):1428–46.

Leger LA, Lambert J. A maximal multistage 20-m shuttle run test to predict VO2 max. Eur J Appl Physiol Occup Physiol. 1982;49(1):1–12.

Mador MJ, Modi K. Comparing various exercise tests for assessing the response to pulmonary rehabilitation in patients with COPD. J Cardiopulm Rehabil Prev. 2016;36(2):132–9.

McKeough ZJ, Leung RW, Alison JA. Shuttle walk tests as outcome measures: are two incremental shuttle walk tests and two endurance shuttle walk tests necessary? Am J Phys Med Rehabil. 2011;90(1):35–9.

Pepin V, Laviolette L, Brouillard C, Sewell L, Singh SJ, Revill SM, Lacasse Y, Maltais F. Significance of changes in endurance shuttle walking performance. Thorax. 2011;66(2):115–20.

Probst VS, Hernandes NA, Teixeira DC, Felcar JM, Mesquita RB, Goncalves CG, Hayashi D, Singh S, Pitta F. Reference values for the incremental shuttle walking test. Respir Med. 2012;106(2):243–8.

Puente-Maestu L, Palange P, Casaburi R, Laveneziana P, Maltais F, Neder JA, O'Donnell DE, Onorati P, Porszasz J, Rabinovich R, Rossiter HB, Singh S, Troosters T, Ward S. Use of exercise testing in the evaluation of interventional efficacy: an official ERS statement. Eur Respir J. 2016. doi: ERJ-00745-2015 [pii];47:429.

Revill SM, Noor MZ, Butcher G, Ward MJ. The endurance shuttle walk test: an alternative to the six-minute walk test for the assessment of ambulatory oxygen. Chron Respir Dis. 2010;7(4):239–45.

Sandland CJ, Morgan MD, Singh SJ. Detecting oxygen desaturation in patients with COPD: incremental versus endurance shuttle walking. Respir Med. 2008;102(8):1148–52.

Singh S, Puhan M, Andrianopoulos V, Hernandes N, Mitchell K, Hill C, Lee A, Camillo C, Troosters T, Spruit M, Carlin B, Wanger J, Pepin V, Saey D, Pitta F, Kaminsky D, MCCormack M, MacIntyre N, Culver B, Sciurba F, REvill S, Delafosse V, Holland A. An official systematic review of the European Respiratory Society / American Thoracic Society: measurement properties of field walking tests in chronic respiratory disease. Eur Respir J. 2014;44(6):1447–78.

Singh SJ, Jones PW, Evans R, Morgan MD. Minimum clinically important improvement for the incremental shuttle walking test. Thorax. 2008;63(9):775–7.

Singh SJ, Morgan MD, Hardman AE, Rowe C, Bardsley PA. Comparison of oxygen uptake during a conventional treadmill test and the shuttle walking test in chronic airflow limitation. Eur Respir J. 1994;7(11):2016–20.

Singh SJ, Morgan MD, Scott S, Walters D, Hardman AE. Development of a shuttle walking test of disability in patients with chronic airways obstruction. Thorax. 1992;47(12):1019–24.

Spruit M, Polkey M, Celli B, Edwards L, Watkins M, Pinto-Plata V, Vestbo J, Calverley P, Tal-Singer R, Agusti A, Coxson H, Lomas D, MacNee W, Rennard S, Silverman E, Crim C, Yates J, Wouters E, investigators EoCltipseEs. Predicting outcomes from 6-minute walk distance in chronic obstructive pulmonary disease. J Am Med Dir Assoc. 2012;13(3):291–7.

Van Gestel A, Clarenbach C, Stowhas A, et al. Prevalence and prediction of exercise-induced oxygen desaturation in patients with chronic obstructive pulmonary disease. Respiration. 2012;84:353–9.

Chapter 11
Integrating the Whole: Cardiopulmonary Exercise Testing

J. Alberto Neder, Andrew R. Tomlinson, Tony G. Babb, and Denis E. O'Donnell

11.1 Introduction

Cardiopulmonary exercise testing (CPET) has evolved in the past four decades as an important tool to confirm the presence and uncover the causes of exercise intolerance in patients with cardiorespiratory diseases. In respiratory practice, CPET is more commonly requested as part of the work-up for dyspnea of unknown origin. In this context, it is instructive to consider three different clinical scenarios involving these patients:

- Dyspnea which is deemed out of proportion to resting lung function impairment in a patient with known respiratory disease (*disproportionate dyspnea*)
- Dyspnea in a patient with multiple comorbidities which could contribute to dyspnea (*unclear dyspnea*)
- Dyspnea in an apparently healthy subject whose previous investigations failed to conclusively isolate an organic abnormality (*unexplained dyspnea*)

J. A. Neder · D. E. O'Donnell (✉)
Respiratory Investigation Unit and Laboratory of Clinical Exercise Physiology, Division of Respirology and Sleep Medicine, Department of Medicine, Queen's University and Kingston General Hospital, Kingston, ON, Canada
e-mail: odonnell@queensu.ca

A. R. Tomlinson · T. G. Babb
Division of Pulmonary and Critical Care Medicine, Department of Internal Medicine, University of Texas Southwestern Medical Center and Institute for Exercise and Environmental Medicine, Texas Health Presbyterian Hospital, Dallas, TX, USA

D. A. Kaminsky, C. G. Irvin (eds.), *Pulmonary Function Testing*,
Respiratory Medicine, https://doi.org/10.1007/978-3-319-94159-2_11

Occasionally, CPET is requested as part of the preoperative assessment of candidates for lung resection surgery and before pulmonary or cardiac rehabilitation (*see* Sect. 11.3.2). As such, CPET may take on various individualized forms by which to simulate the exercise/activity condition(s) that provokes symptoms in the patient. These adaptations (described in detail later in this chapter) to conventional testing protocols make CPET a unique and powerful assessment of functional capacity and physiological responses to exertion.

11.2 Integrated Exercise Physiology: Normal Responses

Exercise (or work) can be described as any contraction of skeletal muscle. The processes involved in generating contraction of skeletal muscle require the integrated function of multiple physiological systems. Broadly, this is generated through delivery of oxygen (O_2) from the environment to skeletal muscle to create energy in the form of adenosine triphosphate (ATP) and the elimination of carbon dioxide (CO_2) produced by cellular respiration.

11.2.1 Metabolic Responses

Skeletal muscle contraction requires the hydrolysis of stored ATP to adenosine diphosphate and the release of energy from this terminal phosphate bond. Only small amounts of ATP are stored in the muscle, and it must therefore be constantly produced or regenerated from its precursors. Phosphocreatine functions as an intermediate storage form for high-energy phosphate bonds allowing the rapid repletion of ATP stores early in exercise. Further muscular contraction, however, requires regeneration of ATP from glycolysis and oxidative metabolism. ATP regeneration is predominantly aerobic at low workloads when energy requirements are lower. In these phases of exercise, metabolism of glycogen stores to pyruvate and then through the tricarboxylic acid cycle results in direct production of ATP, release of CO_2 by-product, and reduction of nicotinamide adenine dinucleotide (NAD^+) to NADH and H^+. CO_2 production by contracting muscles increases PCO_2 in mixed venous blood. Consequently, there is an increase in the rate of CO_2 diffusion from lung capillaries to alveoli which increases pulmonary CO_2 output ($\dot{V}CO_2$). The NADH produced from these pathways is oxidized back to NAD^+ by transfer of the electrons and protons through the electron transport chain, resulting in ATP production and O_2 consumption at the cellular level. As O_2 is utilized by the contracting muscles, its partial pressure in the mixed venous blood decreases. Consequently, there is a corresponding increase in the rate of O_2 diffusion from lung capillaries to alveoli thereby increasing pulmonary O_2 uptake ($\dot{V}O_2$). According to the relative contribution of carbohydrates, lipids, and amino acids in the mixture being metabolized, the $\dot{V}CO_2/\dot{V}O_2$ ratio varies (respiratory exchange ratio, RER): the highest RER values are seen when carbohydrates are the predominant substrate.

When rate of O_2 demand exceeds the aerobic capacity of the electron transport chain or when insufficient O_2 is available (i.e., low O_2 content or low O_2 delivery), NADH is reoxidized by conversion of pyruvate to lactic acid. In other words, even if at low-to-moderate workloads, aerobic metabolism alone may be sufficient to generate necessary ATP, anaerobic glycolysis is typically required at higher workloads. This chemical reaction provides an important additional source of energy as exercise progresses, albeit with less efficient production of ATP per glucose unit. Lactate begins to accumulate in the blood when the rate of lactate production exceeds its clearance by body metabolism. This is sometimes termed the "lactate threshold" (LT) or, assuming that anaerobic metabolism was the trigger for higher lactate release, the "anaerobic threshold." Plasma bicarbonate is the main buffer of lactic acid leading to the formation of carbonic acid which quickly dissociates into CO_2 and water. Although this reaction has the advantage of turning a fixed acid into a volatile gas, this additional CO_2 accelerates the rate of $\dot{V}CO_2$ increase relative to$\dot{V}O_2$ and requires increased ventilation ($\dot{V}_E$) to maintain acid-base equilibrium. Although there is some controversy about this sequence of events, these phenomena underlie the techniques for a noninvasive estimation of the LT (Fig. 11.1, *panels 2, 5, and 6*; see further discussion in Sect. 11.2.3.1).

The body's maximal capacity to take up and utilize O_2 is an important index of overall cardiorespiratory fitness. When the rate of external work performed (power) increases continuously, $\dot{V}O_2$ increases linearly with a slope of ~10 mL/min/W (Fig. 11.1, *panel 1*). At the point of exhaustion in a highly motivated and fit subject, $\dot{V}O_2$max represents the maximal rate that the body can deliver and then utilize O_2 in cellular respiration. This is characterized by the body's inability to increase $\dot{V}O_2$ despite further increase in workload, i.e., a plateau in the $\dot{V}CO_2$-work rate relationship. Nonathletic subjects, however, frequently terminate exercise without developing such a plateau. Thus, this is better named peak $\dot{V}O_2$ (Fig. 11.1, *panel 1*) or, in patients, symptom-limited $\dot{V}O_2$ ($\dot{V}CO_{2SL}$).

11.2.2 Cardiovascular Responses

Increasing contractile activity of the peripheral muscles during progressive exercise indicates increasing needs for O_2. Thus, muscle O_2 utilization during exercise increases through greater O_2 delivery (DO_2) and increased O_2 extraction, i.e., a wider difference between arterial and venous O_2 content:

$$\dot{V}O_2 = DO_2 \times (CaO_2 - CvO_2) \quad (11.1)$$

DO_2, in turn, depends on CaO_2 and cardiac output (CO). The great majority of O_2 is transported bound to hemoglobin (Hb):

$$CaO_2 = (1.34 \times Hb \times SaO_2) + (0.003 \times PaO_2) \quad (11.2)$$

SaO_2 is typically >95% at rest at sea level and, other than in disease or at the extremes of performance, remains relatively stable with exercise (Fig. 11.1, *panel 6*). Thus, DO_2 is increased primarily by an increase in CO, and (Eq. 11.1) can be rewritten as the Fick principle:

$$\dot{V}O_2 = CO \times (CaO_2 - CvO_2) \quad (11.3)$$

or

$$\dot{V}O_2 = (HR \times SV) \times (CaO_2 - CvO_2) \quad (11.4)$$

Fig. 11.1 The key physiological and sensorial responses to incremental CPET. *First row*: power, metabolic, and cardiovascular responses. Peak $\dot{V}O_2$, peak work rate (WR) and submaximal $\dot{V}O_2$-WR relationship in *Graph 1*; *Graph 2* (with confirmatory information from *Graph 5 and Graph 6*) is useful to estimate the lactate threshold by the gas exchange method (GET) as suggested by an upward inflection in CO_2 output ($\dot{V}CO_2$) and respiratory exchange ratio (RER) relative to $\dot{V}O_2$. Heart rate (HR) and O_2 pulse ($\dot{V}O_2$/HR) as a function of $\dot{V}O_2$ are shown in *Graph 3*. *Second row*: variables describing the "quantitative" features of ventilation and its relationship with metabolic and gas exchange determinants. *Graph 4* shows minute ventilation ($\dot{V}_E$) as related to submaximal metabolic demand ($\dot{V}_E$-$\dot{V}CO_2$) up to the respiratory compensation point (RCP). Decrements in ventilatory reserve ((1-($\dot{V}_E$-maximal voluntary ventilation (MVV)) × 100)) are also depicted. *Graph 5* shows $\dot{V}_E$-$\dot{V}O_2$ and $\dot{V}_E$-$\dot{V}CO_2$ ratios as exercise progresses: consequences on end-tidal partial pressures (PET) for O_2 and CO_2 are seen in *Graph 6*. The latter panel also shows the trajectory of oxyhemoblobin saturation by pulse oximetry (SpO_2). *Third row*: variables describing the "qualitative" features of ventilation. *Graph 7* exposes the operating lung volumes as indicated by changes in inspiratory capacity (IC) and potential tidal volume (V_T) constraints (V_T/IC ratio) as $\dot{V}_E$ increases. Inspiratory reserves are appreciated by the end-inspiratory lung volume (EILV)/total lung capacity (TLC) ratio and inspiratory reserve volume (IRV) relative to $\dot{V}_E$ in *Graph 8*. Respiratory rate (RR), tidal volume (V_T), and RR/V_T ratio as a function of $\dot{V}_E$ are seen in *Graph 9*. Subjective responses are shown at the bottom: Borg dyspnea scores are presented in the *left column* as a function of work rate and ventilatory demands (*Graph A* and *Graph B*). Borg leg discomfort scores are analyzed in relation to work rate and metabolic demands ($\dot{V}O_2$) in the *right column* (*Graph C* and *Graph D*). Expected scores for subject's age and gender as established in our laboratory (shaded rectangles) are presented at selected exercise intensities. *Definition of abbreviations and symbols*: pred predicted, LLN lower limit of normal, ULN upper limit of normal, *S* slope, *I* intercept, $\dot{V}O_2$ oxygen uptake, WR work rate, $\dot{V}CO_2$ carbon dioxide output, RER respiratory exchange ratio, HR heart rate, $\dot{V}_E$ minute ventilation, VT_1 first ventilatory threshold, VT_2 second ventilatory threshold, PET end-tidal pressure, SpO_2 oxyhemoglobin saturation by pulse oximetry, IC inspiratory capacity, V_T tidal volume, IRV inspiratory reserve volume, EILV end-inspiratory lung volume, TLC total lung capacity, RR respiratory rate

where HR is heart rate and SV is stroke volume. These considerations demonstrate that the fundamental task of the cardiovascular system (adequate O_2 offer to peripheral tissues) is particularly challenged during exercise.

As expected, CO increases during exercise due to changes in SV and HR. In a young, healthy adult, this is accomplished by early SV augmentation and a continuous increase in HR throughout exercise up to the maximum predicted by age (Fig. 11.1, *panel 3*). Peripheral O_2 delivery is also enhanced by the preferential

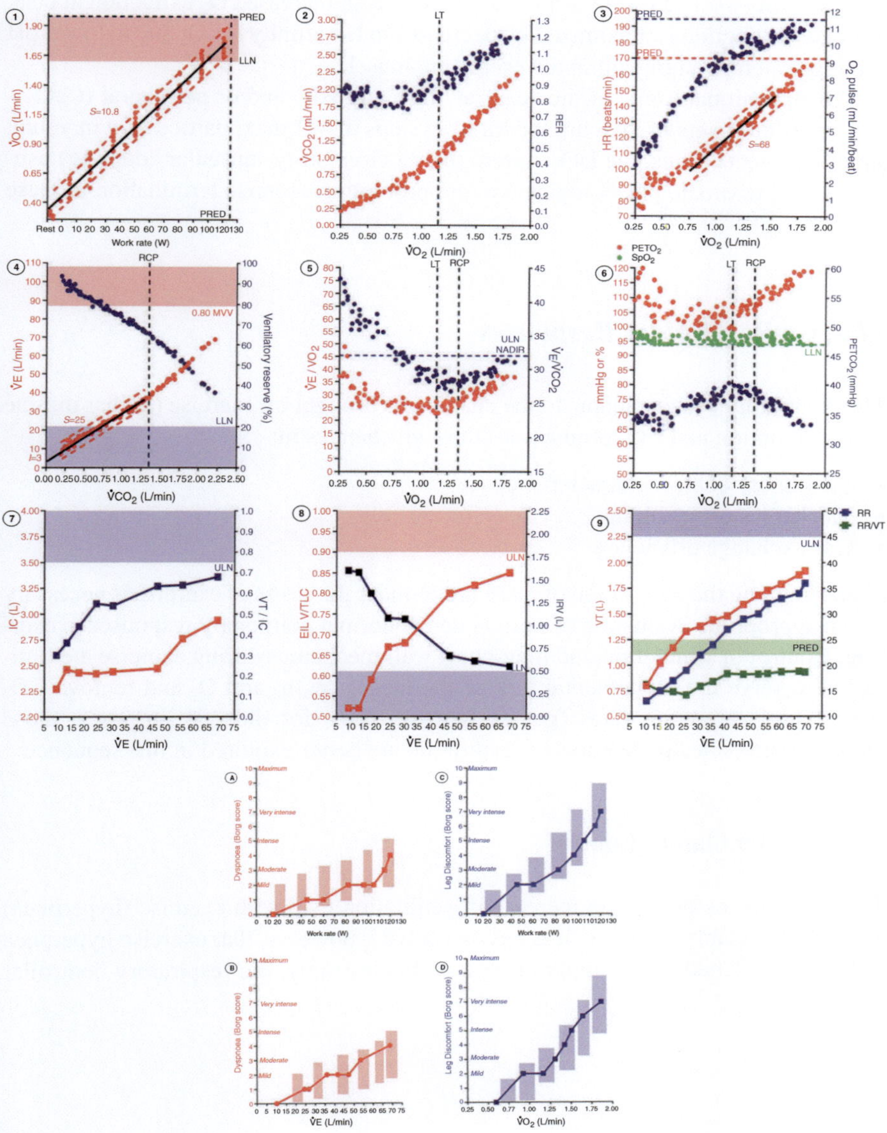

vasodilation of vascular beds supplying exercising muscles. Rearranging (Eq. 11.4) gives how much O_2 is consumed per beat:

$$\dot{V}O_2 / HR = SV \times (CaO_2 - CvO_2) \quad (11.5)$$

It follows that a low $\dot{V}O_2$/HR ratio (O_2 pulse) might be secondary to central hemodynamic abnormalities (such as low SV) and/or poor muscle ability to extract O_2 (low $CaO_2 - CvO_2$). Venous O_2 saturation decreases in exercising muscles from typical values of ~70% at rest to as low as 15–20% with increased O_2 extraction at peak exercise. Extraction is maximized by decreases in Hb affinity for O_2 due to lower pH and higher temperature within the exercising muscle.

The operational limits of the "central" (SV and HR) and/or peripheral (CaO_2 – CvO_2) determinants of DO_2 are the limiting steps of $\dot{V}O_2$max, particularly in young athletic subjects. Thus, the DO_2 system (cardiocirculatory-muscular coupling) usually is the proximate physiological system prompting exercise termination in these subjects.

11.2.3 Respiratory Responses

The respiratory system adapts to the challenges brought by exercise (higher muscle O_2 consumption and CO_2 production) through changes in:

- Ventilatory control characteristics
- Mechanics of breathing
- Gas exchange efficiency

Understanding the integration of these areas under the stress of exercise is necessary for an appropriate evaluation of normal and abnormal pulmonary responses to exertion. Control of ventilation and lung-chest wall mechanics during exercise are optimized to serve the fundamental task of the lungs, i.e., to add O_2 and remove CO_2 from blood at precise rates (gas exchange). Thus, for didactic purposes, those closely interconnected features of respiration are better explored in this sequence.

11.2.3.1 Ventilatory Control

The mechanisms driving an increase in ventilation ($\dot{V}_E$) with exercise (hyperpnea) are understandably complex. It is beyond debate, however, that exercise hyperpnea is closely matched to metabolic demands. Interestingly, the respiratory controller (i.e., pontine-medullary centers and their cortical-limbic connections) more closely follows changes in CO_2 than O_2. Thus, changes in $\dot{V}_E$ impact $\dot{V}CO_2$ more readily than $\dot{V}O_2$. This is largely a result of a much higher CO_2 solubility compared to O_2 and the exquisite sensitivity of the cerebral vasculature to the former. Thus, CO_2 can easily cross the blood-brain barrier allowing rapid access to central chemoreceptors. If CO_2 begins to accumulate in the blood and cerebrospinal fluid, leading to excessive chemo-stimulation, the resulting cerebral vasodilation quickly restores equilibrium. This is important to lessen the ventilatory drive avoiding respiratory alkalosis. Controlling $PaCO_2$ close to the resting value (at least up to the point where it needs to decrease to compensate for lactic acidosis) also provides an important way to limit changes in pH, which can have deleterious systemic effects, e.g., abnormal neural excitability and impaired muscle contraction.

In this context, it is important to consider that $\dot{V}_E$ required to eliminate a given rate of CO_2 production is higher the lower the arterial partial pressure for CO_2 ($PaCO_2$) (as more $\dot{V}_E$ is needed to keep $PaCO_2$ at a low compared to a high value). Increased dead-space ventilation also results in higher ventilatory requirements:

$$\dot{V}E / \dot{V}CO_2 \infty 1 / PaCO_2 \times \left(1 - V_D / V_T\right) \quad (11.6)$$

where $\dot{V}_E/\dot{V}CO_2$ ratio is the ventilatory equivalent for CO_2 and V_D/V_T is the physiological (anatomic plus alveolar) dead-space fraction of tidal volume. This equation shows that the respiratory controller adjusts exercise $\dot{V}_E$ for a given $\dot{V}CO_2$ taking into consideration the prevailing level of CO_2 chemosensitivity (i.e., the inverse of $PaCO_2$) and its access to the alveolar space (i.e., the inverse of V_D/V_T). There are two complementary ways to look at the close relationship between $\dot{V}_E$ and $\dot{V}CO_2$ (frequently called "ventilatory efficiency"):

- Plotting $\dot{V}_E$ against $\dot{V}CO_2$ (Fig. 11.1, *panel 4*) and applying linear regression up to the point it remains a straight line (most commercially available software nowadays allows this calculation to be manually performed by the operator); thus, its starting point is called "intercept," and the inclination is the "slope" (the higher the intercept and/or the slope, the poorer the ventilatory efficiency).
- Plotting $\dot{V}_E/\dot{V}CO_2$ ratio against exercise intensity (e.g., $\dot{V}O_2$) (Fig. 11.1, *panel 5*); thus, the lowest $\dot{V}_E/\dot{V}CO_2$ is called "nadir" (the higher the nadir, the poorer the ventilatory efficiency).

The relationships described above remain relatively constant below the lactate threshold. The advent of the LT has profound implications for the control of ventilation during exercise. Thus, as lactate is buffered by bicarbonate (see Sect. 11.2.1), $\dot{V}CO_2$ increases out of proportion to $\dot{V}O_2$. This is more commonly referred as the *gas exchange threshold* and determined by the V-slope method (Fig. 11.1, *panel* 2). Increase in $\dot{V}CO_2$ parallels $\dot{V}_E$ in direct proportion; thus, $\dot{V}_E/\dot{V}CO_2$ ratio and alveolar CO_2 concentration (reflected by the end-tidal partial pressure for CO_2 ($PETCO_2$)) do not change. Increasing $\dot{V}_E$, however, becomes excessive to $\dot{V}O_2$: the consequent increase in $\dot{V}_E/\dot{V}O_2$ ratio means that more O_2 remains in the alveoli to be expired. Thus, the end-tidal partial pressure for O_2 ($PETO_2$) increases. These findings establish the so-called ventilatory threshold (Fig. 11.1, *panels 5 and 6*). It should be noted that despite reflecting the same phenomenon (lactate buffering), the gas exchange threshold slightly precedes the ventilatory threshold. After the LT, $\dot{V}_E/\dot{V}CO_2$ and $PETCO_2$ remain stable during the period of "isocapnic buffering." However, as more lactate is released with further increases in work rate, the blood pH eventually becomes acidotic. This requires compensatory respiratory alkalosis; in fact, $\dot{V}_E$ increases out of proportion to $\dot{V}CO_2$ leading to alveolar hyperventilation (lower $PETCO_2$) at the respiratory compensation point (RCP in Fig. 11.1, *panels 5 and 6*).

11.2.3.2 Mechanics of Breathing

Increases in $\dot{V}_E$ during exercise are dependent upon changes in V_T and respiratory frequency (*f*). A general rule of thumb is that changes in V_T and *f* are balanced with the goal of minimizing the work of breathing and attendant perceived breathing difficulty (*see* Sect. 11.2.4). Thus, an excessively large V_T increases the work required to distend the lungs (elastic work); conversely, an excessively fast frequency increases the work required to move air in and out through the airways (resistive work). Although both V_T and *f* change almost simultaneously with activity onset, V_T expansion predominates over *f* up to the mid-stages of progressive exercise (note, for instance, the initial decrease in the f/V_T ratio in Fig. 11.1, *panel* 9). End-expiratory lung volume (EELV) reduction by expiratory muscle recruitment during exercise allows V_T expansion to about 50–60% of the vital capacity (VC) by encroachment on both the expiratory and the inspiratory reserve volumes. This helps mitigate the increased elastic work associated with breathing closer to total lung capacity (TLC). As the latter does not change appreciably with exercise, the difference between EELV and TLC (i.e., inspiratory capacity (IC)) increases (Fig. 11.1, *panel 7* and Fig. 11.2, *left panel*). When the rate of V_T increase becomes slower, *f* may accelerate up to 40–50 breaths/min at peak exercise in a young athletic subject. The resistive work is minimized despite high flow rates during exercise by intra- and extrathoracic airway dilatation.

Increase in *f* during exercise means that the total respiratory time per cycle (TTOT) decreases. Higher *f* is almost entirely caused by a shortening in expiratory time (TE) due to recruitment of the abdominal expiratory muscles. In contrast, inspiratory time (TI) remains unchanged or only decreases slightly. It follows that:

$$\dot{V}_E = (V_T / TI) \times (TI / TTOT) \tag{11.7}$$

In other words, $\dot{V}_E$ is the product of the average rate at which air is inspired (V_T/TI or mean inspiratory flow) multiplied by the relative duration of inspiration (TI/TTOT, the inspiratory duty cycle). As TI/TTOT increases only modestly, increase in $\dot{V}_E$ with exercise is strongly dependent on V_T/TI; thus, the latter provides an indirect index of the respiratory neural drive in health.

The capacity of the respiratory system to generate inspiratory and expiratory flows over the total range of the vital capacity is determined by the maximal flow-volume (MFV) loop envelope (Fig. 11.2). Even in a highly fit and motivated young subject, the spontaneous expiratory FV loop at maximal exercise only approaches

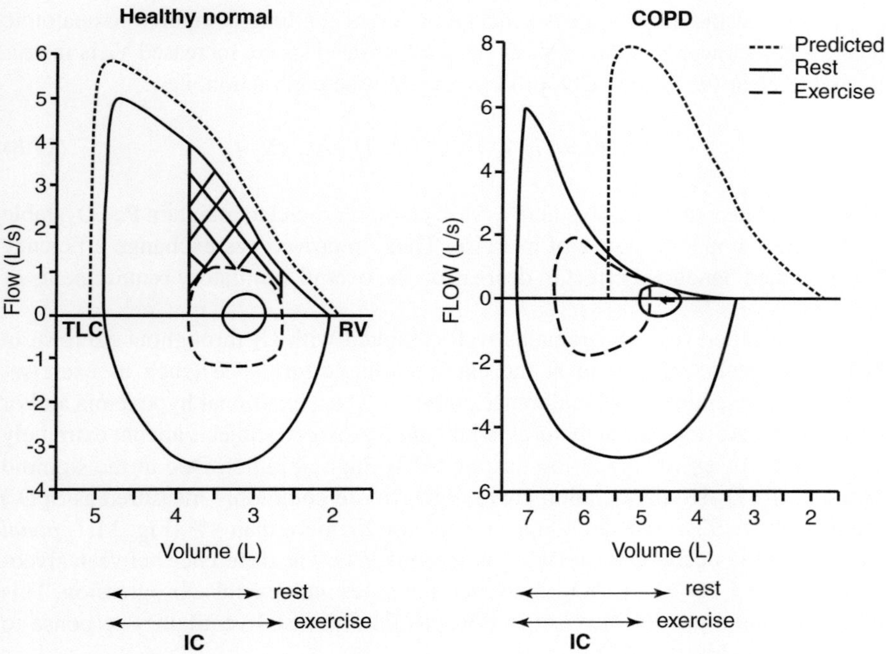

Fig. 11.2 Tidal-to-maximal expiratory flow-volume comparison at rest and during exercise in a healthy subject and a patient with COPD. Shaded region in left panel represents area of flow reserve. Please see text for further elaboration. *Definition of abbreviations*: IC inspiratory capacity, TLC total lung capacity, RV residual volumes

(or, occasionally, exceeds) the MFV over a small fraction of V_T (<25%) (Fig. 11.2, *left panel*). This observation, in addition to the fact that $\dot{V}_E$ at maximal exercise remains a fraction of the maximal sustainable ventilatory capacity (roughly estimated by maximal voluntary ventilation (MVV)) (Fig. 11.1, *panel 4*), underscores the notion that the ventilatory pump does not limit exercise in healthy humans – at least in young to middle-aged subjects who are not extremely well trained.

11.2.3.3 Gas Exchange

Efficiency of intrapulmonary gas exchange (i.e., higher alveolar ventilation ($\dot{V}_A$) due to lower V_D/V_T) is optimized by enhanced $\dot{V}_A$/capillary perfusion (Qc) matching as better ventilated areas have higher alveolar PO_2 leading to local vasodilatation. Higher lung perfusion pressures due to higher CO and lower pulmonary vascular resistance during exercise improve blood flow to the typically less well-perfused upper lung fields. Another key adjustment is the increase in V_T: owing to the higher compliance of the alveolar gas exchange region of the lung compared to anatomic dead space, a lower fraction of V_T is "wasted" as dead space. Increased $\dot{V}_A$ is instrumental to clear the "extra" CO_2 produced by muscle contraction, i.e.,

$$PaCO_2 \propto 1/\left(\dot{V}_E/\dot{V}CO_2\right) \times \left(1 - V_D/V_T\right) \quad (11.8)$$

The parallel decrease in V_D/V_T and $\dot{V}_E/\dot{V}CO_2$ ratio is crucial to maintain $PaCO_2$ stable in the mild–moderate stages of exercise. Thus, improved gas exchange efficiency has a marked beneficial effect in decreasing the overall ventilatory requirements of exercise.

Arterial blood typically remains well saturated with O_2 throughout exercise in healthy subjects, other than at the extremes of performance (such as exercise-induced hypoxemia in elite endurance athletes). Thus, exertional hypoxemia and/or hypercapnia are not normal features in humans – provided subjects are not extremely well trained or exercising at low inspired PO_2 (high altitude). Due to the sigmoid shape of the O_2-Hb dissociation curve, SaO_2 (more commonly measured as SpO_2) remains above 93% and rarely does it decrease by more than 4% (Fig. 11.1, *panel 6*) despite mild decrements in PaO_2 in older subjects. The difference between alveolar and arterial PO_2 ($P(A\text{-}a)O_2$), however, increases with exercise progression. This is largely due a greater increase in $P\bar{A}O_2$ as the increased ventilatory response to lactic acidosis lowers $P\bar{A}CO_2$.

11.2.4 Perceptual Responses

The physiological responses to exercise are optimized to lessen the potentially uncomfortable sensations brought by physical effort. The sense of leg effort rises in tandem with the motor drive required to remain upright and move the body (walking) or overcome the resistance imposed to the pedals (cycling), being also modulated by intramuscular and joint receptors. Similarly, the sense of respiratory effort is influenced by increased central corollary discharge from brainstem and cortical motor centers. Other neural inputs that reach the somatosensory cortex and contribute to respiratory sensations include:

- Afferent information from receptors in the airways (pulmonary stretch receptors, C fibers) and lungs (pulmonary stretch receptors, C fibers, J receptors)
- Peripheral locomotor and respiratory muscles (muscle spindles, Golgi tendon organs, type 3 and 4 afferents)
- Central and peripheral chemoreceptors

In simple terms, the respiratory controller (i.e., pontine-medullary centers and their cortical-limbic connections) continuously asks the following question: *how good* is my breathing? To answer this question, the controller jointly analyzes the responses to three sub-questions: *how much?* (the "quantitative domain"), *how well?* (the "qualitative domain"), and *how adequate?* (the "affective domain").

The *how much* question equates to the respiratory neural drive which is influenced by:

- Chemo-stimulation of central and peripheral receptors
- Efferent motor output to respiratory muscles which is largely dictated by the muscles' elastic loading in addition to feed-forward mechanisms related to peripheral muscle activation

The following abnormalities may increase chemo-stimulation:

- High $\dot{V}_A/Qc$ lung units and increased physiological dead space
- Arterial O_2 desaturation due to increased flow of blood with low mixed venous O_2 pressure through areas with low $\dot{V}_A/Qc$
- Downward displacement of CO_2 set point
- Increased acid-base disturbances (e.g., early metabolic acidosis) due to deconditioning or impaired cardiac function

In the absence of critical mechanical constraints, increased reflex chemo-stimulation translates into excessive ventilatory response relative to metabolic demand. Consequently, when increased drive is the main cause of shortness of breath on exertion (and ventilation is not limited), patients tend to report higher dyspnea for a given work rate but similar dyspnea for a given ventilation compared with normal subjects.

The answer to the *how well* question depends on lung mechanics. Particularly during exercise, this is critically influenced by operating lung volumes and instantaneous compliance of the lung-chest wall unit. This question is negatively answered when V_T becomes positioned close to TLC and the upper reaches of the S-shaped pressure-volume relation of the relaxed respiratory system. Thus, compliance is decreased, the inspiratory muscles are functionally weakened, and intolerable dyspnea quickly ensues. As a corollary, dynamic mechanical constraints lead to higher dyspnea ratings as a function of both work rate and ventilation. Increased respiratory discomfort disproportionate to objective findings (i.e., lack of increased chemostimulation or mechanical-ventilatory constraints) characterizes subjects with a low threshold to negatively answer the *how adequate* question. This is clinically identified by chaotic/dysfunctional breathing pattern accompanied by varied degrees of alveolar hyperventilation.

As expected, the sensation of leg effort and dyspnea increases with exercise intensity in males and females, being higher at a given work rate in older subjects due to greater mechanical constraints and higher ventilation at a given work rate. These sensations increase at a faster rate as exercise progresses; thus, the relationship between symptoms and power output (cycle ergometry) is best described by a power function in which a doubling of power results in ~3.5-fold increase in leg effort and dyspnea. Subjects with a low tolerance for discomfort commonly stop exercise when discomfort is "somewhat severe" (0–10 Borg scale score 4), and more trained (and/or more stoic) subjects may stop exercise at "maximal" (Borg 10). Thus, the motivated healthy subject stops exercise at a symptom intensity close to leg effort's "very severe" (Borg 7–8) and dyspnea's "moderately severe" (Borg 3–4) (Fig. 11.1, *bottom panels*).

A potential limitation of an incremental test to interrogate dyspnea relates to the slower temporal dynamics of respiratory sensations as compared with the physiological responses. Thus, the intensity and quality of respiratory sensations can change as the exercise intensity and ventilatory demands change quickly. Use of submaximal constant workload stages may provide an adequate amount of time at a given exercise intensity to allow the respiratory sensations to reach a temporal steady state.

11.3 Exercise Testing

11.3.1 Overview

Authoritative papers and textbooks have launched the basis for CPET interpretation in the past few decades. The clinical landscape, however, has changed markedly since these initial recommendations were published. The "typical" subject with isolated cardiovascular or respiratory abnormalities has become rare. Today patients usually present with multiple comorbidities. The wide availability of imaging, particularly chest computed tomography and echocardiography, has decreased the prevalence of truly "unexplained dyspnea." Polypharmacy, obesity, and extreme sedentarism further complicate the scenario. Thus, in the context of exercise intolerance, CPET should be seen as an initial *screening* test to guide further investigative efforts. In other words, the test describes patterns of abnormalities; the referring physician should be aware that individual features overlap across diseases. Thus, when appropriately interpreted, it may shorten the list of differential diagnoses rather than providing a single specific diagnosis. Alternatively, results might give reassurance that major organ dysfunction is not currently limiting exercise responses. Importantly, clinical CPET should be interpreted with a solid knowledge of the pretest likelihood of abnormality as inferred from medical history and previous investigations.

11.3.2 Indications

In clinical practice, however, CPET is more frequently requested in the following scenarios:

- As part of the work-up in a patient with *disproportionate dyspnea* or *unclear dyspnea* (as defined in Sect. 11.1) and, less commonly, in *unexplained dyspnea.*
- In early or mild respiratory disease when symptoms are deemed excessive relative to resting lung function impairment.
- In patients with suspected pulmonary vascular disease (e.g., pulmonary arterial hypertension (PAH), chronic thromboembolic pulmonary hypertension (CTEPH)).
- In patients with known chronic cardiac and pulmonary diseases (e.g., heart failure with reduced ejection fraction (HFrEF), chronic obstructive pulmonary disease (COPD), interstitial lung disease (ILD), PAH) to determine whether the observed pattern of abnormalities is consistent with the primary diagnosis or, alternatively, other cause(s) of exercise intolerance should be considered. For instance, persistence of dyspnea and/or exercise intolerance in a patient whose therapy for a given heart or lung disease has been maximized may bring concerns about diagnostic accuracy and confirming, or not, that CPET responses are "within the expected profile" for that specific disease is frequently valuable to the patient's management:
- To guide exercise training intensity pre-rehabilitation (COPD, HFrEF)
- Prognosis evaluation (HFrEF, PAH) and risk assessment for interventions (particularly, thoracic surgery involving parenchymal resection in lung cancer)

11.3.3 Methodology

11.3.3.1 Equipment and Measurements

Most CPETs are currently performed using computerized "metabolic carts." Regardless of the specific technology (bag collection, mixing chamber, breath by breath, etc.), three basic signals are obtained:

- Flow with integration (i.e., area under the flow-time curve) to obtain volume; thus, a calibrated flowmeter is required.
- Respiratory O_2 and CO_2 concentrations, usually measured only in the expired gas; thus, calibrated gas analyzers are required.
- Heart rate from ECG's R-R distance.

Pulse oximetry, systemic blood pressure measurements, and symptom assessment (Borg 0–10 category ratio scale, visual analogue scale) are also mandatory. In some circumstances, arterial blood or, alternatively, arterialized (capillary) blood sampling (including [lactate] measurements) or transcutaneous gas tensions might prove useful. Falsely low pulse oximetry readings are common, particularly in treadmill tests using finger probes. Use of a forehead sensor to minimize motion artifact during exercise and a pulse oximeter that displays a waveform are useful strategies for quality control. Noninvasive measurements of cardiac output (e.g., acetylene rebreathing, impedance cardiography) are usually valuable to help differentiate central cardiac dysfunction from peripheral muscle/metabolic dysfunction.

As in standard ergometry, CPET variables can be measured in response to any exercise modality. Due to better quantification of power (work rate), less data noise, wider availability of reference values, and safety issues, a cycle ergometer is more commonly used than treadmill for clinical CPET. However, arterial O_2 desaturation is greater in response to walking than cycling (see Sect. 11.3.4); moreover, the sense of excessive muscle (leg) effort might prompt earlier termination of a cycle ergometer-based test compared to a treadmill test. However, if needed for specific cases (e.g., athletes), other modes of ergometry can be used to reproduce patient symptoms.

11.3.3.2 Calibration and Quality Control

The flowmeter (using a 3-L syringe using different flows) and gas analyzers (using known gas concentrations at 0–8% CO_2 and 13–21% for O_2) must be calibrated daily. The frequency of repeated calibrations varies according to the manufacturer instructions. It is a good practice, however, to repeat the calibrations (particularly the gas analyzers) every two or three tests. Calibration differs from a control program in that quality control demonstrates the reliability of the measurements not just individual signals. Most labs will collect data on a test subject at a given work rate (sub-LT) periodically to demonstrate the reproducibility of the measurements (e.g., within 10% for metabolic and ventilatory responses).

11.3.3.3 Protocols

Protocols commonly used in cardiac stress test (e.g., Bruce, Naughton) are associated with sudden changes in workload, leading to ample variability in metabolic and ventilatory responses. Thus, they are less well suited to CPET. The most popular protocol is the rapidly incremental test (either following a continuous, "ramp," or

1- to 2-min stepwise increase in work rate) performed on a stationary cycle ergometer, usually electrically braked. The work rate increment usually follows a period (1–3 min) of unloaded, mild exercise. The rate of work rate increase is individually selected aiming at an incremental phase between 8 and 12 min. If a treadmill is used, the modified Balke protocol or a linearized treadmill test (for severely disabled patients) also provides reasonably linear responses. Constant (endurance) tests below the lactate threshold or at ~75% peak are commonly used to assess the sensory and physiological responses under steady-state conditions or to evaluate the efficacy of interventions (e.g., bronchodilators in COPD), respectively.

Exercise at a constant workload may better approximate the physiologic demands of daily living than an incremental protocol. Because respiratory sensations may lag behind the physiological responses of exercise, a longer interval constant workload may be useful in helping to elucidate symptoms, including dyspnea on exertion. In this context, one option is to perform submaximal constant workload stages (one well below and one near the estimated lactate threshold), prior to a typical incremental or graded test. Regardless of the chosen protocol, standard testing contraindications and criteria for test interruption should be observed.

11.3.3.4 Data Presentation

Recorded responses should be presented in both numerical (tabular summary report) and graphical formats: a layout that has been useful in practice is shown in Fig. 11.1. In breath-by-breath systems, shorter averaging intervals should be used in graphic compared to tabular report, e.g., eight to ten breaths and 20–30-s average, respectively. Whatever the chosen graphical report, care should be taken to avoid duplicate information or superfluous variables. The key responses should be presented in a logical sequence, taking care to select adequate scales to express the full range of values of both dependent (y) and independent variables (x). Obtained values should be compared to the theoretical values that best predict the exercise responses of a local sample of non-trained males and females.

11.3.4 General Approach to Clinical Interpretation

Traditional interpretation algorithms have focused on measuring aerobic capacity and on the quantification of an individual's cardiac and ventilatory reserves. One might expand this approach to include evaluation of symptom intensity, together with a simple "noninvasive" assessment of relevant ventilatory control parameters and dynamic respiratory mechanics. In this context, for the physician interested in evaluating the severity of activity-related symptoms and in discovering their cause(s) in the individual patient, a simple ordered interrogation of perceptual and physiological responses to incremental exercise might be used. These include:

- *Metabolic and cardiocirculatory responses*: $\dot{V}O_2$-WR, $\dot{V}CO_2$-$\dot{V}O_2$, HR, and O_2 pulse (Fig. 11.1, *first row*). If available, measurements of cardiac output as a function of $\dot{V}O_2$
- *Ventilatory control and gas exchange*: $\dot{V}_E$, submaximal $\dot{V}_E$/MVV, $\dot{V}_E$-$\dot{V}CO_2$, $\dot{V}_E$-$\dot{V}O_2$, SpO_2, and $PETCO_2$ (Fig. 11.1, *second row*). If available, arterial (or arterialized) blood-gas tensions and [lactate])
- *Dynamic respiratory mechanics*: IC, V_T/IC, EILV/TLC, IRV, V_T, *f*, and *f*/V_T ratio (Fig. 11.1, *third row*). If available, quantitative and qualitative tidal flow-volume loop analysis (Fig. 11.2)
- *Perceptual responses*: dyspnea and leg effort (Borg) ratings (Fig. 11.1, *bottom panels*)

Table 11.1 presents a structured, stepwise approach for gathering key CPET data. Using this framework, selected clusters of findings might allow identification of the following patterns: (a) obesity, (b) O_2 delivery/utilization impairment (which encompasses cardiocirculatory and peripheral muscle abnormalities), (c) mechanical-ventilatory impairment, (d) pulmonary gas exchange impairment, and (e) dysfunctional breathing-hyperventilation (Table 11.2). Some age- and gender-based cutoffs of key variables for clinical interpretation are presented in Table 11.3.

11.3.4.1 Normal Test

The expected physiological responses to incremental exercise have been presented in Sect. 11.2. A normal test is established if the response course (trajectory) follows the expected profile (Fig. 11.1) and discrete values at the estimated lactate threshold

Table 11.1 Standardized sequence of data gathering for CPET interpretation

1. Pre-reading	1.a Review indication and available clinical information 1.b Review reported morbid history and medications 1.c Review technologist's comments: effort, cooperation, events
2. Symptoms	2.a Symptoms at peak, reason (s) for exercise termination 2.b Submaximal dyspnea x WR and dyspnea x $\dot{V}_E$ 2.c Submaximal leg effort x WR and leg effort x $\dot{V}O_2$
3. Exercise capacity	3.a Peak $\dot{V}O_2$: % predicted and absolute values 3.b Peak WR: % predicted and absolute values

4. Respiratory	*Gas exchange* 4.a PcO_2, $PcCO_2$, V_D/V_T: values and trajectory 4.b $PETCO_2$: apex and trajectory 4.c P(c-ET)CO_2: values and trajectory 4.d SpO_2: nadir and trajectory *Mechanical-ventilatory: quantitative domain* 4.e Ventilatory reserve: submaximal and maximal 4.f $\dot{V}_E$-$\dot{V}CO_2$ relationship: slope and intercept 4.g $\dot{V}_E/\dot{V}CO_2$ ratio: nadir and trajectory *Mechanical-ventilatory: qualitative domain* 4.h Operating volumes: IC, V_T/IC, IRV, EILV/TLC values and trajectory 3.i Breathing pattern: Values and trajectory 3.j Tidal flow-volume loop: boundaries and morphology
5. Metabolic/ power	5.a Δ $\dot{V}O_2$ /Δ WR: linearity, slope, up and downward shifts 5.b estimated $\dot{V}O_2$ LT: if identified, express as % predicted peak $\dot{V}O_2$ 5.c If available, [lactate] and C(a-v)O_2 5.d Resting and exercise RER: values and trajectory
6. Cardiovascular	6.a If available, stroke volume and cardiac output 6.b HR reserve and 1-min HR recovery 6.c Δ HR /Δ $\dot{V}O_2$: linearity and slope 6.d O_2 pulse: peak values and trajectory 6.e Review ECG: relate to Δ $\dot{V}O_2$ /Δ WR and O_2 pulse 6.f Review systemic blood pressure values and trajectory
7. Reporting	7.a Group key findings to define the abnormal pattern(s) of dysfunction 7.b Under the light of available information, clearly state how these results might assist in further investigative efforts (if required)

Definition of abbreviations and symbols: WR work rate, $\dot{V}_E$ minute ventilation, $\dot{V}O_2$ oxygen uptake, Pc capillary (arterialized) pressure, V_D dead space, V_T tidal volume, $\dot{V}CO_2$ carbon dioxide output, PET end-tidal pressure, SpO_2 oxyhemoglobin saturation by pulse oximetry, IC inspiratory capacity, IRV inspiratory reserve volume, EILV end-inspiratory lung volume, TLC total lung capacity, LT estimated lactate threshold, Ca arterial content, Cv venous content, RER respiratory exchange ratio, HR heart rate, ECG electrocardiogram.

Table 11.2 Cluster of findings to characterize individual patterns of dysfunction according to CPET

Physiological bases	Key CPET findings	Modifiers and comments
Obesity		
⇑ Metabolic cost of work	⇑ $\dot{V}O_2$ for a given WR	⇑⇑ In weight-bearing exercise
⇔ Work efficiency	⇔ Δ $\dot{V}O_2$ /Δ WR	⇑ In extreme obesity
⇓ End-expiratory lung volume	⇑ IC	⇓ In respiratory muscle weakness
⇑ Work of breathing	⇑ Dyspnea-WR, occasionally ⇑ dyspnea-$\dot{V}_E$	⇑⇑ In weight-bearing exercise
O_2 delivery/utilization impairment		
⇓⇓ O_2 delivery as exercise progresses	⇓ Δ $\dot{V}O_2$ /Δ WR	"Plateau" in severe impairment
Early shift to anaerobiosis	⇓ Estimated lactate threshold	Not always identified

(continued)

Table 11.2 (continued)

Physiological bases	Key CPET findings	Modifiers and comments
Increased anaerobiosis	⇑ [Lactate]	Needs additional measurements to standard, noninvasive CPET
⇑ Reliance on HR to increase CO	⇑ Δ HR/Δ $\dot{V}O_2$	Might be obscured by β-blockers
⇓ Stroke volume and/or ⇓ O_2 extraction	⇓ O_2 pulse	"Plateau" in severe impairment
⇑ Neural drive	⇑ Dyspnea-WR but ⇔ dyspnea-$\dot{V}_E$	Relate to sources of ⇑ drive
Central hemodynamic impairment	⇓ Cardiac output	Needs additional measurements to standard CPET
⇓ O_2 delivery relative to O_2 demand	⇑ $C(a\text{-}v)O_2$	Needs additional measurements to standard, noninvasive CPET
Impaired O_2 extraction	⇓ $C(a\text{-}v)O_2$	Needs additional measurements to standard, noninvasive CPET
Mechanical-ventilatory impairment		
⇓ ventilatory reserve	⇑ Submaximal $\dot{V}_E$ /MVV	MVV might overestimate ceiling
Dynamic hyperinflation	⇓ IC as $\dot{V}_E$ increases	⇔ If IC already ⇓⇓ at rest
⇑ Inspiratory constraints	⇑ V_T/IC, ⇓ IRV, ⇑ EILV/TLC	Adequate IC maneuver is critical
Tidal expiratory flow limitation	Tidal flow-volume loop "overlap"	Trapezoid/concave shape
Impaired lung mechanics	⇑ Dyspnea-WR and ⇑ dyspnea-$\dot{V}_E$	Relate to inspiratory constraints
Gas exchange abnormality		
Hypoxemia	⇓ SpO_2, ⇓ PcO_2	⇓⇓ In walking than cycling
Hypercapnia	⇑ $PETCO_2$, ⇑$PcCO_2$	⇑ As mechanical constraints ⇑
⇑ V_D/V_T or ⇓ $PaCO_2$ set point	⇑ $\dot{V}_E$-$\dot{V}CO_2$ relationship	⇓ As mechanical constraints ⇑
Ventilation/perfusion mismatch	⇓ Negative or positive $P(c\text{-}ET)CO_2$	Trending more informative
⇑ Neural drive	⇑ Dyspnea-WR, occasionally ⇑ dyspnea-$\dot{V}_E$	Relate to sources of ⇑ drive
Dysfunctional breathing-hyperventilation		
Chaotic breathing pattern	⇑ variability in V_T-f relationship	Standardize data averaging
Hyperventilation	⇑ RER, ⇑ $\dot{V}_E/\dot{V}CO_2$, ⇓ $PETCO_2$	Trending more informative
⇑ Neural drive	⇑ Dyspnea-WR but ⇔ dyspnea-$\dot{V}_E$	Relate to sources of ⇑ drive

Definition of abbreviations and symbols: WR work rate, $\dot{V}_E$ minute ventilation, $\dot{V}O_2$ oxygen uptake, Pc capillary (arterialized) pressure, V_D dead space, V_T tidal volume, $\dot{V}CO_2$ carbon dioxide output, PET end-tidal pressure, SpO_2 oxyhemoglobin saturation by pulse oximetry, IC inspiratory capacity, IRV inspiratory reserve volume, EILV end-inspiratory lung volume, TLC total lung capacity, LT estimated lactate threshold, Ca arterial content, Cv venous content, RER respiratory exchange ratio, HR heart rate, ECG electrocardiogram.

Table 11.3 Suggested cutoffs for key variables of interest to clinical CPET interpretation

	20 years		40 years		60 years		80 years	
	Males	Females	Males	Females	Males	Females	Males	Females
Metabolic								
$\dot{V}O_2$ peak (% pred)	>83	>83	>83	>83	>83	>83	>83	>83
$\Delta \dot{V}O_2/\Delta$ WR (mL/min/W)	>9.0	>8.5	>9.0	>8.5	>9.0	>8.5	>9.0	>8.5
$\dot{V}O_2$ at the LT (%$\dot{V}O_2$ peak pred)	>35	>40	>40	>40	>45	>50	>55	>60
Cardiovascular								
HR peak (bpm)	>175	>170	>160	>155	>150	>145	>130	>125
O_2 pulse (mL/min/beat)	>12	>10	>10	>8	>9	>7	>7	>6
$\Delta HR/\Delta \dot{V}O_2$ (beat/L/min)	<60	<85	<70	<90	<80	<100	<90	<105
Ventilatory/gas exchange								
$\dot{V}_E$ peak/MVV	<0.80	<0.75	<0.80	<0.75	<0.80	<0.75	<0.80	<0.75
$\dot{V}_E$ peak/MVV at the LT	<0.35	<0.40	<0.40	<0.40	<0.45	<0.45	<0.50	<0.50
$\Delta \dot{V}_E/\Delta \dot{V}CO_2$	<26	<28	<28	<30	<30	<32	<32	<32
$\dot{V}_E/\dot{V}CO_2$ nadir	<30	<32	<32	<34	<32	<34	<34	<34
f peak (breaths/min)	<50	<50	<50	<50	<45	<50	<45	<45
f/V_T peak	<28	<30	<28	<30	<28	<35	<30	<40
V_T/IC peak	<0.70	<0.75	<0.70	< 0.75	<0.70	< 0.75	<0.70	< 0.75
P_{ET} CO_2 at the LT (mmHg)	>43	>41	>41	>40	>39	>39	>37	>37
SpO_2 peak (%)	>93	>93	>93	>93	>93	>93	>93	>93
SpO_2 rest -peak (%)	<5	<5	<5	<5	<5	<5	<5	<5

Definition of abbreviations and symbols: $\dot{V}O_2$ oxygen uptake, WR work rate, LT estimated lactate threshold, HR heart rate, $\dot{V}_E$ minute ventilation, MVV maximum voluntary ventilation, $\dot{V}CO_2$ carbon dioxide output, *f* breathing frequency, V_T tidal volume, IC inspiratory capacity, PET end-tidal pressure, SpO_2 oxyhemoglobin saturation by pulse oximetry

(if identified) and at peak do not cross the cutoffs suggested in Table 11.3. It should be remembered that peak $\dot{V}O_2$ is usually interpreted as a single point in time. Thus, a "normal" peak $\dot{V}O_2$ does not rule out substantial loss of aerobic capacity in a subject with previous (but unknown) supranormal value. In apparently healthy subjects, it is useful to compare the timing of symptom progression with the development of lactic acidosis: a close temporal association gives an important clue in the genesis of subject's complaints. A test suggesting submaximal effort can be suggested in the presence of the following findings:

- A large HR reserve (peak HR < 85% predicted)
- A large ventilatory reserve (e.g., peak $\dot{V}_E$ / MVV ratio < 0.6)
- Large mechanical reserves (e.g., peak V_T/IC < 0.5, EILV/TLC < 0.8)
- Lack of substantial lactic acidosis (peak [lactate] < 4 mEq/L)
- Low peak RER (<1)
- Low end-exercise symptom burden (peak Borg ratings ≤ 3)

High symptom burden in an otherwise normal CPET should raise concerns on over-interpretation of the sensory consequences of exertion (e.g., chronic sedentarism) or, occasionally, malingering.

11.3.4.2 Obesity

Obesity has become an important cause of dyspnea on exertion. The metabolic ($\dot{V}O_2$ and $\dot{V}CO_2$) and cardiovascular costs of absolute work rate are increased in the obese as the subject needs to move a large body mass against gravity (i.e., even when moving the legs during cycling). The chemical efficiency in regenerating ATP per O_2 molecule (work efficiency), however, is not altered; thus, the absolute rate of increase in $\dot{V}O_2$ as a function of work rate remains close to normal ($\Delta\dot{V}O_2/\Delta WR$ ~ 10 mL/min/W). These considerations explain why there is an upward and parallel shift of $\dot{V}O_2$ as a function of work rate in the obese. The increased mechanical and metabolic costs and higher symptom burden may result in low peak WR. Owing to high $\dot{V}O_2$ for a given work rate, however, absolute peak $\dot{V}O_2$ values (L/min) might be close to normal (Fig. 11.3, *panel 1*). It is conceivable, therefore, that peak work rate gives a better picture of patient's exercise capacity. In weight-bearing exercise (cycle ergometry), simply dividing peak $\dot{V}O_2$ by body weight may underestimate subject's peak aerobic capacity (because body mass is, of course, much higher than leg mass). Expressing peak $\dot{V}O_2$ as % of predicted values based on height or ideal body weight is a fairer alternative. In case of low peak work rate but apparently preserved peak $\dot{V}O_2$, the former is likely to better reflect subject's peak aerobic capacity.

There is also higher than normal ventilation at a given submaximal work rate; however, when corrected to the equally higher metabolic rate ($\dot{V}CO_2$), the former is usually normal (Fig. 11.3, *panel 4*). Obesity is associated with lower EELV in most subjects, which increases the available volume for tidal expansion, albeit at significantly increased work of expanding the chest wall. Consequently, there is a downward shift in the operating lung volumes with relatively preserved inspiratory reserves at exercise cessation (Fig. 11.3, *panel 8*). Due to higher metabolic and ventilatory demands, obese subjects tend to report higher leg effort and dyspnea scores at a given submaximal work rate (Fig. 11.3, *bottom panels*).

In the morbid obese, impaired lung mechanics assume a more prominent role in limiting exercise tolerance. More extensive mechanical-ventilatory constraints result in lower than expected ventilation relatively to the higher metabolic demand, i.e., low $\dot{V}_E$-$\dot{V}CO_2$ slope and $\dot{V}_E/\dot{V}CO_2$ nadir. Thus, higher dyspnea scores are seen both at a given submaximal work rate and at a given ventilation. Patients with obesity hypoventilation syndrome might present with further hypercapnia and hypoxemia on exercise. There is also evidence that some obese women who report higher dyspnea ratings at any given ventilation tend to report greater unpleasantness and anxiety related to breathlessness following exercise. Thus, both the sensory

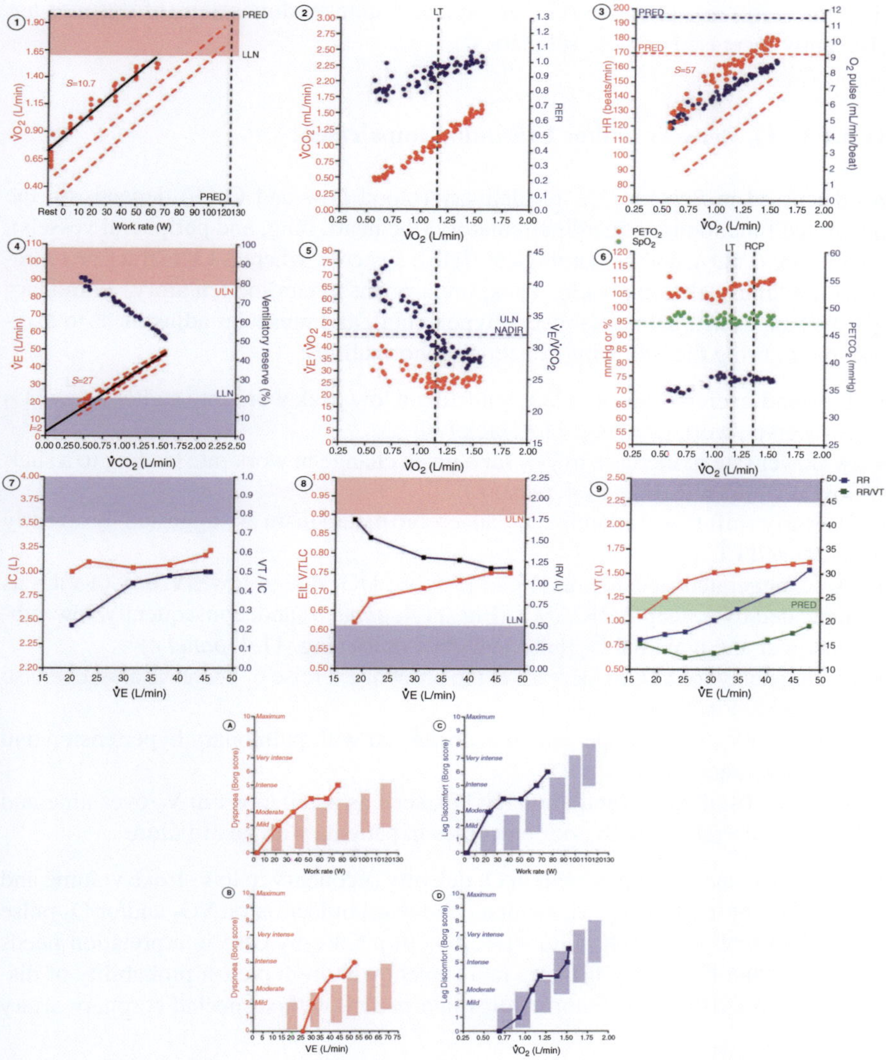

Fig. 11.3 Graphic representation of metabolic-cardiovascular (*first row*), ventilatory-gas exchange (*second row*), lung mechanics-breathing pattern (*third row*), and sensory responses (*bottom panels*) to incremental CPET in a 54-year-old apparently healthy woman, body mass index = 46.4 kg/m^2. Please see text for further elaboration. *Definition of abbreviations and symbols*: pred predicted, LLN lower limit of normal, ULN upper limit of normal, *S* slope, *I* intercept, $\dot{V}O_2$ oxygen uptake, WR work rate, $\dot{V}CO_2$ carbon dioxide output, RER respiratory exchange ratio, GET gas exchange threshold, HR heart rate, $\dot{V}_E$ minute ventilation, VT_1 first ventilatory threshold, PET end-tidal pressure, SpO_2 oxyhemoglobin saturation by pulse oximetry, IC inspiratory capacity, V_T tidal volume, IRV inspiratory reserve volume, EILV end-inspiratory lung volume, TLC total lung capacity, RR respiratory rate

(i.e., intensity) and affective (i.e., emotional response) dimensions of dyspnea are aberrantly increased in these subjects.

11.3.4.3 O_2 Delivery and/or Utilization Impairment

As discussed in Sect. 11.2.2, O_2 delivery (blood flow and CaO_2) depends on the integrated functioning of cardiocirculatory (the heart, lung, and peripheral vessels), respiratory (PaO_2), and hematological ([Hb]) systems, whereas O_2 extraction represents the “muscle” component. Thus, impairment in cardiocirculatory, pulmonary gas exchange (i.e., including severe hypoxemia), and muscular adjustment to exercise might bring the following cluster of abnormalities:

- Low end-exercise (“peak”) $\dot{V}O_2$ reflecting a low peak work rate and/or a low $\dot{V}O_2$ for a given work rate (Fig. 11.4, *panel a*)
- A slower rate of increase in $\dot{V}O_2$ for a given change in work rate leading to a shallow $\Delta\dot{V}O_2/\Delta WR$ (Fig. 11.4, *panel b*)
- An early shift to a predominantly anaerobic metabolism as suggested by an early estimated LT
- An exaggerated reliance on HR to increase DO_2 due to low SV or $C(a\text{-}v)O_2$ as indicated by a steep $\Delta HR/\Delta\dot{V}O_2$ (Fig. 11.4, *panel b*) and, consequently, low submaximal and maximal O_2 pulse ($\dot{V}O_2$/HR ratio) (Fig. 11.4, *panel c*)
- A long delay for $\dot{V}O_2$ to increase at the onset of exercise or decrease after exercise cessation (Fig. 11.4, *panel g*)
- Increased $\dot{V}_E$-$\dot{V}CO_2$ slope, which is correlated with pulmonary hypertension and poor RV function
- Exercise oscillatory ventilation (EOV), seen as oscillations in $\dot{V}_E$ over time and strongly correlated with poor outcomes in patients with heart failure

Of note, pronounced impairment in O_2 delivery secondary to low stroke volume and cardiac output might lead to a sudden downward inflection on $\dot{V}O_2$ and/or O_2 pulse at an abnormally low WR (Fig. 11.4, *panel c*). Case-by-case interpretation needs consideration of ancillary findings in a subject with high pretest probability of disease, e.g., coexistent ST abnormalities in a patient with suspected coronary artery disease.

It is important to recognize that noninvasive CPET without CO measurements is not particularly sensitive to detect mild cardiocirculatory disease. In fact, certain abnormalities (exercise-induced pulmonary hypertension or diastolic dysfunction) can only be reliably detected with invasive hemodynamic studies considering that a sizeable fraction of patients currently referred to clinical CPET have their resting and exertional HR under pharmacological or external control (e.g., β-blockers and pacemakers) or present with chronotropic incompetence, indexes based on HR should be viewed with caution in these patients. A severely blunted, or even flat, $\Delta HR/\Delta\dot{V}O_2$ in a subject expending maximal volitional effort should be clinically

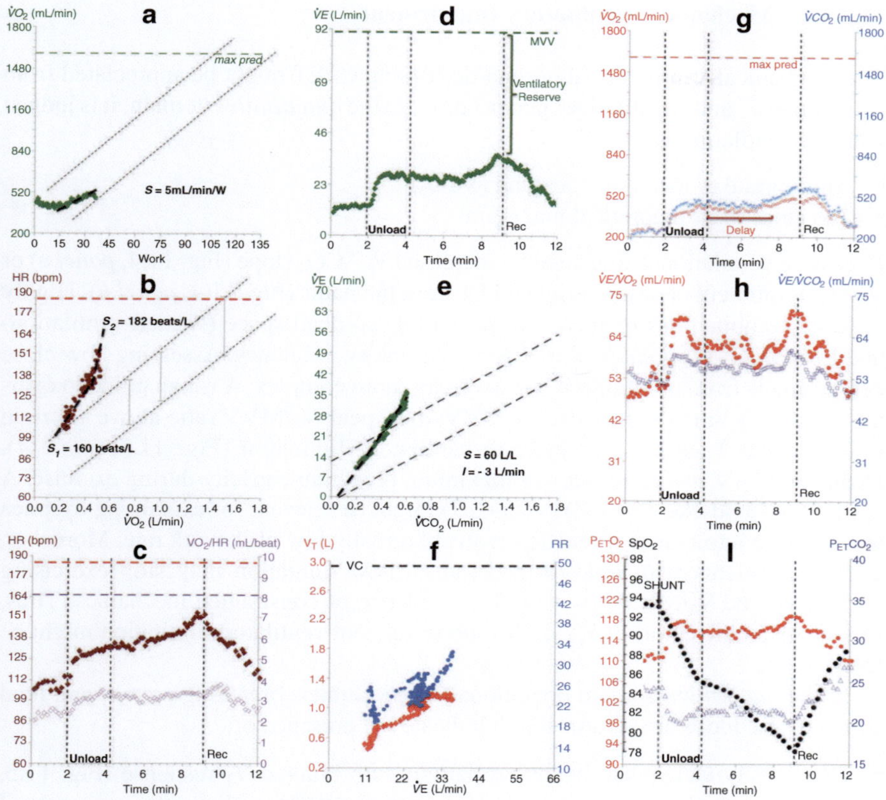

Fig. 11.4 Graphic representation of metabolic (*panels* **a**, **g**), cardiovascular (*panels* **b**, **c**), ventilatory (*panels* **d-f**, **h**), and gas exchange (*panel* **i**) responses to incremental CPET in a 23-year-old woman with combined O_2 delivery/utilization and gas exchange impairment due to pulmonary arterial hypertension (PAH) associated with congenital heart disease (*secundum* atrial septal defect). Please see text for further elaboration. Inspiratory capacity was not measured during exercise precluding assessment of noninvasive mechanics. *Definition of abbreviations and symbols*: S slope, I intercept, rec recovery, unload unloaded exercise, $\dot{V}O_2$ oxygen uptake, HR heart rate, $\dot{V}_E$ minute ventilation, MVV maximal voluntary ventilation, $\dot{V}CO_2$ carbon dioxide output, V_T tidal volume, RR respiratory rate, PET end-tidal pressure, SpO_2 oxyhemoglobin saturation by pulse oximetry. (Reproduced, with permission, from Neder et al. (2015))

valued as a potential source of exercise intolerance. In these cases, the measurement of CO is extremely useful in determining central versus peripheral limitations.

11.3.4.4 Mechanical-Ventilatory Impairment

The mechanical-ventilatory abnormalities during CPET might be appreciated from "quantitative" and "qualitative" perspectives. In the *quantitative* domain, it is judged whether ventilation is:

- Appropriate to metabolic demand ($\dot{V}CO_2$)
- Too close to its theoretical maximum

Excessive ventilation is indicated by increased $\dot{V}_E$-$\dot{V}CO_2$ slope (Fig. 11.4, *panel e*) or $\dot{V}_E/\dot{V}CO_2$ ratio either at the estimated LT or at the nadir (Fig. 11.4, *panel h*). Highly variable combinations of increased physiological dead space (wasted ventilation) and low $PaCO_2$ set point lead to a poor ventilatory efficiency. Assessing how close ventilation is from its ceiling is substantially more complex. A rough guide to overall ventilatory limits is provided by MVV; thus, peak $\dot{V}_E$/MVV ratio above a certain threshold has been used to indicate ventilatory limitation (Fig. 11.5, *panel 4*). However, MVV is a poor index of maximum breathing capacity during exercise. A "preserved" end-exercise $\dot{V}_E$/MVV (<0.7) might be relevant for explaining dyspnea and exercise intolerance if reached at an abnormally low peak work rate. Moreover, dyspneic patients with mild-to-moderate airflow limitation may stop exercising with preserved $\dot{V}_E$/MVV but with clear evidence of constrained mechanics. Thus, relying on single cutoff of $\dot{V}_E$/MVV ratio to rule out ventilatory limitation might be misleading.

In the *qualitative* domain operational lung volumes, breathing pattern and tidal flow-volume loops are scrutinized to indicate the presence of:

- Excessively tachypneic breathing pattern with blunted V_T response (Fig. 11.5, *panel 9*) which, in the right clinical context, might indicate the presence of heightened ventilatory drive and/or mechanical constraints
- Dynamic hyperinflation as indicated by decreases in IC > 0.2 L (Fig. 11.5, *panel 7*)
- Critical mechanical constraints induced by excessively high tidal volumes (e.g., V_T/IC > 0.70, IRV < 0.5 L, and EILV/TLC > 0.9 frequently leading to an early plateau in V_T) (Fig. 11.5, *panel 7 and 8*)
- Tidal expiratory flow-volume loop reaching or surpassing the maximal resting loop and proximity of tidal inspiratory flow to the maximum (Fig. 11.2, *right panel*)
- High dyspnea ratings as a function of WR and ventilation (Fig. 11.5, *bottom panels*)

Special attention should be given to correct technique in performing the IC maneuver during exercise, for instance, a low IC might merely reflect lack of stability in EELV just prior to the maneuver, insufficient inspiratory effort, or, in the right clinical context, exercise-related inspiratory muscle weakness. Patients with severe air trapping at rest may start exercising with low IC which cannot further decrease during exercise. Thus, lack of IC decrease from rest should not be misinterpreted as

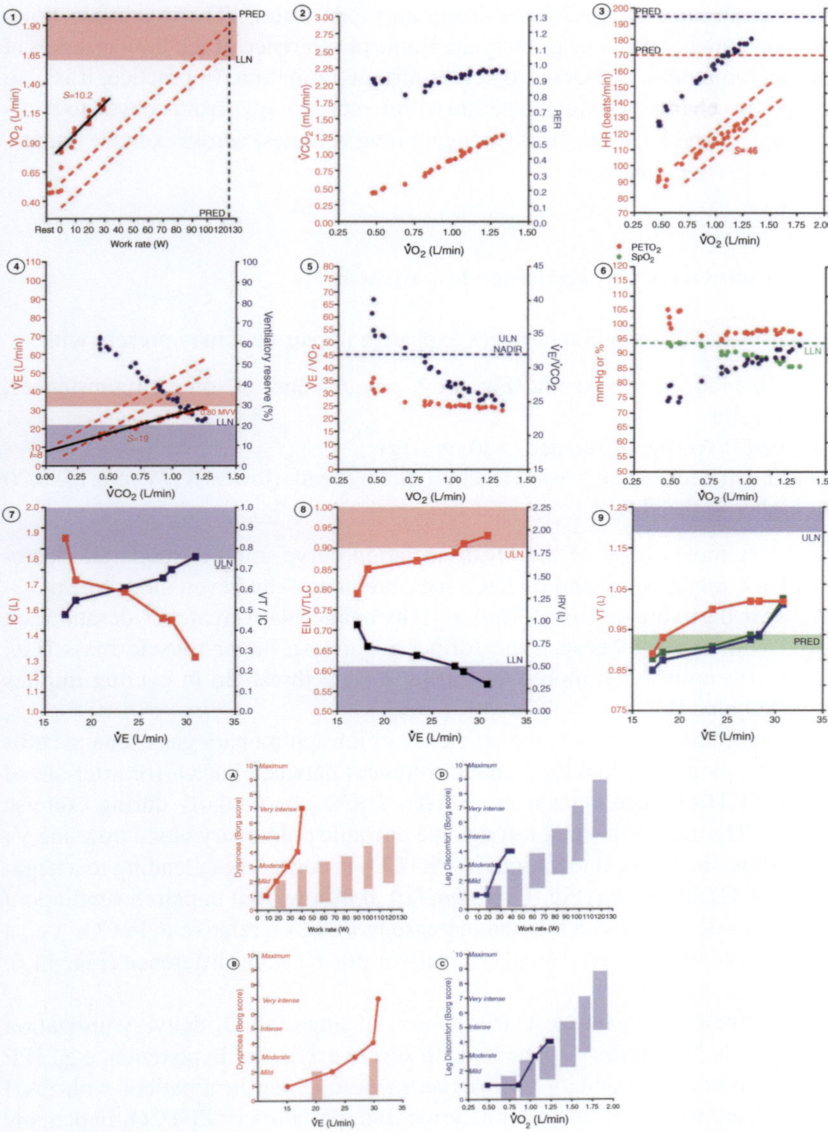

Fig. 11.5 Physiological and sensory responses to incremental CPET in a 53-year-old woman, long-term smoker (68 pack-years) presenting with severe dyspnoea and $FEV_1 = 1.02$ L (53% pred). Note evidences of mechanical-ventilatory impairment and, secondarily, gas exchange impairment. Please see text for further elaboration. *Definition of abbreviations and symbols*: pred predicted, LLN lower limit of normal, ULN upper limit of normal, *S* slope, *I* intercept, $\dot{V}O_2$ oxygen uptake, WR work rate, $\dot{V}CO_2$ carbon dioxide output, RER respiratory exchange ratio, HR heart rate, $\dot{V}_E$ minute ventilation, PET end-tidal pressure, SpO_2 oxyhemoglobin saturation by pulse oximetry, IC inspiratory capacity, V_T tidal volume, IRV inspiratory reserve volume, EILV end-inspiratory lung volume, TLC total lung capacity, RR respiratory rate

indicative of absence of mechanical-inspiratory constraints. The maximum flow-volume loop may not provide an adequate frame of reference of the flow reserves at a given lung volume in moderate-to-severe airflow limitation. In practice, it is also useful to assess changes on tidal expiratory limb morphology (from convex to rectified or concave) and leftward shifts (to higher lung volumes) across exercise intensities (Fig. 11.2, *right panel*).

11.3.4.5 Pulmonary Gas Exchange Impairment

Patients with significant pulmonary gas exchange impairment may present with:

(a) Exercise-induced hypoxemia (Fig. 11.4, *panel i*) and, in some circumstances, hypercapnia
(b) Enlarged $P(A\text{-}a)O_2$ difference (>20 mmHg)
(c) Insufficient decrease in wasted fraction of the breath (lowest V_D/V_T >0.15–0.20 but higher in the elderly)

Due to the sigmoid shape of the O_2 dissociation curve, mild-to-moderate decrements in PaO_2 might be missed by SaO_2 measurements – and even more by SpO_2 – due to noise in the oximetry signal. Walking is associated with greater O_2 desaturation compared with cycling because the former requires a larger muscle mass (i.e., lower mixed venous PO_2); moreover, earlier lactate threshold in cycling implies higher $\dot{V}_E/\dot{V}O_2$ and PAO_2.

Some important insights into the efficiency of intrapulmonary gas exchange efficiency can be gained by looking at the differences between $PaCO_2$ (or arterialized PCO_2) and $PETCO_2$. The latter overestimates $PaCO_2$, particularly during exercise when more CO_2 reaches the lung through the pulsatile pulmonary blood flow and V_T increases: thus, the cyclic fluctuations in $PETCO_2$ become larger, leading to a negative $P(a\text{-}ET)CO_2$ difference (Fig. 11.6, *panel a*). It follows that impaired ventilation/perfusion is associated with a blunted increase in $PETCO_2$ relative to $PaCO_2$, i.e., a trend to less negative (or even frankly positive) $P(a\text{-}ET)CO_2$ difference (Fig. 11.6, *panel d*).

It is important to emphasize that a pattern of impaired O_2 delivery/utilization might be seen in "respiratory" patients with severe exertional hypoxemia, e.g., IPF or right-to-left shunt secondary to *foramen ovale* opening in a patient with PAH (Fig. 11.4). Care should be taken for a correct interpretation of $PETCO_2$ in patients with respiratory diseases: low values may indicate high ventilation/perfusion and/or alveolar hyperventilation (Fig. 11.6, *panel d*). Conversely a high value might either reflect the late emptying of poorly ventilated units with higher $P\bar{A}CO_2$ or alveolar hypoventilation. Thus, "noninvasive" V_D/V_T (using $PETCO_2$) underestimates true V_D/V_T in patients with ventilation-perfusion inequalities and may be significantly inaccurate. Minimally invasive or noninvasive alternatives to $PaCO_2$ include arterialized (capillary) PCO_2 or transcutaneous PCO_2.

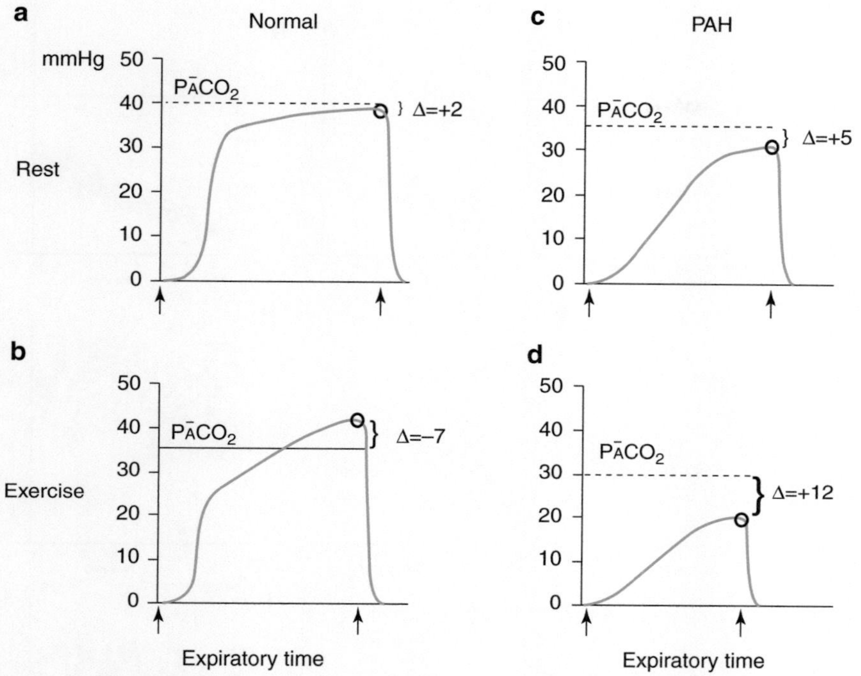

Fig. 11.6 Schematic representation of expiratory partial pressure for CO_2 ($PECO_2$) over a single breath at rest (*upper panels*) and exercise (*lower panels*) in health and disease. "Δ" is the difference between mean alveolar ($\bar{A}$) and end-tidal (ET) CO_2 partial pressures. At very early expiration, $PECO_2$ remains near zero as the first exhaled air comes from the anatomical dead space (with very low CO_2 concentration). Subsequently, $PECO_2$ increases faster: (a) the better CO_2 is washed out from mixed venous blood to the alveoli (better ventilation/perfusion matching) and (b) the more homogeneous the lungs empty. The last part of the exhaled tidal volume is less "contaminated" with the air from dead space; thus, it is biased to reflect alveolar gas which has the highest CO_2 concentration (end-tidal $PECO_2$; $PETCO_2$) (*panel* **a**). During exercise, $PETCO_2$ becomes *greater* than $PaCO_2$ in health (i.e., the $PaCO_2$-$PETCO_2$ difference becomes negative) due to the effects of (a) pulsatile increases in pulmonary perfusion with CO_2-enriched mixed venous blood, (b) faster and more homogenous lung emptying, and (c) a larger tidal volume leading to greater sampling of alveolar gas (*panel* **b**). In the presence of poor pulmonary blood flow (i.e., high ventilation/perfusion due to low perfusion), $PECO_2$ increases slowly thereby leading to a lower $PETCO_2$ (*panel* **c**); thus, $PaCO_2$-$PETCO_2$ difference fails to turn negative during exercise (PAH) (*panel* **d**). As expected, this abnormal response is worsened if a patient develops a shallow and faster breathing pattern as a relatively lesser amount of alveolar gas is sampled and expiratory time becomes too short. Additional decrements in $PETCO_2$ may occur if a PAH patient (alveolar) hyperventilates. (Reproduced, with permission, from Neder et al. (2015))

11.3.4.6 Dysfunctional Breathing-Hyperventilation

Subjects with an abnormal breathing pattern and/or symptoms compatible with hyperventilation are frequently referred for CPET for investigation of unexplained dyspnea. The main features in a typical patient with both disorders include:

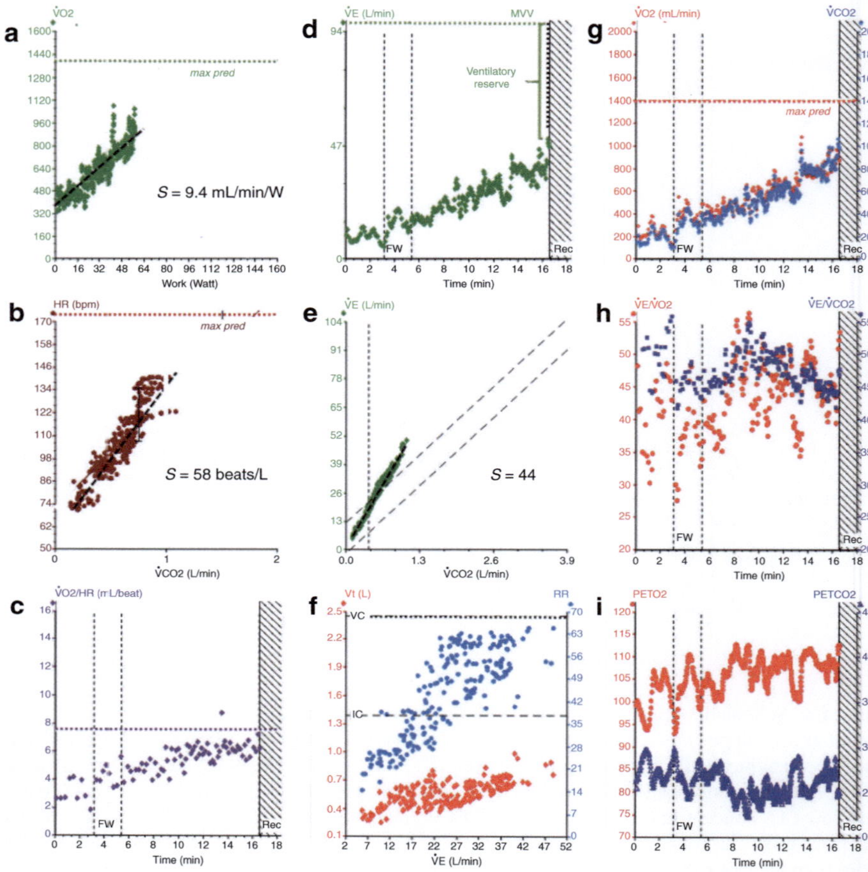

Fig. 11.7 Graphic representation of metabolic (*panels* **a**, **g**), cardiovascular (*panels* **b**, **c**), ventilatory (*panels* **d–f**, **h**), and gas exchange (*panel* **i**) responses to incremental CPET in a 38-year-old apparently healthy woman referred for investigation of shortness of breath of unclear etiology. The pattern of responses is consistent with dysfunctional breathing. Please see text for further elaboration. Inspiratory capacity was not measured during exercise precluding assessment of noninvasive mechanics. *Definition of abbreviations and symbols*: S slope, I intercept, rec recovery, unload unloaded exercise, $\dot{V}O_2$ oxygen uptake, HR heart rate, $\dot{V}_E$ minute ventilation, MVV maximal voluntary ventilation, $\dot{V}CO_2$ carbon dioxide output, V_T tidal volume, RR respiratory rate, PET end-tidal pressure, SpO_2 oxyhemoglobin saturation by pulse oximetry

- A chaotic breathing pattern with a trend to alternating surges of low V_T and high V_T in a background of fast *f* (Fig. 11.7, *panel f*)
- A clear dissociation between ventilation and metabolic demand as indicated by large variations in $\dot{V}_E/\dot{V}CO_2$ and $\dot{V}_E/\dot{V}O_2$ accompanied by similar, but noncyclical, fluctuations in $PETCO_2$ and $PETO_2$ (Fig. 11.7, *panel h and i*)
- High RER (usually, but not always, evident at rest) and steep $\dot{V}_E$-$\dot{V}CO_2$ slope (Fig. 11.7, *panel e*)

- High dyspnea burden for a given WR, occasionally associated with classical symptoms of hyperventilation (tingling, peri-oral numbness, light-headedness) which are largely the result of hypocapnia-induced cerebral vasoconstriction and regional hypoperfusion.

Hyperventilation is less commonly seen than dysfunctional breathing: due to a trend of rapid and shallow breathing pattern, most of the "extra" ventilation is wasted in the dead space and does not reach the alveoli. This explains why many patients with dysfunctional breathing do not present with symptoms of hyperventilation. Differentiating a chaotic breathing pattern from the normal breath-by-breath noise might be complex if the plotted data are not adequately smoothed. Care should be taken to rule out a cyclical pattern of ventilatory oscillation which represents an important sign of cardiovascular disease and/or breathing control instability (periodic breathing in heart failure with reduced ejection fraction).

11.4 Conclusions

This chapter provides the basis for a practical interpretation of CPET based on the identification of cluster of findings indicative of a given syndrome of exercise intolerance (Table 11.2). It should be recognized that those abnormalities commonly overlap in individual cardiorespiratory diseases, sometimes making this testing less useful to pinpoint a specific diagnosis. In the right context, however, careful association of CPET results with other available information (including laboratory and imaging findings) is valuable to answer clinically relevant questions in symptom-limited patients.

Selected References

American Thoracic Society. American College of Chest Physicians. ATS/ACCP statement on cardiopulmonary exercise testing. Am J Respir Crit Care Med. 2003;167:211–77.

ERS Task Force, Palange P, Ward SA, Carlsen K-H, Casaburi R, Gallagher CG, Gosselink R, O'Donnell DE, Puente-Maestu L, Schols AM, Singh S, Whipp BJ. Recommendations on the use of exercise testing in clinical practice. Eur Respir J. 2007;29:185–209.

Babb TG, Rodarte JR. Estimation of ventilatory capacity during submaximal exercise. J Appl Physiol. 1993;74:2016–22.

Babb TG. Exercise ventilatory limitation: the role of expiratory flow limitation. Exerc Sport Sci Rev. 2013;41:11–8.

Bernhardt V, Babb TG. Exertional dyspnoea in obesity. Eur Respir Rev. 2016;25(142):487–95.

Neder JA, Ramos RP, Ota-Arakaki JS, Hirai DM, D'Arsigny CL, O'Donnell D. Exercise intolerance in pulmonary arterial hypertension. The role of cardiopulmonary exercise testing. Ann Am Thorac Soc. 2015;12:604–12.

Neder JA, Berton DC, Arbex FF, Alencar MCN, Rocha A, Sperandio PA, Palange P, O'Donnell DE. Physiological and clinical relevance of exercise ventilatory efficiency in COPD. Eur Respir J. 2017;49(3) pii: 1602036.

O'Donnell DE, Elbehairy AF, Faisal A, Webb KA, Neder JA, Mahler DA. Exertional dyspnoea in COPD: the clinical utility of cardiopulmonary exercise testing. Eur Respir Rev. 2016;25:333–47.

O'Donnell DE, Elbehairy AF, Berton DC, Domnik NJ, Neder JA. Advances in the evaluation of respiratory pathophysiology during exercise in chronic lung diseases. Front Physiol. 2017;8:82.

Ramos RP, Alencar MC, Treptow E, Arbex F, Ferreira EM, Neder JA. Clinical usefulness of response profiles to rapidly incremental cardiopulmonary exercise testing. Pulm Med. 2013;2013:359021. https://doi.org/10.1155/2013/359021.

Whipp BJ. The bioenergetic and gas exchange basis of exercise testing. Clin Chest Med. 1994;15:173–92.

Chapter 12
Special Considerations for Pediatric Patients

Graham L. Hall and Daniel J. Weiner

12.1 Physiologic Considerations: Why Children Are Not Little Adults and Why Infants Are Not Littler Adults

The growth and development of the airways, lung parenchyma, and chest wall (i.e., the respiratory system) begins in utero and is not complete until an individual reaches their early to mid-twenties. Critically the pattern of lung growth and development means that the direct application of evidence from adults to infants, young children, and adolescents is inappropriate. For example, the chest wall develops rapidly over the first 12–18 months of life, and therefore the proportional contribution of the lungs and chest wall to respiratory system mechanics varies over time; accordingly, techniques that assess respiratory system mechanics need to be interpreted in different ways in infants compared to older children and adults. Similarly, work from the Global Lung Function Initiative has demonstrated that spirometry outcomes vary greatly through childhood and puberty and that the lower limit of normal for FEV1, FVC, and FEV1/FVC needs to be adjusted for age, sex, and height to ensure appropriate interpretation of obstruction can occur (readers are directed to Chap. 14 for further details). The following summarizes growth and development of the respiratory system and its potential impact on pulmonary function tests.

G. L. Hall (✉)
Children's Lung Health, Telethon Kids Institute, Subiaco, WA, Australia

School of Physiotherapy and Exercise Science, Faculty of Health Science, Curtin University, Bentley, Perth, WA, Australia
e-mail: graham.hall@telethonkids.org.au

D. J. Weiner
University of Pittsburgh School of Medicine, Pulmonary Function Laboratory, Antonio J. and Janet Palumbo Cystic Fibrosis Center, Children's Hospital of Pittsburgh of UPMC, Pittsburgh, PA, USA
e-mail: Daniel.Weiner@chp.edu

D. A. Kaminsky, C. G. Irvin (eds.), *Pulmonary Function Testing*, Respiratory Medicine, https://doi.org/10.1007/978-3-319-94159-2_12

Prenatal lung development occurs across five stages: embryonic, pseudoglandular, canalicular, saccular, and postnatal. Cartilage-containing airways are generally thought to be formed by 16 weeks of gestation with growth stimulated by fetal breathing movements that commence around week 10 and increase in frequency throughout pregnancy. The parenchyma begins to form by week 16 with rapid differentiation to form bronchioles (saccular stage), thinning of alveolar septa (saccular-alveolar stage) and increasing surfactant secretion, development of pulmonary capillary networks, and development of alveolar spaces (alveolar phase). Exposures that occur during pregnancy will impact on airway and/or alveolar development, dependent on timing, and can affect subsequent lung physiology both in infancy and later in life, with maternal smoking during pregnancy being a prime example.

Postnatal growth can be characterized as containing rapid growth during infancy and linear growth during childhood with further sex-dependent accelerating growth during puberty leading up to the peak of respiratory growth in the early 20s. Infancy sees rapid alveolarization until 2–3 years of age with further increases in lung volume by alveolar expansion, with vital capacity increasing over fourfold in the first 2 years of life. The chest wall rapidly stiffens in the first 18 months of life with progressive ossification until early adulthood. Respiratory growth during childhood is characterized by linear growth in the lung and airways and as a consequence is characterized by tracking of functional outcomes. Puberty sees rapid changes in thoracic dimensions, especially in males, leading to men having significantly higher lung function than women of the same standing height and age. While production of new alveoli is thought to continue until about age 8 years, lung size continues to increase with age reaching a maximum in the early 20s. Such increase in lung size seems to be mainly due to expansion in size of alveoli, although there is evidence that alveolarization and microvascular maturation may continue into young adulthood.

It is critical that pediatric health professionals consider lung growth and development when examining the role of lung function tests in the diagnosis and management of lung disease, the performance of tests and the interpretation of lung function outcomes. It is vital that the relevance of current guidelines for the performance and interpretation of lung function tests are assessed for both the age and disease stage with individual patients. For example, the role of spirometry in the management of a 5-year-old child with cystic fibrosis should consider the child's ability to perform acceptable and repeatable spirometry and the age dependence of lower limits of normal and changes in absolute lung function with age (and therefore the importance of using age-, height-, and sex-corrected predicted values). In addition, the generally milder stage of lung disease influences the relative sensitivity of spirometry to inform the clinician of important changes in clinical status. The following sections highlight specific tests and considerations in infants, preschool children, and school-aged children and adolescents.

12.2 Tests in Infants

12.2.1 General Issues

Infant pulmonary function tests (iPFTs) have many possible applications, which are generally the same as for the testing performed in older children. The most common use is to document the nature of and severity of disease states (e.g., obstructive vs. restrictive disease), to establish the effectiveness of certain therapies (e.g., bronchodilators), and to document the course of the illness overtime (e.g., serial measurements in patients with cystic fibrosis). Finally, utilized as an investigative tool, infant lung function testing can tell us much about normal lung and airway growth, an area which has been poorly understood.

Internationally, infant lung function tests have not been widely utilized clinically for several reasons, including:

(a) The need for specialized and generally expensive equipment
(b) The need for very experienced and specially trained personnel for their performance
(c) The need for sedation
(d) The duration of the test, which can easily exceed 2 h because of the need to administer the sedation and to recover from it
(e) The lack of standardized reference equations and interpretation of results
(f) Highly variable support of the provision of these services from healthcare authorities

The most commonly used infant lung function systems at the time of writing are the MasterScreen BabyBody system (CareFusion, San Diego, CA), the Infant Pulmonary Lab system (IPL, nSpire Health, Longmont, CO) and the Exhalyzer D system (EcoMedics, Duernten, Switzerland). A detailed analysis of the advantages and limitations of each of these systems is beyond the scope of this chapter, and readers are directed to the excellent series of recommendations for the use of and clinical utility of infant PFTs that have been published under the auspices of the American Thoracic Society and the European Respiratory Society. All systems allow the measurement of tidal breathing outcomes (e.g., respiratory rate, tidal volumes and flow), and options to collect forced expiratory maneuvers and static lung volumes are available. Some systems also allow respiratory mechanics (resistance and compliance) to be determined. As commercial systems do change over time and new systems become available, we have not detailed these here. For example, the IPL system from nSpire is no longer supported by the manufacturer but is still in use in some infant laboratories in North America. Specifics of certain techniques will be outlined in other chapters (e.g., refer to Chaps. 4 and 5 for details on the measurement of static lung volumes with plethysmography or gas dilution).

Importantly, most infant lung function techniques require sedation of the infant. In most infant pulmonary function laboratories, this is accomplished using oral chloral hydrate. Recently, however, this has been difficult to obtain in the United States, and alternative sedation strategies have been sought. Additionally, most toddlers find chloral hydrate unpalatable and achieving good sedation as children age can be challenging. As such, the clinician must balance these concerns against the information to be gained from testing and take these factors into account in determining frequency of testing.

Additionally, reference ranges used to allow accurate interpretation have originated from relatively small populations of healthy infants, and these are often equipment specific, limiting their broader use in clinical practice. It has been proposed that a control group of healthy infants always be used in studies utilizing infant lung function for research, but federal research regulations in the United States would typically preclude sedation of healthy infants, and this is not feasible for clinical practice.

12.2.2 Spirometry in Infants: RTC and RV-RTC

Detection of airflow obstruction, by physical examination or by quantitative measurement techniques, is facilitated by increasing expiratory flow rates. Older children or adults are asked to breathe out quickly and forcefully; for toddlers, a gentle "squeeze" of the chest during exhalation may elicit wheeze that is not heard during quiet breathing. In older children performing spirometry, patients are coached to inspire to near total lung capacity (TLC) and then to exhale rapidly and forcefully down to residual volume (RV). The maximal flows thus generated are indicative of airway diameter. Because infants cannot cooperate in this maneuver, other techniques have been utilized. The rapid thoracic compression (RTC) technique involves rapidly inflating a plastic bladder within a jacket that encircles the chest and abdomen of a sedated infant; the inflation is timed to occur at end inspiration. Expiratory flow (and volume by integration) is measured via a facemask and pneumotachograph, and a flow-volume curve over the tidal range of breathing (partial forced expiratory flow) can be constructed (Fig. 12.1).

Jacket pressures are increased until no further increases in expiratory flow occur. Instantaneous flows can be measured, the most common being the flow rate at the functional residual capacity (FRC) point, or end expiration (called V'maxFRC). By increasing flow rates over tidal flow values, the ability to detect abnormal airway function is enhanced. The RTC has been used serially to assess normal and abnormal airway growth and to gain understanding of airway function in a variety of disease states. One major limitation of the RTC technique is that measured flows are dependent on the lung volume at which they are measured. End-expiratory lung volume in infants, however, can vary dramatically because infants actively maintain FRC. Instability of the FRC point will limit the reproducibility of the flow measurements and may decrease the sensitivity of the technique to detect subtle changes in airway mechanics. Additionally, flows are measured over a narrow range of lung

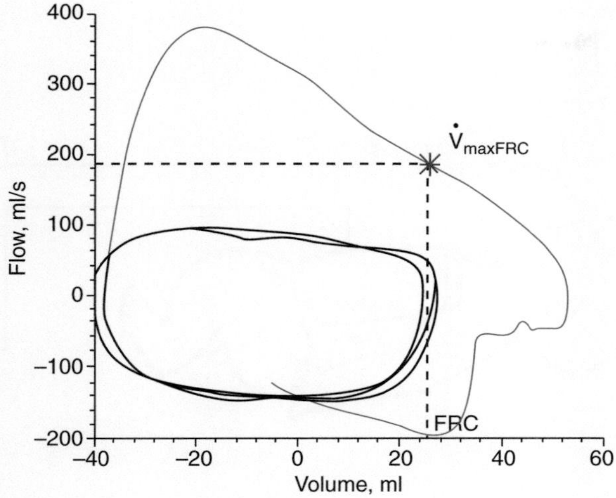

Fig. 12.1 Rapid thoracic compression method for measurement of forced flows. A partial expiratory flow-volume curve is depicted, where maximal flow is quantitated by extrapolating a line from the end-expiratory (FRC) point to the maximal flow curve. (Reprinted with permission of Nova Science Publishers, Inc., from Katsardis C, Koumbourlis A, Anthracopoulos M, Paraskakis EN, editors. Chapter 7. Infant pulmonary function testing. In: Paediatric pulmonary function testing: indications and interpretation. 2015)

volume (from slightly above FRC to slightly below FRC), unlike in traditional spirometry, where flows are measured from TLC to RV.

A modification of the RTC technique has been used to overcome the variability in lung volume at which flow measurements are made. In the raised volume rapid thoracic compression (RV-RTC) technique, the infant's lung is first inflated to a predetermined pressure (typically 30 cm H2O) with bias flow and occluded expiration (Fig. 12.2). The bias flow is directed into the lung by inflation of the expiratory balloon until the preset pressure is achieved. This results in an end-inspiratory lung volume close to total lung capacity (whereas the RTC technique begins measurement close to FRC). The expiratory balloon is then deflated allowing passive exhalation. Several such inflations are performed, resulting in mild hyperventilation and, as a consequence, a brief apneic pause. At this point, after one additional inflation to near-TLC, the plastic bladder is rapidly inflated to achieve maximal exhalation down to residual volume. The resultant flow-volume curves (Fig. 12.2) are highly reproducible with values being reported as timed volumes (e.g., FEV0.5, FEV0.75) in addition to instantaneous flow rates. This technique also allows for flows to be measured over a larger portion of the vital capacity.

Several studies have demonstrated that the RV-RTC technique is more sensitive than the RTC maneuver in detecting diminished pulmonary function in young infants. Moreover, the results from this technique are strictly analogous to the flow-volume curves obtained in cooperative children during standard spirometry testing and may help track or predict future lung function in children with cystic fibrosis.

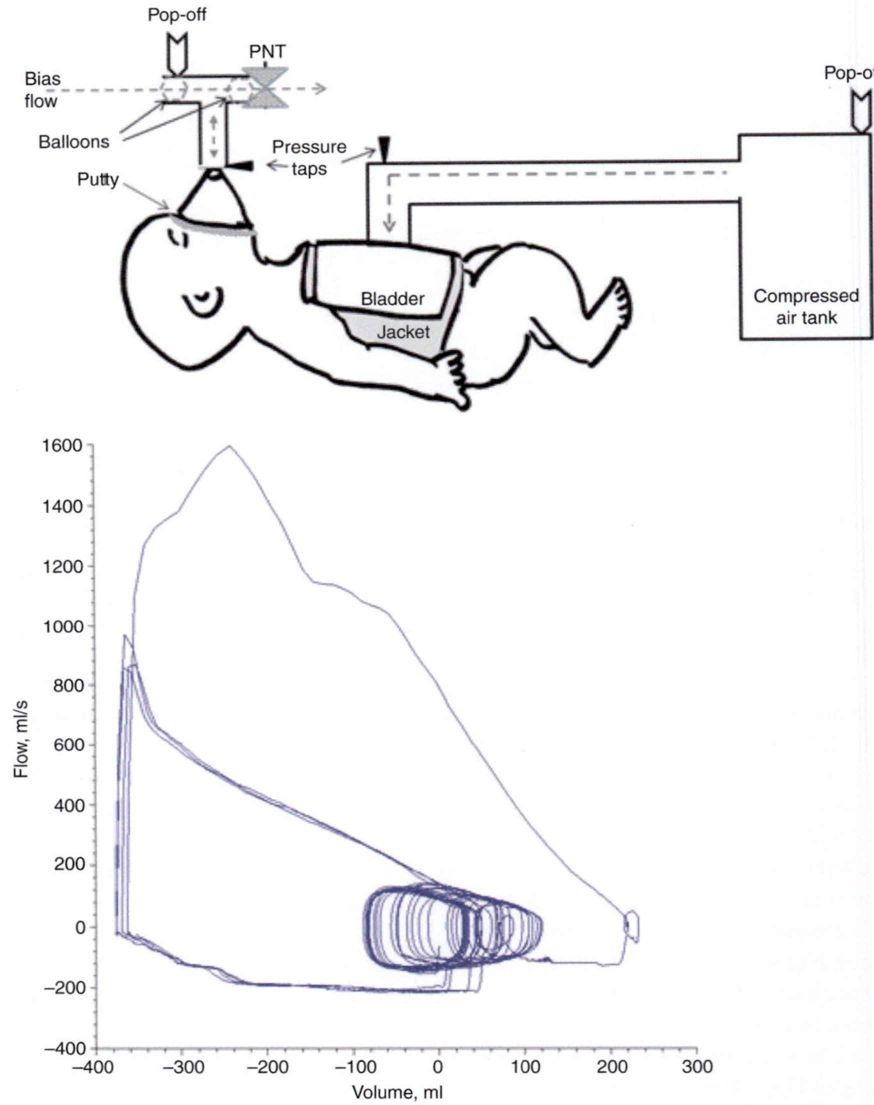

Fig. 12.2 Raised volume rapid thoracic compression method for measurement of forced flows. Above, configuration of patient, pneumotachometer (PNT), balloons and pressure taps, inflatable jacket, and inspiratory bias flow. Below, a full expiratory flow-volume curve. The largest curve represents maximal flow from a raised lung volume. The smaller curves represent passive exhalation after inflation. The numerous small curves depict tidal breathing before and after the raised volume maneuver. (Reprinted with permission of Nova Science Publishers, Inc., from Katsardis C, Koumbourlis A, Anthracopoulos M, Paraskakis EN, editors. Chapter 7. Infant pulmonary function testing. In: Paediatric pulmonary function testing: indications and interpretation. 2015)

12.2.3 Static Lung Volumes

Static lung volumes, most notably FRC, can be measured by dilutional techniques or body plethysmography in infants and young children. Theoretically, both techniques can be utilized to measure any lung volume (from residual volume to total lung capacity), but in practice, the lung volume measured is the resting end-expiratory lung volume (functional residual capacity, FRC) with some systems allowing TLC and RV to also be determined when combined with the RV-RTC technique as outlined above.

Gas dilution involves having the infant breathe, through a facemask, a gas mixture from a closed circuit with volume V1, containing a known concentration (C1) of an inert gas (e.g., helium, sulfur hexafluoride (SF6)) not taken up across the alveolar-capillary membrane. After an equilibration period, the final concentration of tracer gas is measured in the breathing circuit, and the principle of conservation of mass ($C1 \times V1 = C2 \times V2$) is used to calculate the volume that was added to the circuit (that in the lung of the infant, $V2 = V1 + Vlung$). Leaks in the circuit (especially at the facemask) will result in overestimation of the lung volume (as the final concentration of helium will be artifactually low). Also, non-communicating portions of the lung volume (e.g., due to airway obstruction) will not be measured, and dilutional techniques may underestimate the true lung volume in these cases.

The calculation of plethysmographic measurements of lung volume involves application of Boyle's Law: $(P1 \times V1) = (P1 + \Delta P) \times (V1 - \Delta V)$, where P1 is mouth pressure, V1 is infant's resting lung volume, and ΔP and ΔV are the pressure and volume changes during breathing efforts against an occluded airway. For these measurements, the infant is placed within a rigid closed container of fixed volume. The infant breathes through a facemask connected to an airway pressure gauge and a pneumotach to measure flow and volume. A shutter within the facemask can briefly occlude the infant's airway; continued respiratory efforts alternately compress and rarify the gas within the lung. Since airflow is absent when the shutter occludes the airway, pressure measurements made at the mask (airway opening) are reflective of alveolar pressure. By relating alveolar pressure changes to the volume changes in the plethysmograph (which are equal and opposite to those in the infant's lung), the volume of gas within the lung can be calculated. Plethysmographic measurements would include any gas in the thorax, including that in lung units subtended by obstructed airways.

Both approaches can be applied across the infant age range. One potential advantage of the gas dilution technique is that it can be performed during unsedated quiet sleep and therefore can facilitate the measurement of FRC and ventilation distribution (see below) across a wider range of ages than lung function tests that require more active effort. However, the potential decreased feasibility at older ages is a trade-off of unsedated lung function testing.

12.2.4 Tidal Mechanics

These techniques involve measurement of total respiratory system mechanics (compliance and resistance) during a passive exhalation. Compliance is defined as the volume change resulting from a change in pressure (*dV*/*dP*), while resistance is the amount of pressure required for a given flow rate (*dP*/*V*′). If the pressure is measured only at the airway opening (i.e., at the facemask in a sedated infant), the mechanics measurements are those for the respiratory system as a whole (including the airways, lung, and chest wall). These measurements do require that the respiratory muscles be completely relaxed.

The most common way of achieving respiratory muscle relaxation is by eliciting the Hering-Breuer (inspiratory) reflex. In the single-breath occlusion technique, the airway is very briefly occluded (typically 400–500 ms) by inflating a balloon on the expiratory side of a valve proximal to the facemask, while the infant is breathing at a lung volume above functional residual capacity (FRC), such as at end inspiration. Exhaling against the occluded airway, a brief apnea is induced and the muscles of respiration relax. The balloon is then deflated, allowing exhalation, and the lung empties passively due to its elastic recoil. The resultant passive expiratory flow is measured and plotted against exhaled volume (Fig. 12.3). This flow-volume curve can be used to calculate compliance (exhaled volume, extrapolated to zero flow, divided by airway occlusion pressure), resistance, and the time constant of the entire respiratory system (airways, lung parenchyma, and chest wall).

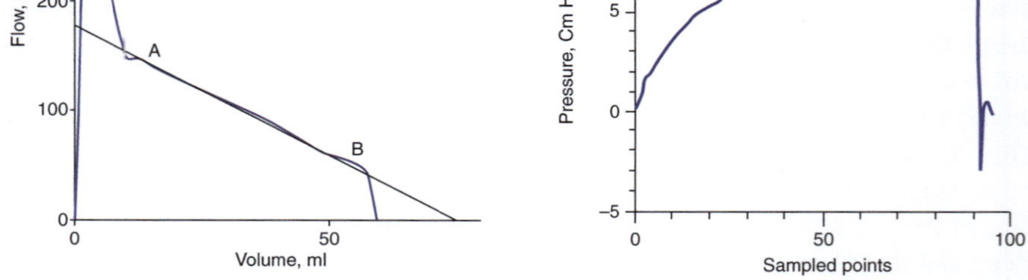

Fig. 12.3 The passive flow-volume curve (left) can be obtained by occluding the airway at end inspiration to invoke the Hering-Breuer reflex. A plateau in pressure must be observed for a minimum of 100 ms (right). Data is acquired at 200 samples per second, and sample number is displayed as a surrogate of acquisition time. The slope of the line A-B is the negative reciprocal of the time constant (τ). (Reprinted with permission of Nova Science Publishers, Inc., from Katsardis C, Koumbourlis A, Anthracopoulos M, Paraskakis EN, editors. Chapter 7. Infant pulmonary function testing. In: Paediatric pulmonary function testing: indications and interpretation. 2015)

This technique assumes that alveolar pressure equilibrates with airway opening (mouth) pressure during occlusions; this assumption may not be valid in the presence of severe lower airway obstruction. This technique also assumes that the entire lung behaves as a single compartment that empties uniformly. The time constant (τ), which is the product of resistance (cm H_2O/L/s) and compliance (mL/cm H_2O), describes how quickly the lung empties. It is calculated as the reciprocal of the slope of the descending limb of the passive flow-volume curve (mL/mL/s), thus yielding units of seconds. Longer time constants imply slower lung emptying. The resistance of the respiratory system can then be calculated by dividing the time constant by compliance. Limitations of this technique include failure to invoke the Hering-Breuer reflex and violation of the one compartment assumption, both of which can occur in infants with severe obstructive lung disease.

The forced oscillation technique has also been applied in infant populations. However, there is no commercially available equipment for use within this age range, and its use is generally limited to specialized research laboratories.

12.2.5 Ventilation Distribution

Measurements of gas mixing and ventilation distribution during infancy have been reported for many decades. However, it is only with the advent of commercially available equipment that the technique is gaining more widespread use in this age group. These tests utilize the tidal breathing of an inert gas (such as helium or SF6 – see Chap. 5 for full details) and can assess the evenness of ventilation distribution. Unlike in older age groups measurements cannot be performed using 100% oxygen washout, as the prolonged hyperoxia alters tidal breathing and resting lung volumes. One advantage of this measurement approach is that sedation is not required, and therefore this facilitates its use across a broader range of environments including epidemiological field studies. Similar to other infant PFTs, reference values are poorly defined and limit the accurate application of these tests to individual patients. Research groups using this technique have reported increases in the lung clearance index (LCI, a global marker of ventilation distribution) in infants with CF that worsens with pulmonary infection (Fig. 12.4) and structural lung disease. Early data suggest that outcomes of ventilation distribution may not be clinically useful in infants with recurrent wheeze or in infants born preterm.

12.2.6 Clinical Utility

The utility of testing in infants has long been debated, and in general the following have been seen as barriers to routine and widespread introduction of infant PFTs into clinical practice: (i) access to appropriate facilities, expertise and equipment, (ii) need for sedation, (iii) lack of reference ranges, and (iv) limited understanding of

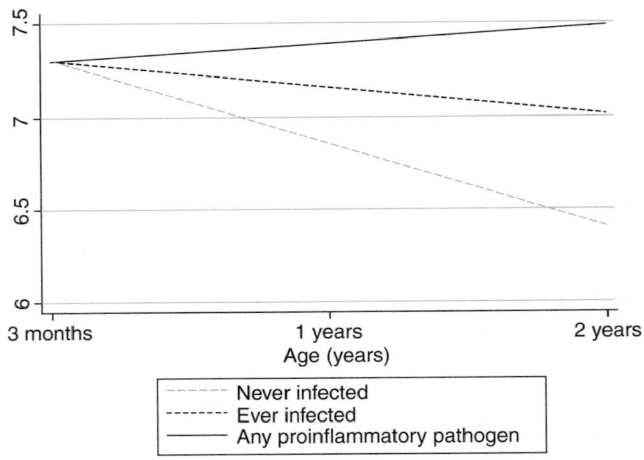

Fig. 12.4 The change in lung clearance index (LCI) over the first 2 years of life in children with cystic fibrosis. Linear mixed effects models were used to predict the association between LCI and the presence of pulmonary pathogens. (Reprinted with permission from Simpson et al. Progressive ventilation inhomogeneity in infants with cystic fibrosis after pulmonary infection. European Respiratory Journal. 2015;46(6):1680–90)

minimally clinically important differences in lung function outcomes with treatment or disease progression. Despite these limitations infant PFTs are used clinically and Godfrey and colleagues proposed the following indications for infant PFT in 2003:

(a) "The infant who presents with unexplained tachypnea, hypoxia, cough, or respiratory distress in whom a definitive diagnosis is not apparent from physical examination and other, less difficult investigations.
(b) The infant with severe, continuous, chronic obstructive lung disease who does not respond to an adequate clinical trial of combined corticosteroid and bronchodilator therapy.
(c) The infant with known respiratory disease of uncertain severity in whom there is need to justify management decisions."

As an example of this, Godfrey listed infants with tracheal stenosis for whom thoracic surgery was being considered. Much more common, however, might be infants with cystic fibrosis where management decisions might include hospitalization for intravenous antibiotics or initiation of mucolytic therapies. Several examples are included below to highlight how the testing can be used in clinical decision making.

12.2.7 Clinical Cases of Infant Lung Function

Case 1

An infant was diagnosed with cystic fibrosis by newborn screening (dF508/W1282X). She had several admissions in her first year of life due to poor growth and had a difficult social situation that including ongoing tobacco smoke exposure.

She presented for a pulmonary function test at 15 months of age. There were no crackles on examination or hypoxemia. This testing demonstrated marked reduction in flows, especially at lower lung volume ($FEV_{0.5}$ 45%, FEF_{75} 20%, FEF_{85} 14% predicted), as well as a decrease in vital capacity that may be due to air trapping (RV 145% predicted, RV/TLC 210% predicted). Following hospitalization, flows improved substantially ($FEV_{0.5}$ 77%, FEF_{85} 54%). In this situation, iPFT demonstrated that the severity of lung disease was worse than initially suspected clinically (prompting aggressive treatment with intravenous antibiotics). This testing could, in theory, also be used to determine duration of therapy as it is in older children; in this case, lung function did not completely normalize after 21 days of antibiotics.

Case 2

An infant presented at 8 months of age with inspiratory crackles and subcostal retractions. Hyperinflation was noted on chest radiography. She was initially evaluated for gastroesophageal reflux and aspiration which was negative. Computed tomography of the chest demonstrated patchy areas of ground glass opacity in the right middle lobe and lingula. Infant pulmonary function testing demonstrated a restrictive pattern on spirometry (FVC 53%, $FEV_{0.5}$ 56%), a normal TLC (80%), and marked air trapping (RV 170%, RV/TLC 205%). She subsequently underwent a thoracoscopic lung biopsy which revealed neuroendocrine hyperplasia of infancy (NEHI). The iPFT findings of this interstitial lung disease have recently been characterized, and some experts feel that classical findings of this disorder that include a characteristic CT scan and pulmonary function test obviate the need for an invasive biopsy.

Case 3

An 18-month-old infant with bronchopulmonary dysplasia (former 26-week EGA), pulmonary hypertension, and poor growth presented for infant lung function testing. This demonstrated severe obstructive disease ($FEV_{0.5}$ 57%, FEF_{85} 17%) with significant bronchodilator responsiveness ($FEV_{0.5}$ increased 31% after bronchodilator). She was treated with inhaled corticosteroids given the bronchodilator responsiveness, which was eliminated on subsequent testing. Her partial forced expiratory curves demonstrated that her forced expiratory flows were not very different than her tidal flows (i.e. she was flow limited during quiet breathing at rest). It was felt that her work of breathing was the likely explanation for her failure to thrive (wt-for-age <3rd %ile), and a gastrostomy tube was placed resulting in better growth.

12.3 Tests in Preschool Children

Preschool children (often considered those between 2 and 6 years of age) present unique challenges. They may be too large or difficult to sedate for infant/toddler techniques and too young to cooperate with traditional lung function maneuvers. In 2007 a statement on testing preschool children was jointly published by the American Thoracic Society, and European Respiratory Society reviews multiple techniques described below in detail, and readers are highly recommended to consult this and other more recent publications in this area.

12.3.1 Spirometry

Many studies have demonstrated that preschool children are able to perform spirometric maneuvers. Modifications of quality control criteria are needed to accommodate differences in children as younger children have lung volumes smaller than older children/adults and airways that are relatively larger for their lung volume. This results in more rapid emptying of lung volume (often in less than 1 s). As such, modifications to end of test criteria are required for preschoolers (no minimum exhalation time, but flow should decrease to less than 10% of peak flow prior to termination of effort). Many investigators have used timed lung volumes (FEVt) at times less than 1 s (e.g., $FEV_{0.4}$, $FEV_{0.5}$). Additionally, it has been suggested that back extrapolated volume up to 80 ml or 12.5% of FVC be considered acceptable (compared to 150 ml or 5% of FVC for adults). Some laboratories routinely employ graphical incentives with preschool patients, although there are conflicting reports about whether this is helpful and may instead distract young children. A learning effect is common in young children and significant improvements between successive test sessions are often noted. Respiratory scientists and pediatricians should be especially vigilant if individual children demonstrate significant responses to bronchodilators on spirometry that appear unsupported by other clinical data (see clinical case 4).

It is vital that suitable reference equations are used to allow appropriate interpretation of spirometry results. The most appropriate reference equations for spirometry are the equations published by the Global Lung Function Initiative in 2012. These equations commence at 3 years of age and extend beyond 90 years. Age-height-sex-specific equations for different ethnic groups are available, and these have been validated in a number of populations – see Chap. 13 for more details.

Bronchodilator responsiveness in young children can be assessed using spirometry using similar protocols to older children, and further details can be found in Chap. 7. It is thought that with the smaller lung volumes of young children a change in FEV of >150 mL and 12% may be inappropriate in this age group. As a result, a change in FEV1 of 10% is often considered to be clinically relevant; however it should be noted that there is little evidence on which to base this. Inhaled challenge tests using spirometry have been reported in young children, but the combination of effort required for spirometry and the time limits associated with most challenge test protocols severely limits the application of spirometry in this way.

12.3.2 Respiratory Mechanics

Respiratory mechanics in preschool children can be measured in a variety of ways including inductance plethysmography, the forced oscillation technique, and the interrupter technique. Of these the forced oscillation technique (FOT) and interrupter technique are the most commonly used in this age group.

Respiratory inductive plethysmography (RIP) is a well-established noninvasive technique that does not require any cooperation and assesses relative changes in thoracic and abdominal volumes, and the derivative of these volume changes can provide information about flow limitation. This technology remains a core feature of traditional polysomnography. The technique can allow for prolonged data collection and has been studied in a variety of diseases without sedation. However, it may be affected significantly by the chest wall and is not likely very sensitive to small airway dysfunction. There are no commercial systems available for performing RIP.

The forced oscillation technique (FOT) is a noninvasive measurement performed during tidal breathing that has been studied in preschool children. The equipment needed to assess respiratory mechanics using the FOT has advanced from research prototypes to being commercially available across a number of vendors. Most commercial systems apply an external pressure wave, across a range of frequencies, at the mouth, and the resulting pressure-flow relationship is analyzed in terms of respiratory impedance (Zrs) which includes frictional (resistive), elastic, and inertial loads. The respiratory system impedance is comprised of the respiratory resistance (Rrs) and reactance (Xrs) across the applied frequencies. The resistance includes the airways, lung, and chest wall, while the Xrs includes both the elastic properties of the lung at lower frequencies and the inertive properties of the airways at higher frequencies. Readers seeking detailed information on technical aspects of the technique are directed to Chap. 7.

Measurements using FOT measurements are performed in a sitting upright position with the child's head in the midline. Children maintain normal tidal breathing through a mouthpiece (usually incorporating a bacterial filter) while wearing a nose clip. The cheeks and floor of the mouth need to be firmly supported to minimize artifact, and in young children, this is best performed by a staff member to maximize test quality.

Measurements of FOT have been reported in children as young as 2 years of age with feasibility increasing from <50% in children under 3 years to over 90% by 5 years of age. Outcomes vary with lung growth, and appropriate reference values are essential. The forced oscillation technique can be used to assess reversible airway obstruction or airway reactivity. It has been reported to be useful in children with asthma and to assess changes on lung function in children born preterm. More recently its role in young children with cystic fibrosis has been questioned, and other preschool tests, such as the multiple breath washout technique, may be more appropriate in this patient population.

The interrupter technique allows the measurement of the resistance of the respiratory system, including the airway tree, lung tissue, and chest wall. Similar to the FOT, the main benefit of the interrupter technique is that it requires minimal patient cooperation. There are commercially available systems and methodological guidelines for its use in young children. The interrupter technique involves the rapid occlusion of the airway opening and the measurement of the flow immediately preceding the interruption and the changes in airway opening pressure (Pao) following the interruption. The interrupter resistance (Rint) is derived from the change in Pao by the flow. For full details of the technique, readers are directed to Chap. 7. Measurement of Rint assumes a rapid equilibration of alveolar and airway opening pressure and that the measured increase in Pao reflects the pressure drop across the whole airway tree.

Measurements are made with the child seated and looking directly ahead while breathing through a mouthpiece and with a nose clip in place and the cheeks firmly supported. The airway is occluded during expiration with the interrupter valve for a period of 100 ms at a flow equating to the peak tidal expiratory flow. A minimum of ten interruptions should be obtained with at least five acceptable measurements retained. Reference equations are available; however, these are equipment dependent and users should assess the compatibility of the methods used in the reference equation study to their own protocols.

Changes in Rint with short-acting bronchodilators have been quantified, and a decrease in Rint of >2.5 hPa.s/L or >30–35% of baseline is considered to confirm bronchodilator responsiveness. The interrupter technique has been combined with exercise tests and with inhaled challenge tests using methacholine and other challenge agents. While feasible in these settings, the most clinically relevant cutoffs to define airway hyperresponsiveness are not well known.

The clinical role of Rint in preschool children has been extensively reviewed, and readers are directed to the American Thoracic Society workshop report on optimal lung function tests in young children for details. The primary clinical role for Rint is thought to be in children with asthma, recurrent wheeze, or persistent cough. Similar to FOT, differences in young children born preterm have been reported, and its role in children with CF has been questioned.

12.3.3 Multiple Breath Washout (MBW)

The MBW method is used to assess ventilation distribution in the lungs and to measure the FRC, and full details of the physiology and technical aspects of the technique can be found in Chap. 5. The most commonly applied method in young children is the nitrogen washout approach, in which children breathe 100% oxygen via a mouthpiece or facemask until the resident nitrogen in the lung is washed out. Indices obtained from MBW include the FRC and measures of ventilation distribution, of which the lung clearance index (LCI) is the most commonly reported (elevated values indicate increased ventilation heterogeneity). Commercial systems are now available, and the American Thoracic Society and the European Respiratory Society have recently released guidelines for its use in young children.

The feasibility of MBW in young children increases with age and is generally >75–80% in children aged >5 years with more variable success in younger children. Reference values for FRC are available and are essential for appropriate interpretation. The LCI appears to be stable in most age groups including young children, and an upper limit of normal of ~7.6 has been reported, although further work in larger cohorts of children is required.

Measurements of MBW are gaining popularity in assessing young children with cystic fibrosis for several reasons, including that (i) it requires only tidal breathing, and as such can be performed in young children, (ii) the LCI derived from MBW appears to be more sensitive to bronchiectasis than traditional spirometry, and (iii) the changes in LCI with age are much smaller than changes that occur with other lung function measures.

There is a significant body of work supporting the role of LCI in clinical studies in cystic fibrosis. MBW is currently being used as an outcome measure in a study of hypertonic saline in preschool children with cystic fibrosis and has also been used to assess response to CFTR modulators. Early data suggests that MBW and LCI may be clinically helpful in young children with recurrent wheeze, although significant work is still required in this clinical population.

12.3.4 Clinical Cases in Preschool Children

Case 4

A 6-year-old girl is referred for lung function testing (spirometry pre- and post-salbutamol) and a clinical question of "query asthma." Parents report recurrent wheeze for 2+ years and diaphragmatic hernia that was "fixed" as an infant and no longer causes problems (Fig. 12.5).

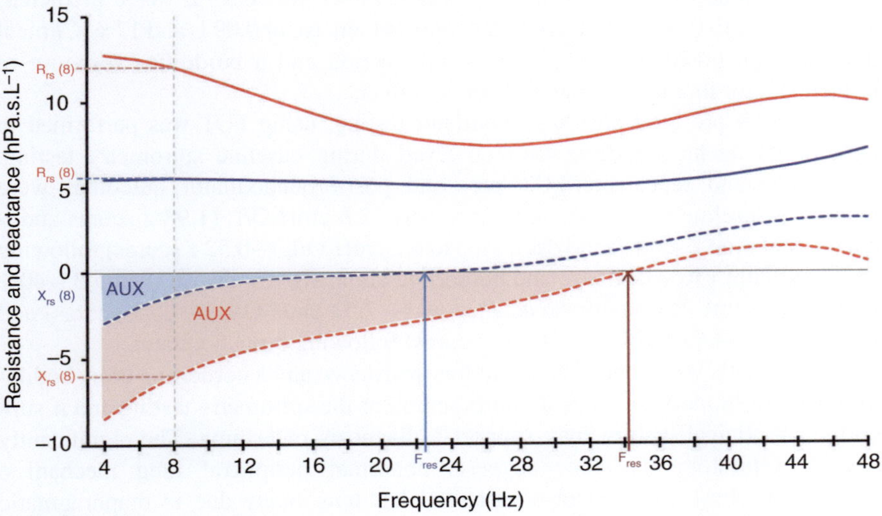

Fig. 12.5 Respiratory resistance (Rrs, solid lines) and reactance (Xrs, dashed lines) in a 4-year-old healthy child (blue lines) and an age- and height-matched child with chronic lung disease (red lines). Lung disease is typically seen to increase resistance and cause a downward and right shift in reactance resulting in an increased area under the reactance curve (AUX) and an increase in the frequency at which Xrs equals zero, which is termed the resonant frequency (Fres)

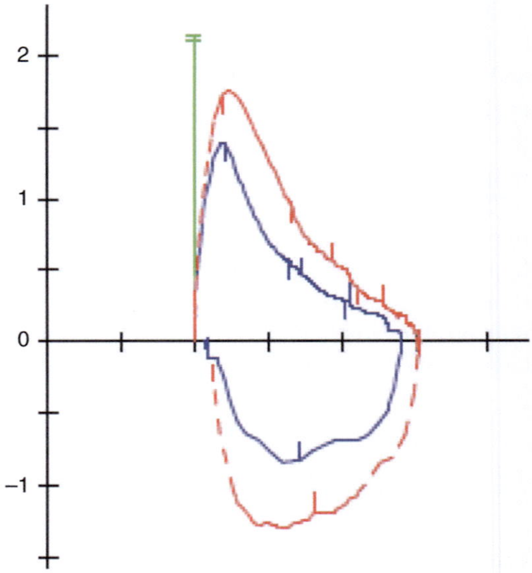

Fig. 12.6 Spirometry on patient in Case 4

Spirometry is attempted and acceptable and repeatable FEV but not FVC obtained pre- (blue) and post-salbutamol (red) (Fig. 12.6). FVC measures were limited by active inspiration at low lung volumes. The technical report from the laboratory correctly identifies that FVC should not be used and that technique improved following bronchodilator. Pre-bronchodilator FEV1 was 0.57 L (81% predicted) and increased to 0.66 L (94% predicted) and an increase of 0.09 L and 17%. Clinical interpretation noted some evidence of obstruction and a borderline response to bronchodilator that may be due to learning effect.

In parallel pre- and post-bronchodilator testing, using FOT was performed in light of the technique difficulties observed during baseline spirometry testing. Acceptable and repeatable FOT pre- and post-bronchodilator outcomes were obtained. Baseline respiratory resistance was 12.8 cmH_2O/L (1.98 z scores and > the ULN of 1.64 z scores) and decreased to 8.2 cmH_2O/L (−0.52 z scores) following bronchodilator (36% decrease and borderline clinically responsive (being 35–40% in the literature). Respiratory reactance was −7.53 cmH_2O/L (−4.5 z scores) and increased to −4.4 cmH_2O/L (−1.38 z scores) following bronchodilator.

These results with abnormal respiratory resistance and a borderline bronchodilator response support the clinical interpretation of the spirometry testing and if supported by clinical history may support a diagnosis of asthma. The significantly altered respiratory reactance suggests abnormal peripheral lung mechanics. Subsequent chest x-ray noted compressed left lung likely due to diaphragmatic hernia.

The use of measures of tidal breathing tests, such as forced oscillation or the interrupter technique in children in whom spirometry is problematic can provide supportive evidence or as in this cases provide additional physiological information of relevance to clinical management.

12.4 Tests in Children and Young People

12.4.1 How Practice and Collection of Standard PFTs Differ in Children and Adolescents When Compared to Adults

For most school-aged children and young people, completing lung function tests using the same equipment and protocols as adults is feasible and is routine practice. Clearly those children aged 6–8 years may find some tests more difficult to complete, for example, inhaled challenge test. However, with appropriately trained staff and space, most will succeed if additional attempts at a 2nd or possibly 3rd visit can be accommodated.

It should not be assumed that the staff training and resources and physical space appropriate in an adult service will be appropriate for children and young people. Engagement with children and families and having an open and welcoming environment are essential. Respiratory services should consider developing environments that allow for younger and older children to have space between them; laboratory designs that are open and airy and have access to natural light will be more welcoming and increase engagement with children and their families. Testing areas need to allow for multiple family members, while retaining privacy between families. Similarly, artwork and educational material should all be age appropriate.

Staff working within pediatric respiratory laboratories should have all appropriate qualifications as required for adult services. However, approaches that work for adults may not and often do not work in children or young people. Staff involved in lung function testing with children will need to be highly engaging; to be open to active role playing, especially in young children; and to have an ability to be at the child's level. It is not uncommon to have to ask parents to leave the testing suite to get the best out of a child, and this requires tact and diplomacy.

Testing standards and definitions of acceptability and repeatability are generally based on evidence from adults and in many cases from older adults with advanced lung disease. It is critical therefore that senior respiratory scientists and their medical directors carefully consider current guidelines for all lung function tests that are offered and ensure that these are age appropriate.

12.4.2 Considerations for Reference Values and Impact of Puberty

Historically, reference values have been developed for separate pediatric and adult populations. While this facilitated appropriate data in the respective age groups, it often created problems at the age at which individuals switched from one equation to the next. Further to this was low numbers of individuals across puberty and thus a highly variable approach to statistical modeling of regression equations through this period of rapid growth.

The advent of the Global Lung Function Initiative reference equations for spirometry in 2012 and gas transfer in 2017 has significantly advanced the appropriate interpretation of lung function in adolescent patients. However, until similar data are available for other lung function tests, health professionals will need to be vigilant when tracking individual patients across puberty and ensure that changes in predicted lung function are not over-interpreted to be related to disease severity in the absence of other clinical signs and symptoms.

Further details on reference values and their application are available in Chap. 13.

12.4.3 Limited Evidence of Interpretation and Relevance in These Age Groups

Much of our data as it relates to the interpretation of lung function outcomes, and their use in the management of children and young people with lung disease, is based on evidence derived from older adults. Considerations as to the impact of age on lung function outcomes, including puberty and the progression of lung disease and differences in the pathophysiology of disease in children, are vital.

As an example, definitions of bronchodilator responsiveness as being >12% and >150 mL increase in FEV_1 are derived from large cohorts of older adults. Studies in children have suggested that a change of ~10% may be more appropriate, and the use of a percent increase matched with an absolute change (150 mL) in children, and especially younger children, has been questioned.

As such while basing practice on current guidelines is essential, the evidence base within these guidelines should be assessed carefully and their application to children and the specific referral population of the individual pediatric lung function service formally tested.

In summary, there are a range of established and emerging lung function tests that can be used in infants, preschool, and school-aged children. These offer new insights in the diagnosis and management of lung disease in the pediatric age range. Health professionals in pediatric respiratory science and medicine should continually assess the evidence base and ensure that their practice suits their own clinical service.

Selected References

American Thoracic Society, European Respiratory Society. ATS/ERS statement: raised volume forced expirations in infants: guidelines for current practice. Am J Respir Crit Care Med. 2005;172(11):1463–71.

Aurora P. Multiple-breath inert gas washout test and early cystic fibrosis lung disease. Thorax. 2010;65(5):373–4.

Aurora P, Bush A, Gustafsson P, Oliver C, Wallis C, Price J, et al. Multiple-breath washout as a marker of lung disease in preschool children with cystic fibrosis. Am J Respir Crit Care Med. 2005;171(3):249–56.

Bar-Yishay E, Springer C, Hevroni A, Godfrey S. Relation between partial and raised volume forced expiratory flows in sick infants. Pediatr Pulmonol. 2011;46(5):458–63.

Bates JH, Schmalisch G, Filbrun D, Stocks J. Tidal breath analysis for infant pulmonary function testing. ERS/ATS task force on standards for infant respiratory function testing. European Respiratory Society/American Thoracic Society. Eur Respir J. 2000;16(6):1180–92.

Bonner R, Lum S, Stocks J, Kirkby J, Wade A, Sonnappa S. Applicability of the global lung function spirometry equations in contemporary multiethnic children. Am J Respir Crit Care Med. 2013;188(4):515–6.

Cooper BG, Stocks J, Hall GL, Culver B, Steenbruggen I, Carter KW, et al. The global lung function initiative (GLI) network: bringing the world's respiratory reference values together. Breathe (Sheff). 2017;13(3):e56–64.

Davis SD, Rosenfeld M, Kerby GS, Brumback L, Kloster MH, Acton JD, et al. Multicenter evaluation of infant lung function tests as cystic fibrosis clinical trial endpoints. Am J Respir Crit Care Med. 2010;182(11):1387–97.

Dundas I, Beardsmore C, Wellman T, Stocks J. A collaborative study of infant respiratory function testing. Eur Respir J. 1998;12(4):944–53.

Fauroux B, Khirani S. Neuromuscular disease and respiratory physiology in children: putting lung function into perspective. Respirology. 2014;19(6):782–91.

Frey U, Stocks J, Coates A, Sly P, Bates J. Specifications for equipment used for infant pulmonary function testing. ERS/ATS task force on standards for infant respiratory function testing. European Respiratory Society/American Thoracic Society. Eur Respir J. 2000a;16(4):731–40.

Frey U, Stocks J, Sly P, Bates J. Specification for signal processing and data handling used for infant pulmonary function testing. ERS/ATS task force on standards for infant respiratory function testing. European Respiratory Society/American Thoracic Society. Eur Respir J. 2000b;16(5):1016–22.

Godfrey S, Bar-Yishay E, Avital A, Springer C. What is the role of tests of lung function in the management of infants with lung disease? Pediatr Pulmonol. 2003;36(1):1–9.

Gustafsson PM. Inert gas washout in preschool children. Paediatr Respir Rev. 2005;6(4):239–45.

Gustafsson PM, De Jong PA, Tiddens HA, Lindblad A. Multiple-breath inert gas washout and spirometry versus structural lung disease in cystic fibrosis. Thorax. 2008;63(2):129–34.

Hall GL, Thompson BR, Stanojevic S, Abramson MJ, Beasley R, Coates A, et al. The global lung initiative 2012 reference values reflect contemporary Australasian spirometry. Respirology. 2012;17(7):1150–1.

Hayden MJ, Devadason SG, Sly PD, Wildhaber JH, LeSouef PN. Methacholine responsiveness using the raised volume forced expiration technique in infants. Am J Respir Crit Care Med. 1997a;155(5):1670–5.

Hayden MJ, Sly PD, Devadason SG, Gurrin LC, Wildhaber JH, LeSouef PN. Influence of driving pressure on raised-volume forced expiration in infants. Am J Respir Crit Care Med. 1997b;156(6):1876–83.

Hayden MJ, Wildhaber JH, LeSouef PN. Bronchodilator responsiveness testing using raised volume forced expiration in recurrently wheezing infants. Pediatr Pulmonol. 1998;26(1):35–41.

Irvin CG, Hall GL. An epilogue to lung function and lung disease: state-of-the-art 2015. Respirology. 2015;20(7):1008–9.

Khirani S, Dabaj I, Amaddeo A, Ramirez A, Quijano-Roy S, Fauroux B. The value of respiratory muscle testing in a child with congenital muscular dystrophy. Respirol Case Rep. 2014;2(3):95–8.

Lai SH, Liao SL, Yao TC, Tsai MH, Hua MC, Chiu CY, et al. Raised-volume forced expiratory flow-volume curve in healthy Taiwanese infants. Sci Rep. 2017;7(1):6314.

Linnane BM, Hall GL, Nolan G, Brennan S, Stick SM, Sly PD, et al. Lung function in infants with cystic fibrosis diagnosed by newborn screening. Am J Respir Crit Care Med. 2008;178(12):1238–44.

Lum S, Hoo AF, Stocks J. Effect of airway inflation pressure on forced expiratory maneuvers from raised lung volume in infants. Pediatr Pulmonol. 2002a;33(2):130–4.

Lum S, Hoo AF, Stocks J. Influence of jacket tightness and pressure on raised lung volume forced expiratory maneuvers in infants. Pediatr Pulmonol. 2002b;34(5):361–8.

Morris MG. Comprehensive integrated spirometry using raised volume passive and forced expirations and multiple-breath nitrogen washout in infants. Respir Physiol Neurobiol. 2010;170(2):123–40.

Morris MG. Nasal versus oronasal raised volume forced expirations in infants – a real physiologic challenge. Pediatr Pulmonol. 2012;47(8):780–94.

Morris MG, Gustafsson P, Tepper R, Gappa M, Stocks J, ERS/ATS Task Force on Standards for Infant Respiratory Function Testing. The bias flow nitrogen washout technique for measuring the functional residual capacity in infants. ERS/ATS Task Force on Standards for Infant Respiratory Function Testing. Eur Respir J. 2001;17(3):529–36.

Peterson-Carmichael SL, Rosenfeld M, Ascher SB, Hornik CP, Arets HG, Davis SD, et al. Survey of clinical infant lung function testing practices. Pediatr Pulmonol. 2014;49(2):126–31.

Pillarisetti N, Williamson E, Linnane B, Skoric B, Robertson CF, Robinson P, et al. Infection, inflammation, and lung function decline in infants with cystic fibrosis. Am J Respir Crit Care Med. 2011;184(1):75–81.

Pillow JJ, Frerichs I, Stocks J. Lung function tests in neonates and infants with chronic lung disease: global and regional ventilation inhomogeneity. Pediatr Pulmonol. 2006;41(2):105–21.

Quanjer PH, Stocks J, Cole TJ, Hall GL, Stanojevic S, Global Lungs I. Influence of secular trends and sample size on reference equations for lung function tests. Eur Respir J. 2011;37(3):658–64.

Quanjer PH, Stanojevic S, Cole TJ, Baur X, Hall GL, Culver BH, et al. Multi-ethnic reference values for spirometry for the 3-95-yr age range: the global lung function 2012 equations. Eur Respir J. 2012;40(6):1324–43.

Ramsey KA, Ranganathan S. Interpretation of lung function in infants and young children with cystic fibrosis. Respirology. 2014;19(6):792–9.

Ramsey KA, Ranganathan S, Park J, Skoric B, Adams AM, Simpson SJ, et al. Early respiratory infection is associated with reduced spirometry in children with cystic fibrosis. Am J Respir Crit Care Med. 2014;190(10):1111–6.

Ramsey KA, Ranganathan SC, Gangell CL, Turkovic L, Park J, Skoric B, et al. Impact of lung disease on respiratory impedance in young children with cystic fibrosis. Eur Respir J. 2015a;46(6):1672–9.

Ramsey KA, Schultz A, Stick SM. Biomarkers in paediatric cystic fibrosis lung disease. Paediatr Respir Rev. 2015b;16(4):213–8.

Ramsey KA, Rosenow T, Turkovic L, Skoric B, Banton G, Adams AM, et al. Lung clearance index and structural lung disease on computed tomography in early cystic fibrosis. Am J Respir Crit Care Med. 2016;193(1):60–7.

Ranganathan SC, Hoo AF, Lum SY, Goetz I, Castle RA, Stocks J. Exploring the relationship between forced maximal flow at functional residual capacity and parameters of forced expiration from raised lung volume in healthy infants. Pediatr Pulmonol. 2002;33(6):419–28.

Ranganathan SC, Hall GL, Sly PD, Stick SM, Douglas TA, Australian Respiratory Early Surveillance Team for Cystic Fibrosis. Early lung disease in infants and preschool children with cystic fibrosis. What have we learned and what should we do about it? Am J Respir Crit Care Med. 2017;195(12):1567–75.

Robinson PD, Latzin P, Verbanck S, Hall GL, Horsley A, Gappa M, et al. Consensus statement for inert gas washout measurement using multiple- and single- breath tests. Eur Respir J. 2013;41(3):507–22.

Robinson PD, Latzin P, Ramsey KA, Stanojevic S, Aurora P, Davis SD, et al. Preschool multiple-breath washout testing. An Official American Thoracic Society Technical Statement. Am J Respir Crit Care Med. 2018;197(5):e1–e19.

Rosenfeld M, Allen J, Arets BH, Aurora P, Beydon N, Calogero C, et al. An official American Thoracic Society workshop report: optimal lung function tests for monitoring cystic fibrosis, bronchopulmonary dysplasia, and recurrent wheezing in children less than 6 years of age. Ann Am Thorac Soc. 2013;10(2):S1–S11.

Rosenow T, Ramsey K, Turkovic L, Murray CP, Mok LC, Hall GL, et al. Air trapping in early cystic fibrosis lung disease-does CT tell the full story? Pediatr Pulmonol. 2017;52(9):1150–6.

Schibler A, Hall GL, Businger F, Reinmann B, Wildhaber JH, Cernelc M, et al. Measurement of lung volume and ventilation distribution with an ultrasonic flow meter in healthy infants. Eur Respir J. 2002;20(4):912–8.

Schittny JC. Development of the lung. Cell Tissue Res. 2017;367:427–44.

Schmalisch G, Schmidt M, Foitzik B. Novel technique to average breathing loops for infant respiratory function testing. Med Biol Eng Comput. 2001;39(6):688–93.

Schulzke SM, Hall GL, Nathan EA, Simmer K, Nolan G, Pillow JJ. Lung volume and ventilation inhomogeneity in preterm infants at 15-18 months corrected age. J Pediatr. 2010;156(4):542–9.e2.

Simpson SJ, Hall GL, Wilson AC. Lung function following very preterm birth in the era of 'new' bronchopulmonary dysplasia. Respirology. 2015;20(4):535–40.

Simpson SJ, Logie KM, O'Dea CA, Banton GL, Murray C, Wilson AC, et al. Altered lung structure and function in mid-childhood survivors of very preterm birth. Thorax. 2017;72(8):702–11.

Sly PD, Tepper R, Henschen M, Gappa M, Stocks J. Tidal forced expirations. ERS/ATS task force on standards for infant respiratory function testing. European Respiratory Society/American Thoracic Society. Eur Respir J. 2000;16(4):741–8.

Stanojevic S, Stocks J, Bountziouka V, Aurora P, Kirkby J, Bourke S, et al. The impact of switching to the new global lung function initiative equations on spirometry results in the UK CF registry. J Cyst Fibros. 2014;13(3):319–27.

Stanojevic S, Bilton D, McDonald A, Stocks J, Aurora P, Prasad A, et al. Global lung function initiative equations improve interpretation of FEV1 decline among patients with cystic fibrosis. Eur Respir J. 2015;46(1):262–4.

Stanojevic S, Graham BL, Cooper BG, Thompson BR, Carter KW, Francis RW, et al. Official ERS technical standards: global lung function initiative reference values for the carbon monoxide transfer factor for Caucasians. Eur Respir J. 2017;50(3):1700010.

Stocks J. Infant respiratory function testing: is it worth all the effort? Paediatr Anaesth. 2004;14(7):537–40.

Stocks J, Quanjer PH. Reference values for residual volume, functional residual capacity and total lung capacity. ATS Workshop on Lung Volume Measurements. Official Statement of the European Respiratory Society. Eur Respir J. 1995;8(3):492–506.

Stocks J, Sly PD, Morris MG, Frey U. Standards for infant respiratory function testing: what(ever) next? Eur Respir J. 2000;16(4):581–4.

Stocks J, Godfrey S, Beardsmore C, Bar-Yishay E, Castile R, ERS/ATS Task Force on Standards for Infant Respiratory Function Testing. Plethysmographic measurements of lung volume and airway resistance. Eur Respir J. 2001;17(2):302–12.

Subbarao P, Milla C, Aurora P, Davies JC, Davis SD, Hall GL, et al. Multiple-breath washout as a lung function test in cystic fibrosis. A Cystic Fibrosis Foundation Workshop Report. Ann Am Thorac Soc. 2015;12(6):932–9.

Turner DJ, Lanteri CJ, LeSouef PN, Sly PD. Improved detection of abnormal respiratory function using forced expiration from raised lung volume in infants with cystic fibrosis. Eur Respir J. 1994;7(11):1995–9.

Turner DJ, Stick SM, Lesouef KL, Sly PD, Lesouef PN. A new technique to generate and assess forced expiration from raised lung volume in infants. Am J Respir Crit Care Med. 1995;151(5):1441–50.

van den Wijngaart LS, Roukema J, Merkus PJ. Respiratory disease and respiratory physiology: putting lung function into perspective: paediatric asthma. Respirology. 2015a;20(3):379–88.

van den Wijngaart LS, Roukema J, Merkus PJ. The value of spirometry and exercise challenge test to diagnose and monitor children with asthma. Respirol Case Rep. 2015b;3(1):25–8.

Chapter 13
Reference Equations for Pulmonary Function Tests

Bruce H. Culver and Sanja Stanojevic

13.1 Introduction

The vast majority of clinical laboratory tests are interpreted using a single range of normal values, which apply for all individuals. The range of values considered normal for pulmonary function tests are not as straightforward and require consideration of body size (typically height, which is a proxy for chest size), age (an indicator of maturity and aging), sex, and ethnicity. To accurately interpret a pulmonary function test result, and distinguish between health and disease, reference equations derived from healthy individuals are necessary. The healthy individuals used to derive the reference equation typically exclude anyone with a smoking history, history of respiratory disease, or chronic health condition. However, historically there have been numerous approaches used to define pulmonary function reference equations, and as a consequence, an individual result can be interpreted differently depending on the approach used.

13.2 Evolution of Reference Equations

The need for reference equations to interpret pulmonary function test results has been well recognized for many decades. In early studies, the reference population was often a sample of convenience and may have included smokers or a specific

B. H. Culver
Pulmonary, Critical Care and Sleep Medicine, University of Washington School of Medicine, Seattle, WA, USA
e-mail: bculver@uw.edu

S. Stanojevic (✉)
Translational Medicine, The Hospital for Sick Children, Toronto, ON, Canada
e-mail: sanja.stanojevic@sickkids.ca

D. A. Kaminsky, C. G. Irvin (eds.), *Pulmonary Function Testing*,
Respiratory Medicine, https://doi.org/10.1007/978-3-319-94159-2_13

subset of the population (e.g., male military recruits, coal miners). Notably, the European Coal and Steel Community equations, widely used across Europe even today, were based upon a compilation of relatively small samples of men with some inclusion of smokers, while the equations for females were based on a fixed adjustment of 80% of the male equations. In later decades (1970–1990), a greater emphasis was placed on the exclusion of smokers and other conditions that may affect lung health. The first ATS Snowbird Statement (1979) on the standardization of spirometry recommended inclusion of only healthy individuals to define a normal range of values, which limited the population to lifelong non-smokers without a history of disease that affected the respiratory system or circulatory problems. Consequently, reference equations were often derived from a small sample of adults, and differences between published reference equations were attributed to differences in population characteristics. It was thus recommended that individual pulmonary function laboratories collect normative data to guide selection of equations representative of their patient population.

Although it was recognized that pulmonary function was dependent on sex, height as well as age, it was assumed that the spread of values around the mean was uniform, such that the lower limit of normal was commonly taken to be a fixed percentage of the predicted values. In their influential 1971 textbook, Bates and Christie introduced the 80% predicted "handy rule of thumb" for the lower limit of normal, which is still widely, but inappropriately, used today. Since the reference population often included a limited age range of subjects, many early reference equations were derived using a simple linear regression to describe the relationship between sex, height, age, and pulmonary function, and the assumption that the spread of values around the mean was uniform was reasonable (Fig. 13.1a). However, this is not necessarily true when data across the span of childhood and adulthood are considered (Fig. 13.1b), and if the 80% predicted cutoff is extended to all ages, and all pulmonary function outcomes, this results in an underdiagnosis of abnormalities in younger, taller individuals and overdiagnosis in older, shorter individuals.

The vast majority of early reference equations for pulmonary function tests were available only for adults (older than 16–20 years of age), or limited to children (6–12 years of age), with no reference equations available to seamlessly monitor patients from childhood into old age. During puberty, lung growth is rapid and not always synchronized with somatic growth. Switching between pediatric and adult equations, especially during puberty, often resulted in artificial jumps and drops in predicted values between consecutive measurements in the same patient, which can cause misinterpretation of results.

In the 1990s, reference equations for pulmonary function measurements started to take on a more sophisticated approach to accurately describe the relationship between growth and aging. Importantly, women and children were now included in the reference population, although some of the previous assumptions and limits of normal persisted despite new evidence. The inclusion of children in the reference population made derivation of reference equations more complicated since lung growth increases with height and age in children but declines with age in adults

(Fig. 13.1b). The NHANES III equations (Hankinson et al. 1999) were the first set of comprehensive extended-age equations, ranging from 8 to 80 years of age, and were derived using two equations joined at age 20 for males (Fig. 13.1c) or 18 for

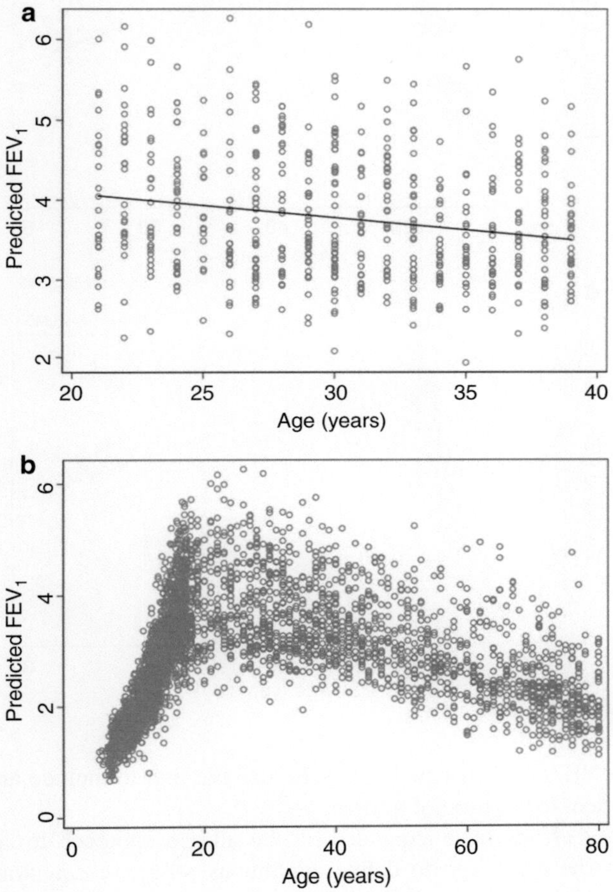

Fig. 13.1 (**a**) Observed FEV_1 values with age in males 20–40 years of age demonstrating uniform spread of values around the predicted value. (**b**) Observed FEV_1 values with age in males 3–80 years of age, demonstrating the nonlinear relationship between pulmonary function and age, as well as the nonuniform spread of values at different ages. (**c**) Polynomial regression equations (NHANES III) predicted values for FEV_1 with age. (**d**) Continuous LMS method ("all-age") predicted values for FEV_1 with age. (Figs. 13.1b, c and d are reprinted with permission of the American Thoracic Society. Copyright © 2017 American Thoracic Society. Stanojevic S, Wade A, Stocks J, Hankinson J, Coates AL, Pan H, Rosenthal M, Corey M, Lebecque P, Cole TJ. Reference ranges for spirometry across all ages. Am J Respir Crit Care Med. 2008;177:253–260. The *American Journal of Respiratory and Critical Care Medicine* is an official journal of the American Thoracic Society)

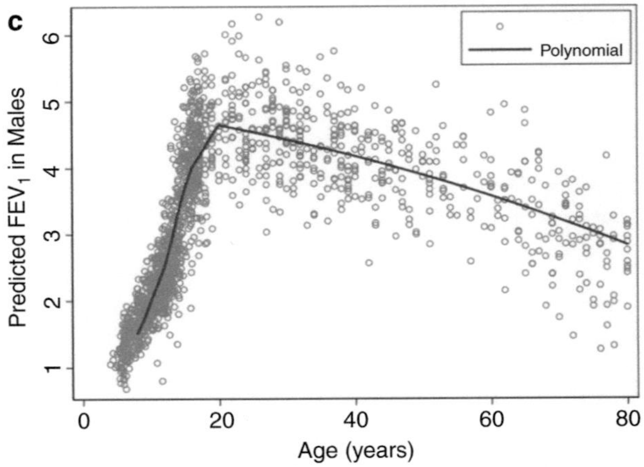

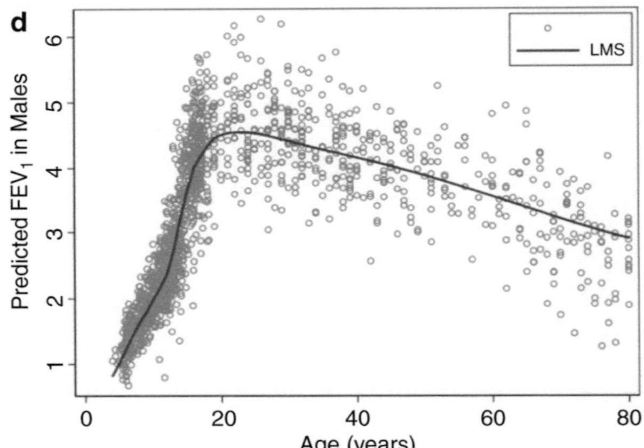

Fig. 13.1 (continued)

females. The NHANES III equations were also the first to include an appropriate height-dependent lower limit of normal.

More recent efforts have expanded on the all-age approach to apply smooth curves across the age range to define continuous reference equations from 3 to 95 years of age which capture the rapid growth of the lungs observed in childhood and the slow decline observed in adults (Fig. 13.1c). Statistical methods specifically designed to define population reference equations (e.g., lambda-mu-sigma) are used, where at each age, a median (mu), variability (sigma), and skewness (lambda) parameter is estimated to define a predicted value and lower limit of normal for an individual of a specific age, height, sex, and ethnicity. The methodological approach transforms the distribution of values to be a normal distribution, to more accurately define the lower limit of normal or the 5th percentile.

13.3 Choice of Reference Equations

Given the historical context of how reference equations for pulmonary function tests evolved, it is not surprising that there are over 400 reference equations for spirometry alone. Logistically it is challenging to recruit a large and representative healthy population for each pulmonary function laboratory, city, or even country, which meant that dozens of reference equations were published for small and often biased samples. Individual laboratories were left to choose from one of these equations, or derive their own, and in many cases, default equations set by manufacturers were never changed. In addition, many pulmonary function laboratories are not aware of which reference equation is selected within their equipment, or whether it is appropriate for their patient population.

Several studies have shown how the use of inappropriate reference equations can lead to serious errors in both under- and overdiagnosis, with its associated burden in terms of financial and human costs. A large proportion of the differences observed between different reference equations can be explained by how the sample of healthy individuals was selected and how many healthy individuals are included. With current technology, factors such as equipment or software differences contribute minimally to the observed differences, and temporal changes in populations are not commonly observed in resource-rich countries. However, rapid changes in environmental and socioeconomic conditions in resource-poor countries have been shown to affect both somatic growth (i.e., height) as well as pulmonary function, with younger generations demonstrating significantly better pulmonary function relative to older cohorts. Similar changes may be seen in immigrant populations in more developed countries.

13.4 Currently Recommended Reference Equations

13.4.1 Spirometry

Both the ATS and ERS have endorsed the Global Lung Function Initiative spirometry equations (GLI-2012), as have several regional respiratory societies. In North America, given the similarities between GLI-2012, NHANES III, and recently published Canadian equations, the ATS has recommended all three for use.

The GLI-2012 reference equations, based on nearly 100,000 healthy nonsmokers, were developed using the LMS method and have the advantage of continuous data over a wide age range and inclusion of multiple ethnic groups. The GLI spirometry equations are available for *Caucasians* (n = 57,395), which include people from Europe, Israel, Australia, the United States, Canada, Brazil, Chile, Mexico, Uruguay, Venezuela, Algeria, and Tunisia and Mexican Americans,

African-Americans ($n = 3545$), *Southeast Asians* ($n = 8255$), which include people from Thailand, Taiwan, and China (including Hong Kong) south of the Huaihe River and Qinling Mountains, and *Northeast Asians* ($n = 4992$), which include people from Korea and China north of the Huaihe River and Qinling Mountains. In addition, since many individuals were either not represented by these four groups or were of mixed ethnic origin, a composite equation was derived as the average of available data to facilitate interpretation until a more appropriate solution is developed with adequate high-quality data. One important observation from the GLI spirometry equations is that ethnic differences in FEV_1 and FVC differed proportionally between Caucasians and other ethnic groups, such that FEV_1/FVC remained virtually independent of ethnic group. The inclusion of preschool children in the GLI-2012 equations is also advantageous for children with chronic respiratory conditions, such as cystic fibrosis, where early detection of disease offers an opportunity to intervene before permanent damage occurs. Another advantage of these equations is that pulmonary function is expressed as a function of both height and age, such that during periods of rapid growth, a younger individual will have a smaller predicted value than an older individual of the same height.

13.4.2 Diffusing Capacity

Appropriate reference equations for diffusing capacity (DLCO), also referred to as the transfer factor for carbon monoxide (TLCO), have been a long-standing problem in respiratory medicine. Although the DLCO test is widely used to both diagnose and distinguish respiratory conditions, as well as to determine eligibility for certain treatments (e.g., chemotherapy, surgery), there have been a limited number of reference equations published for the test. Comparisons of published studies have found that differences between predicted values have been reported to vary by as much as 40%. Furthermore, the majority of the available reference equations are outdated and based on equipment and protocols that are no longer available or used today. New recommendations and standards for the DLCO test methodology have recently become available, but there is still considerable variability between laboratories in terms of how the test is performed. Other factors such as the gas concentrations and partial pressure of oxygen, which is dependent on the altitude of the laboratory as well as daily fluctuations in humidity, can also influence results, as can an individual's hemoglobin levels, which are seldom measured and used to interpret results.

The GLI has recently completed reference equations for Caucasians aged 4–80 years for DLCO, carbon monoxide transfer coefficient (*KCO*), and alveolar volume (V_A). The advantages of the GLI DLCO reference equations are that they are based on the largest collection of data from healthy individuals and are corrected for major methodological differences that may influence interpretation. Another advantage is that the pulmonary function of the study population aligns closely with that of the GLI-2012 spirometry population, such that the spirometry and DLCO equations can be used together, despite being based upon different individuals. Although these represent a major step forward toward the standardization of reporting and interpretation of test results, there are several limitations that still need to be addressed. The new GLI DLCO equations are limited to Caucasian subjects, which makes it challenging to determine whether there are ethnic differences in DLCO and, if so, how big the offset is.

13.4.3 Lung Volumes

Reference equations for lung volumes are quite a different story, with fewer published studies available. The vast majority that are available are outdated and not appropriate for modern equipment and protocols. A previous summary of available reference equations for lung volumes, published in 2005, found most published studies included a very small number of healthy subjects and were often specific for an ethnic group and the vast majority were from European populations. An even earlier review, published in 1995, made similar conclusions and highlighted the major limitations of what was available and published.

In Europe, the reference equations most commonly used for lung volumes are those of the European Coal and Steel Community (ECSC), which were first published in 1983 and resulted from summarizing many previously published studies, with data collected in the 1960s and 1970s. Unlike the recent GLI collations, which use original data, the ECSC equations were mathematically developed from the prior published equations, a method which adds an additional layer of uncertainty, particularly to the normal range. An alternative set of equations are those published by Crapo et al. (1982), which have the advantage of having measured spirometry and DLCO in the same population. The TLC was obtained from the single-breath helium dilution of the diffusing capacity test, and the number studied (123 M, 122 F) was marginal but was well distributed over the age range. Equations available in some equipment still include those published by Goldman and Becklake in 1959, which are based on fewer than 100 subjects (44 M, 50 F) from Johannesburg, South Africa, with no mention of the smoking history of participants. There are some newer, larger data sets available, reporting lung volumes of healthy non-smoking Caucasian adults from the Barcelona area, Canada, and New Zealand and of children from the Netherlands.

None of the existing reference equations for lung volumes are fully satisfactory, and caution should be applied when using these to interpret results. There is currently a GLI project underway to collate existing lung volume data from healthy individuals measured with a variety of techniques (e.g., single or multiple breath, quiet or forced rebreathing, nitrogen or helium dilution, multiple indicator gases, body plethysmography). Data are being collected separately for each technique and will be investigated for agreement. By collating the available data, there is hope for better lung volume reference data.

13.5 Interpretation of Results

Interpretation of pulmonary function results relies on the accurate comparison of the measured value against an expected range of normal values. It is generally accepted that the values observed in healthy individuals should have a normal distribution (i.e., bell-shaped curve) and that the normal range of values includes 95% of the healthy population (+/−1.96 standard deviations), thereby accepting the risk that 5% of a healthy population will be mislabeled as abnormal (i.e., false positive). Typically, 2.5% of these are below the normal range and 2.5% are above it, but for most pulmonary function tests, we identify only individuals with low pulmonary function as abnormal, so the 5th percentile (−1.645 standard deviations) is often used to define the lower limit of normal (LLN). The use of the 5th percentile as an LLN has been recommended since the early 1980s, and consistently recommended by ATS and ERS since then, but has yet to be uniformly implemented in clinical PFT laboratories.

In some instances, such as when pulmonary function tests are used to screen the general population for lung disease, or in pediatrics, where we may want to be more certain before identifying lung disease, the 2.5th percentile of the normal distribution might be more appropriate. A normal range of 2.5–97.5 percentile is also appropriate for outcomes where both high and low values can be abnormal (e.g., total lung capacity, functional residual capacity, etc.).

Measured values are commonly compared to the predicted value, (i.e., the midpoint of the reference population), by calculating the percentage of the predicted value ([observed/predicted] *100). This percent predicted is a readily understood indicator of the magnitude of any impairment but has shortcomings when used in place of a true LLN to identify abnormal values. The percent predicted does not take into account the variability of values in the normal population, which depends on the age, height, and sex of the patient, and on the outcome being interpreted. For example, the statistically determined LLN for vital capacity of an average-height middle-aged man may correspond to 79–80% predicted, but for a younger taller man, it could be 84% predicted, and for an older woman, it could be 74% predicted, so applying the commonly used value of 80% predicted to all, in place of the true LLN for each individual, invariably leads to under- or overdiagnosis of abnormality. And for some tests, notably the FEF_{25-75}, the variability in the normal population is much higher, so that the 5th percentile LLN corresponds to 50–60% predicted for most and as low as 35% predicted for older individuals. Notably, underestimation of the wide variability of mid-expiratory flows has largely contributed to the overemphasis of their sensitivity to identify disease. While using the 80% predicted "rule of thumb" is easy, its errors can be readily avoided by simply including the 5th percentile LLN, calculated from the prediction equations, next to the observed values on the form for interpretation or reporting of PFT results. The report format should be standardized according to recent guidelines published by the American Thoracic Society.

The percent predicted is more appropriately used to indicate nearness to the predicted value and the magnitude or severity of any impairment. Various guidelines

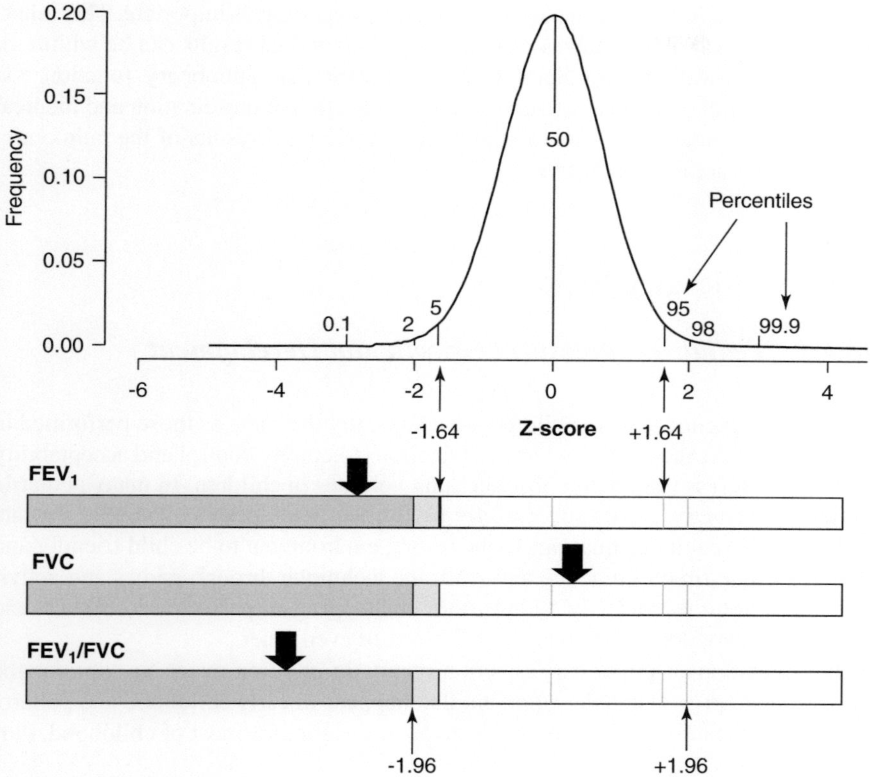

Fig. 13.2 Graphical representation of the normal distribution, z-scores, and percentile and how this visual representation can be used to interpret the magnitude of pulmonary function impairment for individual pulmonary function test results. (Adapted with permission from Levy et al. 2009)

for interpretation or disease management have selected arbitrary cut points of percent predicted to describe levels of impairment. An alternative is to show how many standard deviations from the predicted value an observation is. This is also called a z-score with negative numbers showing low values. Similar to percent predicted, the further away an observed value is from the center of the normal distribution, the less likely it is compatible with health, and the more likely an indication of disease (Fig. 13.2). One advantage of using standard deviations (or z-scores) is that, unlike percent predicted, the same limit of normal (−1.645 for the 5th percentile) applies for all outcomes and all ages. Although increasingly being used, numerically or in a visual scale, to show the placement of a result relative to the normal range, there is as yet limited literature describing the use of z-scores to grade disease severity. The number of standard deviations an observation is from the predicted value tells us how likely, or unlikely, this value would be in a normal population, but it is not intrinsically related to the impact of the disease.

Regardless of which approach is used to interpret pulmonary function tests, an appreciation that pulmonary function tests show variability between individuals, and even within individuals measured repeatedly over time, is important. This inherent biological variability means that by chance, individual results can be within, or outside, the lower limit of normal. The application of pulmonary function test results to an individual needs to consider both the clinical presentation and medical history of the patient and should include repeat testing if results of the pulmonary function tests are not conclusive.

13.6 Challenging Topics

13.6.1 Pediatric-Adolescent Growth and Development

Pulmonary function tests in children are technically the same as those performed in adults, with the exception of a few modifications to quality control and acceptability criteria to address the smaller absolute lung volumes in children. In many pediatric centers, spirometry can be successfully performed in children as young as 3 years of age but do require adaptations to the testing environment to be child friendly and should include time to practice and learn the technique through games and activities. Lung volumes and DLCO are more challenging to perform in children and typically are not done until the age of 6 years, or even older.

Interpretation of pulmonary function results in children needs to consider the rapid somatic growth and development that happens in early childhood and puberty (Fig. 13.3). While somatic and lung growth are parallel for most of childhood, dur-

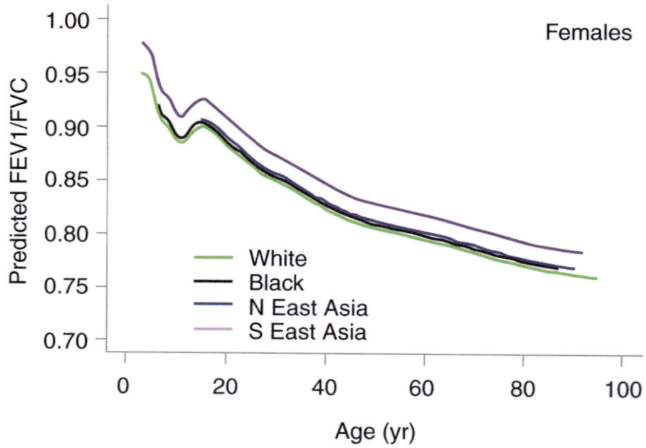

Fig. 13.3 Desynapsis between somatic and lung growth is particularly evident for the FEV_1/FVC ratio during puberty. During early childhood, FEV_1 and FVC are similar; the lungs are small and the vital capacity can easily be expired in 1 second or less. For this reason, $FEV_{0.75}$ is reported in children under the age of 6, and even older children with smaller lung volumes. Thereafter, FVC typically outgrows FEV_1, leading to a gradual fall in FEV_1/FVC. The opposite occurs during puberty, when changes in FEV_1 outpace FVC, leading to a kink in predicted FEV_1/FVC ratio. (Reproduced with permission from the ©ERS 2012. *Eur Respir J.* 2012, 40(6):1324–1343. https://doi.org/10.1183/09031936.00080312)

ing these periods of rapid growth, somatic growth often outpaces lung growth, which can lead to misdiagnosis of abnormal pulmonary function. For this reason, it is recommended that the calculation of predicted values in children and adolescents be based on age to the nearest tenth (e.g., 6.5 years).

For the vast majority of children and young adults, the LLN for the FEV_1/FVC ratio will be greater than 0.70, so airflow obstruction will not be identified using that fixed ratio cutoff. It is important to identify those that have FEV_1/FVC below the lower limit of normal or with early signs of obstructive disease. This is particularly relevant given the recent evidence that suggests adult lung diseases such as COPD have origins in early life and that exposures in childhood are strongly associated with later pulmonary function and disease incidence.

13.6.2 Predicting Pulmonary Function in the Elderly

Predicted values and normal limits for older individuals require special consideration for several reasons. Earlier reference data often was collected on individuals only to age 60 or 70, so the resulting equations could be considered valid only to that age. However, lacking better data, predicted values were often extrapolated to higher ages with a resulting increase in the uncertainty of their accuracy. Such an extrapolation assumes that trends established in mid-age will continue unchanged in the elderly. However, living 90-year-olds represent only a fraction of the cohort alive at 60 and are more likely to come from the healthier portion of that cohort with better than average values for many health parameters, including pulmonary function, a so-called survivor effect. On the other hand, the elderly have had more years for small but cumulative effects of detrimental environmental factors or the consequences of intercurrent illness to become manifest so some may have lower than expected pulmonary function. There are also concerns about the technical adequacy of pulmonary function test performance in the elderly. These factors also affect reference data collected on healthy elderly subjects resulting in increased scatter of the values, which, along with the smaller numbers available for testing, cause the confidence intervals of the normal range to be wider in the elderly. A comparison of predicted values from the NHANES III equations extrapolated beyond age 80 with those from GLI-2012 which did include a modest number of subjects age 80–95 showed close agreement in the mid-age range, but in the very elderly and especially at extremes of height, the predicted values could vary significantly. As yet, there is no independent standard to judge which is more accurate. Increased representation of persons aged greater than 75 years in the reference populations is needed to further improve diagnostic accuracy. Therefore caution is required when interpreting pulmonary function in older individuals. There is also a need for more data in older subjects to develop age-appropriate criteria regarding the adequacy of test performance and to evaluate alternative measures of pulmonary function. These improvements may broaden the generalizability of respiratory test results in geriatric practice.

An issue that is of particular concern in the elderly, although it also affects younger individuals, is the inappropriate use of a fixed value of the FEV_1/FVC ratio, such as 0.70 (or 70%), to define airflow limitation. In an effort to increase awareness and recognition of chronic obstructive pulmonary disease (COPD) particularly in less developed areas of the world, the Global Initiative for Chronic Obstructive Lung Disease (GOLD) group (unrelated to the Global Lung Function Initiative) has defined airflow limitation in COPD as a post-bronchodilator FEV_1/FVC ratio of 0.70. This fixed cutoff approximates the LLN in the mid-range of age, where screening or case-finding for COPD is most likely to be helpful, but the true LLN of this ratio increases with growth then decreases with age, crossing 0.70 at about age 46 in men and 54 in women. This fixed ratio has been commonly applied to younger and older individuals, and the use of this definition by other COPD guidelines has led some clinicians to inappropriately consider this to be a generally applicable definition of airflow limitation. It has been widely reported that use of this definition results in under-recognition of obstructive disease in young individuals and overdiagnosis in older individuals. Normal FEV_1/FVC values are higher in women than men so the fixed cutoff also creates a sex bias, with young women more likely to be under-recognized and older men more likely to be overdiagnosed. One study (Hardie et al. 2002) showed that one third of healthy, never-smoking older men met this flawed criterion for COPD, which can lead to inappropriate medication and concern. In another study of men and women above age 80 (Turkeshi et al. 2015), two thirds of the individuals with an FEV_1/FVC <0.70 had values above the true LLN for their age and, importantly, did not show an increase in subsequent mortality or hospitalization.

The elderly have an increased likelihood of alternate explanations for common presenting symptoms, such as dyspnea. Indeed, patients with respiratory symptoms and FEV_1/FVC <0.70 but above the true LLN have an increased risk of subsequent adverse cardiovascular events. Accordingly, among older persons with respiratory symptoms, high diagnostic accuracy is a necessity when attributing the underlying mechanism to a respiratory impairment. By reducing the misidentification of normal-for-age pulmonary function as a respiratory impairment, the use of an age-specific LLN may avoid the use of inappropriate and potentially harmful respiratory medications in older persons, as well as delays in considering other diagnoses among older persons with respiratory symptoms.

13.6.3 Consideration of Obesity in Pulmonary Function Prediction and Interpretation

As the prevalence of obesity is increasing in North America and elsewhere, the effect of body weight on both the prediction and interpretation of pulmonary function becomes increasingly important. A recent international compilation of over 10,000 otherwise healthy individuals of broad age range found 27% to be obese, i.e., exceeding a BMI of 30 kg/m^2 in adults or the 85th percentile in children and adolescents (Stanojevic et al. 2017). Excess weight does cause clear physiologic

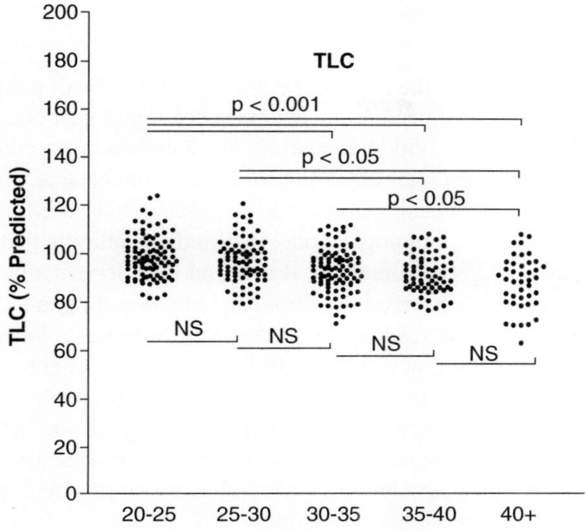

Fig. 13.4 Scattergrams of TLC (% predicted) measurements versus BMI. There is a downtrend in values with increasing weight, but even at BMI >40 most of the values still overlap those of normal weight individuals. (Reproduced with permission from Jones and Nzekwu 2006)

changes in thoracoabdominal function, but these can be quite variable among individuals and the effects on the primary measurements used to define abnormal pulmonary function are modest. Increased weight and adiposity within the chest wall and abdomen shifts the balance of forces within the relaxed chest so that the end-expiratory lung volume, the functional residual capacity, is reduced and, because the residual volume is largely determined by airway closure and changes little, the expiratory reserve volume can be quite markedly reduced. These effects are greatest in the supine position when the abdominal contents press up on the diaphragm and may contribute to postural hypoxemia, but clinical PFTs are done sitting or standing, and key values such as VC and TLC are measured with maximal effort, so the effect on these is much smaller. While it is common to attribute low values of VC or TLC to obesity, studies have shown that this does not become likely until rather extreme degrees of obesity. Figure 13.4 shows the spread of data from one such study (Jones and Nzekwu 2006). While there is a significant downtrend in TLC and VC values with increasing BMI, the great majority of individuals still fall within the normal range even at a BMI of >40. In addition to these direct mechanical effects, there is an increasing literature on the interactions of obesity with asthma and on the systemic inflammatory role of obesity and the metabolic syndrome with COPD.

Obesity has not commonly been listed as an exclusion for the use of data in pulmonary function predicted equations, and weight, when considered, has not been found to add significantly to height as a body size indicator. This will need to be reevaluated in future reference data for spirometry and particularly for lung volumes. The recently published GLI reference data for DLCO/TLCO did address this and found that including subjects with a BMI > 30 did not significantly affect these prediction equations.

13.6.4 Ethnicity

Disentangling the effects of ethnicity from those of geography, environmental exposures, and socioeconomic factors is challenging and depends on the specific population studied. Within resource-rich countries, true ethnic differences can best be distinguished after adjusting for generational status, and socioeconomic status, but even the best designed studies are prone to bias as ethnicity is as much a social construct as it is a biological one. In a study examining genetic ancestry and pulmonary function, genetic ancestry was found to independently explain a proportion of the differences observed in pulmonary function. In general, individuals of African and Asian descent tend to have lower lung volumes relative to Caucasians of the same height. Differences in somatic growth are thought to explain differences in the dimensions of the chest wall and strength of the chest wall muscles. The trunk-leg ratio has also been found to explain about one half of the observed differences in pulmonary function, but clearly there are other factors at play, especially socioeconomic status and the risk factors that are often associated with both socioeconomic status and pulmonary function.

Given the potential influences of ethnicity on pulmonary function in healthy individuals, it is important to take this into consideration when interpreting results. There have been past recommendations that a fixed percentage between 12% and 15% be deducted from Caucasian equations when interpreting results from African-Americans. However, the ethnic-specific NHANES III or GLI-2012 reference equations are more appropriate, given that the differences between ethnic groups are not constant for males and females, nor for all outcomes. Despite the availability of equations for multiple ethnic groups, many of the world's largest populations are still not adequately represented (e.g., African continent, South Asia and India, and Latin America). The spirometry reference equations derived for the Asian population may be biased by cohort effects, as recent studies have shown both cohort and migration effects on pulmonary function in these populations. An additional consideration is that ethnicity itself is difficult to define and often self-reported. Furthermore, the proportion of individuals who identify as mixed ethnicity is growing, making it more challenging to identify an appropriate reference equation for each individual. Often, equipment software also does not allow for individualized equations to be applied and default to specific set of values without notifying the user.

13.6.5 Accepting Uncertainty

Among large and well-represented reference populations, there will be small differences in the LLN for FEV_1/FVC and other pulmonary function parameters. However, one need not overemphasize the exact value of any LLN as there will always be some uncertainty around this point, and the interpreter would be wise to consider a range on either side of any cut point to represent a "borderline value" rather than clearly normal or indicative of disease.

The interpreter faces much greater uncertainties than the exact LLN to apply to a particular individual's PFT results. There are the issues of whether a particular reference equation matches the patient, the laboratory equipment, or the skills of the technicians, but a bigger issue is the clinical meaning of a value near the LLN in this individual. A 5th percentile LLN means that 95% of healthy non-smokers would have higher values, but that does not indicate the likelihood that this person is normal or has disease. For that, the interpreter would need to estimate the pretest probability of disease in this individual or among the population seen in the laboratory. If testing an asymptomatic non-smoker at a screening event, then a result near or just below the LLN may, more likely than not, be "normal." However, in a hospital-based referral lab, those with FEV_1/FVC at or even a few points above the LLN may be quite likely to have early airflow obstruction, even though statistically "within normal limits."

Uncertainty in PFT interpretation has always been present, even if not acknowledged. In discussing this uncertainty, one physician 50 years ago noted that a common response "is toward cautiously noncommittal overinterpretation in language replete with modifiers." A publication of the California Thoracic Society in 1982 stated that "the large and inherent overlap between normalcy and disease states will persist as a limitation in pulmonary function test interpretation."

13.6.6 Future Directions

An ATS update in 1994 described two related, but distinct, tasks for the user of pulmonary function data:

1. The classification of the derived values with respect to a reference population
2. The integration of the values into the diagnosis, therapy, and prognosis for an individual patient

In the years since that publication, there has been good and continuing progress in the first of these tasks with availability of the newer, larger, broadly applicable reference sources discussed in this chapter and with renewed attention to the use of appropriate limits of normal. The second and more important task, however, is still left largely to the judgment of the individual practitioner with little guidance from the literature. That is beginning to change as studies appear analyzing how pulmonary function test results relate to subsequent health outcomes. Earlier identification of patients progressing toward clinically important lung disease, such as COPD, may become possible with better understanding of the outcomes of patient groups with known spirometry values and with well-characterized risk factors.

The seminal long-term study of Fletcher and Peto showed that the development of airflow limitation in COPD was characterized by a slow progressive fall in FEV_1, averaging only about twice the expected decline of normal aging. The wide normal range of spirometry values (as shown in Fig. 13.1a, b above) and the relative insensitivity of forced airflow measurements to increases in small airway resistance mean that early stages of disease will inevitably be present before the FEV_1/FVC ratio falls below the population LLN. This has prompted many efforts to identify a more sensitive indicator of airflow limitation. One important study (Cosio et al. 1978) performed a battery of pulmonary function tests on individuals scheduled for resection of small lung lesions and then analyzed lung parenchymal tissue, remote from the lesion, for evidence of small airway disease. As the pathology score increased from grade 1, minimal, to grade 4 abnormalities, there was a stepwise decline in mean FEV_1/FVC, but it did not become significantly different from those with no small airway disease until grade 3 pathology was present. And, of five tests thought to be potentially more sensitive to small airway dysfunction, none outperformed the FEV_1/FVC ratio. The presence of emphysema has also been demonstrated by computed tomography while spirometry remains within normal limits, but this is not practical for disease screening.

A different approach to confirming suspected COPD at an early stage would be to use a more sensitive criterion for airflow limitation in higher-risk individuals, just as different cutoffs are used for tuberculin skin testing: 5, 10, or 15 mm for high-, moderate-, and low-risk individuals. For example, in individuals judged to be at high risk for COPD, the LLN might be raised from the 5th percentile to the 7.5th or 10th. This possibility has been examined (Vaz Fragoso et al. 2010) by comparing the outcomes of individuals with FEV_1/FVC <5th percentile to those at progressively higher percentile strata, 5th to 10th, 10th to 15th, etc., with those at or above the 25th percentile serving as the reference population. As expected, those below the 5th percentile LLN had increased subsequent all-cause mortality while there was no indication of this for those above the 10th percentile. The borderline strata between the 5th and 10th percentile had a risk of mortality, calculated including such known risks as smoking and age, that was 60% greater than the group with normal spirometry. Any increase in diagnostic sensitivity gained from adjusting the LLN upward is inevitably accompanied by a loss of specificity so, to minimize false positives, it is essential to evaluate any risk stratified cut points with outcomes in appropriate populations.

The outcome study noted above and most others recently available have been based upon general populations with a relatively low prevalence of airway disease, but the situation facing a practitioner in a clinical pulmonary function laboratory is quite different. When spirometry is done on patients with symptoms or relevant risk factors, the pretest probability of airway disease is much higher than in a general population so that spirometry values clearly above the healthy population LLN still may indicate a significant likelihood of early airway disease. It should now be routine to readily and accurately classify spirometry values with respect to a reference population: however, to integrate these values into the diagnosis, therapy, and prognosis for an individual patient is a more complex judgment. The pulmonary field needs to move beyond a simple choice of normal vs. abnormal and develop the risk profiles and outcome data that would allow a rational statement about the probability of disease at any point on the spectrum of FEV_1/FVC from mid-normal down to the LLN and below. With this, pulmonary function reference equation could provide not just the predicted value and LLN but also a prognostic index for a wide range of observed values.

Selected References

Guidelines and Statements

American Thoracic Society. Snowbird workshop on standardization of spirometry. Am Rev Respir Dis. 1979;119:831–8.

American Thoracic Society. Lung function testing: selection of reference values and interpretative strategies. Am Rev Respir Dis. 1991;144:1202–18.

American Thoracic Society. Standardization of Spirometry,1994 update. Am J Respir Crit Care Med. 1995;152:1107–36.

Stocks J, Quanjer PH. Reference values for residual volume, functional residual capacity and total lung capacity. ATS workshop on lung volume measurement. Official statement of the ERS. Eur Respir J. 1995;8:492–506.

Pellegrino R, Viegi G, Brusasco V, Crapo RO, Burgos F, Casaburi R, Coates AL, van der Grinten CP, Gustafsson PM, Hankinson JL, Jensen RL, Johnson DC, MacIntyre NR, McKay RT, Miller MR, Navajas D, Pedersen OF, Wanger JK. Interpretative strategies for lung function tests. Eur Respir J. 2005;26:948–68.

Graham BL, Brusasco V, Burgos F, Cooper BG, Jensen R, Kendrick AH, MacIntyre NR, Thompson BR, Wanger J. ERS/ATS standards for single-breath carbon monoxide uptake in the lung. Eur Respir J. 2017;49:1600016. https://doi.org/10.1183/13993003.00016-2016.

Culver BH, Graham BL, Coates AL, JWanger J, Berry CE, Clarke PK, Hallstrand TS, Hankinson JL, Kaminsky DA, MacIntyre NR, McCormack MC, Rosenfeld R, Stanojevic S, Weiner DJ. Recommendations for a standardized pulmonary function report: an official ATSTechnical statement. Am J Respir Crit Care Med. 2017;196:1463–72.

Pauwels RA, Buist AS, Calverley PM, Jenkins CR, Hurd SS. On behalf of the GOLD scientific committee. Global strategy for the diagnosis, management, and prevention of chronic obstructive pulmonary disease: NHLBI/WHO global initiative for chronic obstructive lung disease (GOLD) workshop summary. Am J Respir Crit Care Med. 2001;163:1256–76.

Spirometry Reference Equation Sources

GLI-2012

Quanjer PH, Stanojevic S, Cole TJ, Baur X, Hall GL, Culver BH, Enright PL, Hankinson JL, Ip MSM, Zheng J, Stocks J. ERS global lung function initiative. Multi-ethnic reference values for spirometry for the 3-95 year age range: the global lung function 2012 equations. Eur Respir J. 2012;40:1324–43.

NHANES III

Hankinson JL, Odencrantz JR, Fedan KB. Spirometric reference values from a sample of the general US population. Am J Respir Crit Care Med. 1999;159:179–87.

Canada

Coates AL, Wong SL, Tremblay C, Hankinson JL. Reference equations for spirometry in the Canadian population. Ann Am Thorac Soc. 2016;13:833–41.

Comparisons of GLI-2012 to Earlier Sources

Brazzale DJ, Hall GL, Pretto JJ. Effects of adopting the new global lung function initiative 2012 reference equations on the interpretation of spirometry. Respiration. 2013;86:183–9.
Quanjer PH, Brazzale DJ, Boros PW, Pretto JJ. Implications of adopting the global lungs initiative 2012 all-age reference equations for spirometry. Eur Respir J. 2013;42:1046–54.
Quanjer PH, Weiner DJ. Interpretative consequences of adopting the global lungs 2012 reference equations for spirometry for children and adolescents. Pediatr Pulmonol. 2014;49:118–25.
Linares-Perdomo O, Hegewald M, Collingridge DS, Blagev D, Jensen RL, Hankinson J, Morris AH. Comparison of NHANES III and ERS/GLI-2012 for airway obstruction and severity. Eur Respir J. 2016;48:133–41.
Swanney MP, Miller M. Adopting universal lung function reference equations. Eur Respir J. 2013;42:901–3.
Miller MR. Choosing and using lung function prediction equations. Eur Respir J. 2016;48:1535–7.

Diffusing Capacity Reference Equations

Stanojevic S, Graham BL, Cooper BG, Thompson B, Carter K, Francis R, Hall GL. Official ERS technical standards: global lung function initiative reference values for the carbon monoxide transfer factor for Caucasians. Eur Respir J. 2017; in press

Lung Volume Reference Equations

Goldman HI, Becklake MR. Respiratory function tests: normal values at median altitudes and the prediction of normal results. Am Rev Tuberc. 1959;79:457467.
Crapo RO, Morris AH, Clayton PD, Nixon CR. Lung volumes in healthy nonsmoking adults. Bull Eur Physiopathol Respir. 1982;18(3):419–25.
Quanjer PH, Tammeling GJ, Cotes JE, Pedersen OF, Peslin R, Yemault JC. Standardization of lung function tests: lung volumes and ventilatory flows. Report working party. European Community for steel and coal and European Respiratory Society. Eur Respir J. 1993;6(Suppl.16):5–40.

Roca J, Burgos F, Barbera J, Sunyer J, Rodriguez-Roisin R, Castellsague J, et al. Prediction equations for plethysmographic lung volumes. Respir Med. 1998;92(3):454–60.
Gutierrez C, Ghezzo RH, Abboud RT, Cosio MG, Dill JR, Martin RR, McCarthy DS, Morse JLC, Zamel N. Reference values of pulmonary function tests for Canadian Caucasians. Can Respir J. 2004;11:414–24.
Marsh S, Aldington S, Williams M, Weatherall M, Shirtcliffe P, McNaughton A, et al. Complete reference ranges for pulmonary function tests from a single New Zealand population. N Z Med J. 2006;119(1244):U2281.
Koopman M, et al. Reference values for paediatric pulmonary function testing: the Utrecht dataset. Respir Med. 2011;105(1):15–23.

Limits of Normal and Interpretation

Fletcher C, Peto R. The natural history of chronic airflow obstruction. Br Med J. 1977;1(6077):1645–8.
Cosio M, Ghezzo H, Hogg JC, Corbin R, Loveland M, Dosman J, et al. The relation between structural changes in small airways and pulmonary function tests. N Engl J Med. 1978;298:1277–81.
Clausen JL. Prediction of normal values. In: Clausen JL, editor. Pulmonaryfunction testing: guidelines and controversies. New York: Academic Press; 1980.
Hardie JA, Buist AS, Vollmer WM, Ellingsen I, Bakke PS, Morkve O. Risk of over-diagnosis of COPD in asymptomatic elderly never-smokers. Eur Respir J. 2002;20:1117–22.
Levy ML, Quanjer PH, Booker R, Cooper BG, Holmes S, Small IR. Diagnostic spirometry in primary care: proposed standards for general practice compliant with ATS and ERS recommendations. Prim Care Respir J. 2009;18:130–47.
Vaz Fragoso CA, Concato J, McAvay G, Van Ness PH, Rochester CL, Yaggi HK, Gill TM. The ratio of FEV1 to FVC as a basis for establishing chronic obstructive pulmonary disease. Am J Respir Crit Care Med 2010; 181:446–451.
Turkeshi E, Vaes B, Andreva E, Mather C, et al. Airflow limitation by the global lungs initiative equations in a cohort of very old adults. Eur Respir J. 2015;46(1):123–32.
Vaz Fragoso CA, McAvay G, Van Ness PH, Casaburi R, Jensen RL, MacIntyre N, Gill TM, Yaggi HK, Concato J. Phenotype of normal spirometry in an aging population. Am J Respir Crit Care Med. 2015;192:817–25.
Jones RL, Nzekwu MMU. The effects of body mass index on lung volumes. Chest. 2006;130:827–33.
Bates JHT, Poynter ME, Frodella CM, Peters U, Dixon AE, Suratt BT. Pathophysiology to phenotype in the asthma of obesity. Ann Am Thorac Soc. 2017;14(Suppl 5):S395–8.
Wouters EFM. Obesity and metabolic abnormalities in chronic ObstructivePulmonary disease. Ann Am Thorac Soc. 2017;14(Suppl 5):S389–94.
Harik-Khan RI, Fleg JL, Muller DC, Wise RA. 2001. The effect of anthropometric and socioeconomic factors on the racial difference in lung function. Am J Respir Crit Care Med. 2001;164:1647–54.

Chapter 14
Management of and Quality Control in the Pulmonary Function Laboratory

Susan Blonshine, Jeffrey Haynes, and Katrina Hynes

14.1 Introduction

The importance of proper management of the PFL cannot be overstated. Poorly managed laboratories can be expected to report data collected from poorly maintained equipment and improperly conducted tests. Physicians may unknowingly draw the wrong conclusions, misdiagnose, and prescribe inappropriate therapy when furnished with spurious PFT data. The medical director of the PFL is responsible for ensuring that the laboratory is properly managed and must therefore be closely involved in the management of the laboratory. This chapter will review the key components of PFL management.

14.2 Pulmonary Function Laboratory Personnel

A PFL must function as a team. The team consists of three distinct components: medical director, management team, and technologists. The size of the laboratory will dictate the structure of each component. For example, a very large laboratory

S. Blonshine (✉)
TechEd Consultants, Inc., Mason, MI, USA
e-mail: sblonshine@techedconsultants.com

J. Haynes
Pulmonary Function Laboratory, St. Joseph Hospital, Nashua, NH, USA
e-mail: jhaynes3@comcast.net

K. Hynes
Pulmonary Function Laboratory, Mayo Clinic, Rochester, MN, USA
e-mail: Hynes.Katrina@mayo.edu

D. A. Kaminsky, C. G. Irvin (eds.), *Pulmonary Function Testing*,
Respiratory Medicine, https://doi.org/10.1007/978-3-319-94159-2_14

may require assistant medical directors and several management team members [e.g., manager, supervisor, chief technologist].

14.2.1 Medical Director

It is recommended that the medical director of the PFL be board certified in pulmonary medicine. The medical director should also have received specific training in the management of a PFL and PFT interpretation. However, a PFL internship for pulmonary medicine trainees is not universally required. In one study, pulmonologists who did not complete an internship in a PFT laboratory were found to have inferior PFT interpretation skills. In small hospitals, clinics, and office-based laboratories, a board-certified pulmonologist may not be available to serve as medical director. In this setting, a physician board certified in internal medicine with a strong interest in pulmonary function testing should be selected. Alternatively, an off-site pulmonologist may be recruited to serve as medical director.

The ideal medical director of a PFL is both competent and willing to provide supportive oversight and education for the rest of the team. Specific medical director responsibilities have been outlined by several societies. The responsibilities include the supervision and education of staff, providing oversight of policy and procedure documents, determining which tests will be offered, quality system management, and oversight of interpreting physicians. According to the 2005 ATS/ERS guidelines, the medical director must provide specific directives on test interpretation to provide ordering physicians with a consistent interpretation style. In most laboratories, due to time constraints, the medical director will need to delegate some of these duties to the laboratory management team (e.g., manager, supervisor, chief technologist) while providing oversight and functioning as the final decision-maker.

14.2.2 Management Team

As mentioned earlier, the structure of the management team is dependent on the size of the laboratory. In large laboratories, a multilayer bureaucracy may be necessary, while a small laboratory may only require a single person to serve as supervisor or chief technologist. The management component of the laboratory is vital to the success of the laboratory.

The ATS recommends that laboratory management personnel should have a bachelor's degree or higher in respiratory care or a healthcare-related field. In the United States, for PFLs which include a blood-gas laboratory (moderately complex laboratory), the Clinical Laboratory Improvement Amendments (CLIA) requires any individual serving as a technical consultant to the medical director to possess a bachelor's degree in laboratory science or medical technology (includes nursing and respiratory care). Four years of testing experience should be completed prior to filling a management position in which time a pulmonary function testing credential should be obtained. In North America, the National Board for Respiratory Care (NBRC) offers the certified pulmonary function technologist (CPFT) and the more advanced registered pulmonary function technologist (RPFT) credentials. The Australian and New Zealand Society of Respiratory Science (ANZSRS) offers the certified respiratory function scientist (CRFS) credential. In Great Britain, the Association for Respiratory Technology and Physiology (ARTP) offers a practitioner-level examination.

It must be recognized that being a competent and effective clinical technologist does not guarantee success as a member of the management team. Management team members must expand their knowledge beyond the clinical environment and learn the business-side of a PFL including leadership, budgeting, inventory management, regulatory compliance, data management, planning, quality systems, and human resource management.

14.2.3 Technologists

The skill and conscientiousness of the technologist is perhaps the most important long-term determinant of test quality. Many studies have shown that over 90% of patients can perform high-quality tests when properly coached by a knowledgeable and motivated technologist. A high level of scrutiny must be given to the applicant wishing to practice in the PFL since only a quality technologist can be relied upon to produce quality data. Studying for the credential exams listed above is an excellent educational opportunity, and passing the examination demonstrates job-specific aptitude. The ATS/ERS guidelines recommend, and the NBRC requires, that technologists complete a minimum of 2 years of college education with an emphasis on health-related sciences. In addition, the ATS/ERS guidelines recommend that technologists, "need to be familiar with the theory and practical aspects of all commonly applied techniques, measurements, calibrations, hygiene, quality control and other aspects of testing, as well as having a basic background knowledge in lung physiology and pathology."

Qualifications alone are unable to accurately predict future job performance. The aptitude and personality traits of technologists may also have an enormous impact on test quality and patient satisfaction. Indeed, standardized testing of aptitude, personality traits, and workplace behavior to identify the best candidates for hire is commonplace in the business world. While highly effective pulmonary function technologists often have a "type A" or "perfectionist" personality, there are no data specific to pulmonary function technologists from standardized personality testing currently available. However, there are at least three important measurable traits that a technologist should possess: high cognitive aptitude, conscientiousness, and critical thinking skills.

Cognitive aptitude, the ability to learn, is an important trait for pulmonary function technologists. However, while cognitive aptitude correlates well with transitional stages of work (learning new tasks), it does not predict good job performance in maintenance stages of work (repetitive completion of routine tasks). Pulmonary function testing can be clearly classified as a maintenance stage of work. Technologists in a busy laboratory perform the same basic tests (e.g., spirometry, diffusing capacity, lung volumes) hundreds of times per year. The personality trait that correlates best with job performance during maintenance stages of work is conscientiousness. Individuals with high conscientiousness scores are reliable, manage time well, set their own goals, and exhibit perseverance when faced with difficult tasks. Pulmonary function technologists must also possess critical thinking skills. Critical thinking skills allow for more efficient problem solving and the ability to make better clinical decisions. Pulmonary function technologists must be able to solve problems quickly and independently.

Appropriate orientation and training of new technologists is critically important to technologist and laboratory success. A structured checklist helps to ensure that all technologists receive the same information during orientation. Orientation is an excellent opportunity to promote practice uniformity and reduce technologist-related testing variability. Training time is generally dependent on a technologist's knowledge, experience, and aptitude. Familiarization with the pulmonary function equipment including calibration should precede patient testing. The laboratory management team should provide continuing education for the staff and promote a culture of continuous performance improvement.

One of the most powerful tools to achieve and maintain high-quality testing is a technologist performance monitoring and feedback program. Multiple studies in epidemiologic and clinical settings have shown that high-quality testing can be achieved and maintained when technologists are regularly given feedback on the quality of the tests they submit for interpretation. Figure 14.1 shows a marked improvement in spirometry test quality in a clinical laboratory after a technologist monitoring and feedback program was instituted.

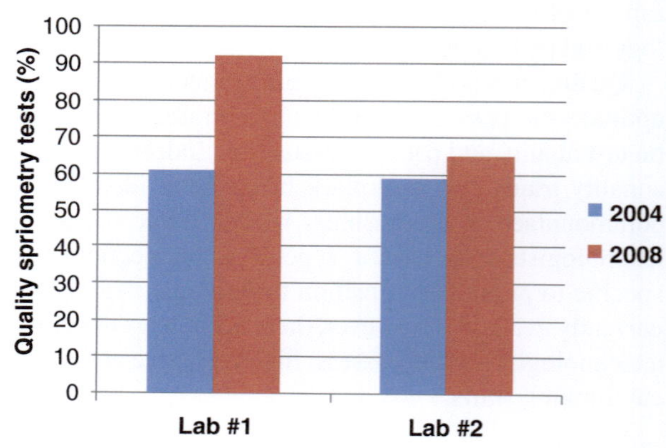

Fig. 14.1 The impact of technologist performance monitoring and feedback on test quality in an accredited PFT laboratory. Baseline data were collected in 2004. After the collection of baseline data, laboratory #1 instituted a technologist monitoring and feedback program and laboratory #2 served as the control. (Adapted from Borg et al. 2012)

14.3 The PFL Quality Management System

The Clinical and Laboratory Standards Institute (CLSI) developed a quality system approach for clinical laboratories that also applies to the PFL. The system includes 12 Quality System Essentials (QSEs) that provide a framework for a well-managed pulmonary laboratory that meets regulatory and accreditation standards. The QSEs include documents and records, organization, equipment, process management, personnel, purchasing and inventory, nonconforming event management, assessment (internal and external), continual improvement, customer focus, facilities and safety, and information management. In addition, the system includes a list of workflow activities for pretesting, testing, and posttesting that should be outlined for each testing method. The QSEs and path of workflow for each test method are included in the *ATS Pulmonary Function Laboratory Management and Procedure Manual.*

14.3.1 Equipment Selection and Installation

The equipment selected, installed, and used in each PFL has a significant impact on workflow processes, efficiency, and data integrity. Every QSE includes some component related to the equipment. The equipment selection and installation process should be outlined and documented for future reference. During the equipment selection process, it is helpful to develop a list of needs or requirements specific to the healthcare system or setting. The medical director and staff should be included in the process of determining the needs and capabilities of the laboratory. The requirements list may include items such as data management options, electronic medical record connectivity, available test methods, software updates, training, technical support, quality control (QC) software and statistical support, equipment maintenance support, reference equation availability, the ability to perform testing in accordance with ATS/ERS standards, the patient population (adult and/or pediatric), and ease-of-use. The frequency, cost, and ease of software updates are also important considerations. Historically, the life of system hardware is approximately 10 years. Consequently, an ill-advised PFT system purchase can impact the laboratory and the staff for an extended period of time. Inclusion of calibration and/or QC devices should also be considered in the selection of PFT equipment. A critical component of the equipment selection process is an on-site evaluation of the equipment by staff.

Once equipment is selected, the planning for installation and staff training should begin. The experience and skill of the technologists should be considered when planning training intensity and time required to achieve competency.

Steps for equipment installation include a biomedical evaluation, selection of reference equations appropriate for the patient population, specific decisions related to user-defined configuration files, report formatting, and a complete equipment quality control evaluation to include a system validation and verification process. Developing and maintaining an installation manual for each piece of equipment serves as a functionality and troubleshooting resource for current and future staff members. The installation manual should include pre- and post installation equipment validation records. The PFL should also maintain a record of all QC completed immediately after installation to serve as a benchmark for future assessments of equipment functionality. A printout of all user-defined files and the selected reference equations for the patient population tested is highly recommended. All reference equations selected need to be approved by the medical director and adhere to ATS/ERS standards. The Global Lung Function Initiative (GLI) all-age equations are recommended to avoid shifts in the predicted values as a patient ages (See Chapter 13). The placement of equipment, particularly a whole-body plethysmograph, in the laboratory space should be carefully considered since exposure to fluctuations in ambient gas flow and pressure can potentially impact the function of the equipment.

There is known variation in measured results between and within equipment manufacturers. For this reason, it is advisable to run the new equipment in parallel with the old equipment for at least 2 weeks to evaluate any changes in the biologic QC standards. The interpreting physicians need to be informed of any shifts in data related to the new equipment or software upgrade.

14.3.2 Quality Control Methods

The ATS/ERS has described minimal calibration and QC requirements for each test method. Calibration is defined as the process of configuring an instrument to provide a result within an acceptable range for a specific input. An example of a calibration check is directing 3 L of gas in and out of a spirometer with a calibration syringe. To pass the calibration check, the spirometer must report a value of 3 L ± 3.5% (2.9–3.1 L). QC is the process of monitoring both the precision and accuracy of the procedure. Precision or repeatability is the ability to get the same result when completing QC test methods. The two most common methods of QC include mechanical models and biologic standards. Table 14.1 describes the minimum ATS/ERS requirements for each test method as provided for the ATS Pulmonary Function Lab Accreditation Program. The QC program is essential to obtain valid reproducible results regardless of the specific test method and is a requirement for accreditation.

14.3.3 Equipment Quality Control: Mechanical Models or Control Material

Mechanical controls may include validated calibration syringes (e.g., 3 L, 7 L), isothermal lung analog, diffusion capacity of the lung for carbon monoxide (DL_{CO}) simulator, sine-wave rotary pump, computerized syringe, computer-driven syringe,

Table 14.1 Quality control requirements and recommendations

Test method	Biologic QC	Mechanical QC	Frequency
Spirometry	Monthly	Linearity check	Weekly
DLCO	Weekly	Syringe DLCO	Weekly
DLCO	NA	Gas analyzer linearity check (e.g., DLCO simulation or other syringe dilution method)	Quarterly
Plethysmography lung volumes	Monthly	Isothermal bottle	NA
Airway resistance	Monthly	NA	NA
Helium dilution	Monthly	NA	NA
Nitrogen washout	Monthly	NA	NA
Exercise with gas exchange	Monthly	NA	NA
Treadmill	NA	Check slope and speed	Monthly
Lung clearance index	Monthly	NA	NA

NA not applicable

and explosive decompression devices. Liquid control materials are used for blood-gas analyzers.

Calibration syringes should be validated at predetermined intervals by an outside source based on the manufacturer's recommendation and current ATS/ERS standards. Validation intervals may vary between 1 and 3 years. Calibration syringe validation should be performed if the syringe has been dropped and/or does not function properly. Monthly leak testing of calibration syringes is also required. The calibration syringe is used both for calibration of devices and QC procedures. For this reason, it is helpful to have at least two syringes to eliminate calibration syringe errors that may occur in the calibration procedure from influencing the QC measurements. The ATS/ERS standards require weekly linearity testing on the flow-based spirometers and a syringe DL_{CO} test on the DL_{CO} system. Both methods require a validated 3 L calibration syringe. An example of each is displayed in Figs. 14.2 and 14.3. The linearity check is completed by using a 3-L syringe at slow, medium, and fast flows, simulating a patient test. The volume measured should be the same regardless of the flow. In Fig. 14.2, the volume varies by 0.04 L. Typically, 0.09 L or less is considered acceptable.

The linearity of the DL_{CO} gas analyzers should be checked quarterly. The ATS/ERS DL_{CO} technical standards describe methods to verify analyzer linearity. A DL_{CO} simulator simulates patient testing and assesses the entire measurement system. The DL_{CO} simulator uses precision gases and a calibrated syringe to allow measurement of DL_{CO} across the measuring range expected in a patient population. The simulator can also be used to replace the weekly biologic QC. A DL_{CO} simulator is helpful to establish the source of an error or validate equipment on installation. Previous studies have found that DL_{CO} equipment problems were present in approximately 25% of the devices tested, and nearly all of the issues were resolved once identified. Potential problems with DL_{CO} systems include faulty demand valves, inaccurate medical gases, lack of regular maintenance, exhausted sample drying lines, electronics failures, and CO analyzer malfunction.

Fig. 14.2 Linearity check on flow-based spirometer

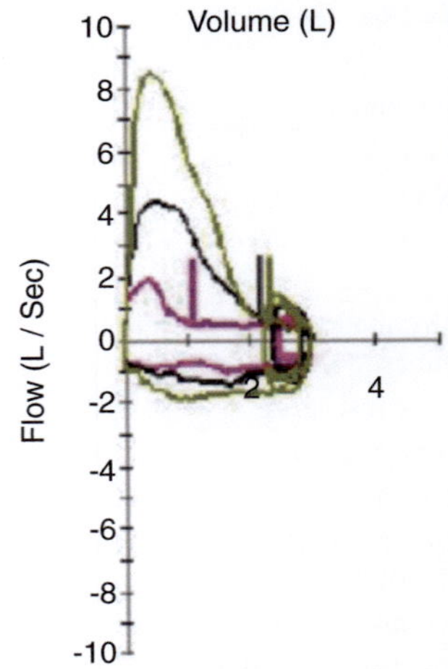

Volume measured (L)	Peak flow (L/sec)
3.01	8.44
3.03	4.32
2.99	1.92

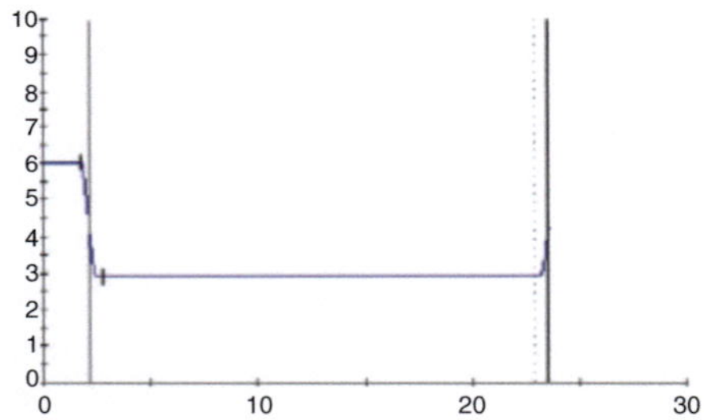

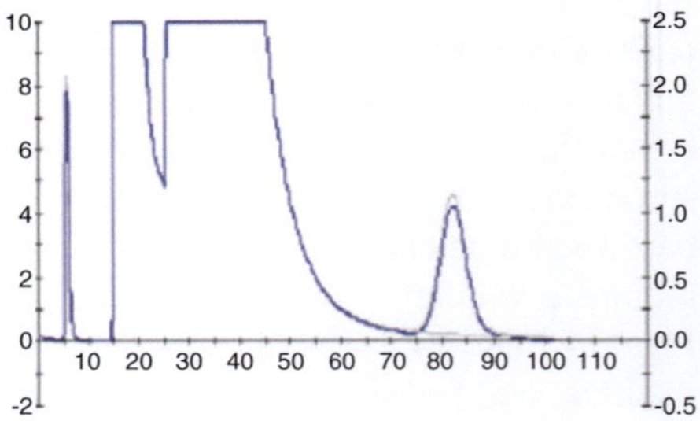

	Measured	Expected
DL_{co} (ml/min/mmHg)	0.30	<0.5 or <0.166 SI Units
IVC (L)	3.00	3.00
VA (L)	3.03	Within 300 ml of 3.00 L (Note the deadspace of the calibration syringe should also be included)

Fig. 14.3 Syringe DL_{CO} completed with 3-liter calibration syringe simulating a patient test. Volumes are converted to ATPS

An isothermal lung analog is used to verify the measured functional residual capacity (FRC) obtained from a body plethysmograph. An isothermal lung analog is an airtight device with a known volume, which is used to simulate the closed-shutter breathing performed by patients. Unfortunately, isothermal lung analogs are not easily available.

The CLSI document C46-A2 is the standard that outlines the QC program for blood-gas instruments. The goal of QC is to evaluate analyzer performance in terms of inaccuracy and imprecision. The CLSI document C24-A4 can be referenced for day-to-day QC guidance. There are two types of QC: surrogate and non-surrogate. A surrogate sample control, as described by CLSI, "is a stable liquid sample designed to simulate a patient sample and is analyzed the same as patient samples." Non-surrogate (alternative) QC refers to all other forms of QC. Blood-gas laboratories must follow governmental regulations for clinical laboratory medicine.

14.3.4 Equipment Quality Control: Biologic Standards

Biologic standards are included as a QC method for spirometry, DL_{CO}, lung volumes, and gas analysis with exercise. A biologic standard is a healthy subject who completes each required test according to the ATS/ERS standards. The data is collected using the same process as patient testing. After repeated measurement over time, longitudinal data is used as the standard for each individual. Control charts are used to monitor the mean, coefficient of variation (CV) and SD of the recorded data. An upper and lower limit is established using the 2 SD range and 95% confidence interval. Westgard rules may be applied to the data like clinical laboratory QC. Figure 14.4 is an example of a spreadsheet for initial biologic QC for spirometry and DL_{CO}. An example of a biologic QC control chart is displayed in (Fig. 14.5).

Date	Time	FEV1	FVC	DLCO	IVC	VA	SVC
10/1/17	17:00	2.52	3.08	22.81	2.97	3.98	3.08
10/2/17	17:13	2.6	3.19	21.42	3.02	3.99	3.31
10/3/17	16.57	2.53	3.04	21.45	2.83	3.8	3.11
10/6/17	17.00	2.48	3.03	23.7	2.96	3.92	3.03
10/8/17	17.28	2.46	3	21.19	2.8	3.69	3.1
10/10/17	13.04	2.51	3.05	22.51	2.85	3.84	3.06
10/14/17	16.48	2.49	2.93	21.79	2.77	3.76	3.04
10/15/17	18.15	2.58	3.2	22.49	2.97	3.95	3.25
10/16/17	18.08	2.6	3.15	22.25	2.89	3.89	3.14
10/17/18	16.34	2.53	3	22.85	2.83	3.85	3.12
Statistical Data							
Mean		2.53	3.07	22.25	2.89	3.87	3.11
Standard Deviation (SD)		0.05	0.09	0.79	0.08	0.1	0.1
2 SD		0.1	0.18	1.58	0.16	0.2	0.2
Coefficient of Variation		1.95	2.88	3.53	2.96	2.53	3.09
Acceptable Range Based on 2 SD							
Low Limit (-2 SD)		2.43	2.89	20.67	2.73	3.67	2.91
High Limit (+2 SD)		2.63	3.25	23.83	3.05	4.07	3.31

Fig. 14.4 Spreadsheet to develop biologic control ranges for spirometry and diffusing capacity

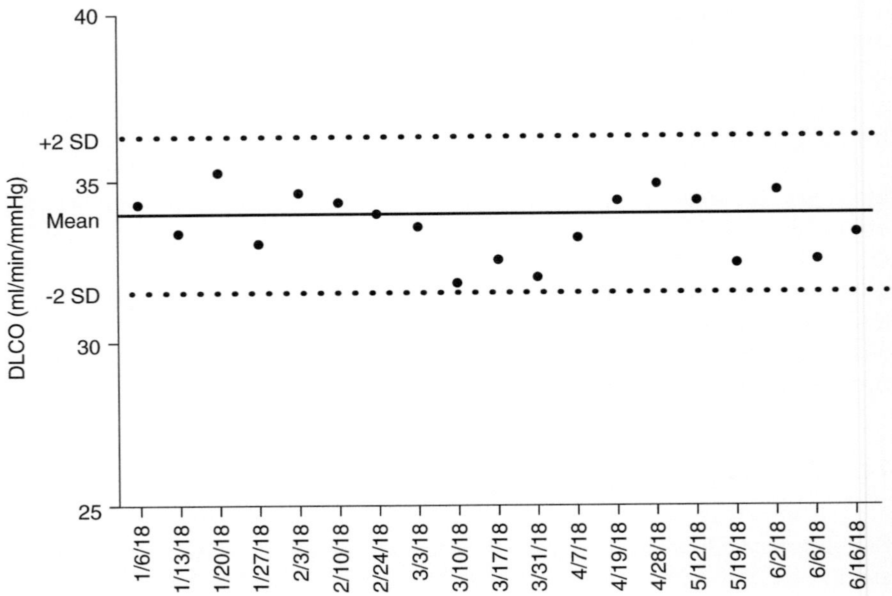

Fig. 14.5 Levey-Jennings plot of diffusing capacity values in a biologic control subject

Biologic testing for gas exchange with exercise is done on at least two workloads with a 50-watt difference and below the anaerobic threshold for the individual. An example for exercise with an ergometer may include 6 min of unloaded cycling, 6 min at 25 watts, and 6 min at 75 watts. The approximate expected oxygen uptake between 25 and 75 watts is 500 ml. Generally, five tests completed over a short period of time can be used to develop the initial mean and SD for minute ventilation ($\dot{V}E$), oxygen consumption ($\dot{V}O_2$), and carbon dioxide production ($\dot{V}CO_2$). Coefficient of variation values for $\dot{V}O_2$ should not differ by more than 5% and approximately 7% for $\dot{V}CO_2$ and $\dot{V}_E$ at the higher workload.

14.3.5 Quality Control Analysis

The analysis and process for out-of-control results for each method of QC collected should be established in a standard operating procedure document. The specific QC method is evaluated in relation to an expected standard for each test method. For example, the 2017 ERS/ATS DL_{CO} standard defines syringe simulation acceptability as a DL_{CO} less than 0.5 ml/min/mmHg or 0.667 SI and the alveolar volume (V_A) should be 3.0 ± 0.3 L. QC documents should be reviewed and signed by the medical director or designee.

14.3.6 *Additional Components of the Quality Management System Plan*

A laboratory's quality system plan should include equipment preventive maintenance (PM) and repair, technologist monitoring, and patient/provider surveys. Equipment maintenance can be documented in the system software or in a maintenance log. PM and corrective activities should be documented including the date, time, maintenance details, identified problems, steps taken to achieve problem resolution, and the attending technologist. Manufacturer recommendations should always be followed. Confirmation of acceptable equipment function following maintenance or repair is highly recommended with both mechanical and biologic QC methods.

14.3.7 *ATS PFL Registry and Accreditation*

The ATS supports a PFL registry for American and international laboratories. The ATS PFL registry is an inclusion and acknowledgment program for laboratories that complete the registry application and commit to following the ATS/ERS standards for lung function testing. Laboratories that have completed all required components of the registry process will receive a certificate that is valid for 5 years. The ATS PFL registry program is the first step toward PFL accreditation in the United States. The accreditation of PFLs has existed for many years in Australia, New Zealand, and several Canadian provinces. More recently, the United Kingdom, Netherlands, and United States have either initiated an accreditation program or are in the process of program development. Accreditation checklists for these programs can be accessed at the respective country or accreditation sponsor Internet site. An ATS accreditation checklist will soon be available as part of the registry process.

14.4 Equipment, Procedures, and Clinical Considerations in a PFL

The medical director and management team must decide which tests will be performed in a PFL. This decision should be dictated by clinical impact, provider demand, test complexity, cost, and the ability of the technologists to perform the tests correctly. Tests that have an important impact on the management of patients are typically in high demand by the practitioners that the PFL serves and therefore must be offered. Tests that are very expensive, difficult for the technologists and/or patients to perform correctly, infrequently ordered, and have questionable impact on patient care must undergo greater scrutiny. The medical director and management team must monitor the performance of the technologists to ensure that all testing regimens that are offered are performed in accordance with ATS/ERS and manufacturer recommendations.

14.4.1 Spirometry

Spirometry is considered the most basic lung function test and is performed using a flow or volume spirometer. Spirometry measures several key values including vital capacity (VC), forced vital capacity (FVC), forced expiratory volume in the first second (FEV_1), peak expiratory flow (PEF), and various derivatives (e.g., FEF_{25-75}). Spirometry is performed to identify the presence of lung disease, identify responsiveness to bronchodilators, and perform bronchoprovocation studies.

14.4.2 Lung Volumes

Lung volume testing determines functional residual capacity (FRC), total lung capacity (TLC), and residual volumes (RV). While the clinical utility of routine lung volume testing has been questioned, lung volume determination can distinguish between obstructive and restrictive disease, reveal air trapping, and identify patients with the non-specific pattern (normal TLC, restriction on spirometry). There are three common tests used to measure lung volumes: body plethysmography, helium dilution, and nitrogen washout.

Plethysmography is considered by many to be the ideal method because it can account for trapped gas, can be repeated without delay, and allows for the measurement of airway resistance. However, many laboratories will offer more than one method of lung volume testing for patients who cannot perform plethysmography correctly or experience claustrophobia with the cabin door closed. In addition, nitrogen washout also allows the measurement of lung clearance index.

14.4.3 Diffusing Capacity DL_{CO}

DL_{CO} [also described as transfer factor (TL_{CO})], is a very important PFT. DL_{CO} is affected by several factors including lung volume, alveolar surface area, alveolar capillary membrane thickness, cardiac output, hemoglobin and carboxyhemoglobin concentration, alveolar oxygen pressure, and ventilation-perfusion matching. Although there are several methods to measure the uptake of CO from the lungs, the single-breath technique is the most widespread methodology used. DL_{CO} can differentiate between different types of obstructive lung disease; evaluate cardiovascular diseases such as primary pulmonary hypertension; evaluate parenchymal lung disease, pulmonary involvement in systemic diseases, and pulmonary toxicity; and be followed longitudinally.

Another method to assess pulmonary diffusion is the diffusing capacity of the lung for nitric oxide (DL_{NO}). While DL_{NO} possesses technical advantages when compared to DL_{CO} (e.g., not clinically affected by hemoglobin, carboxyhemoglobin, or alveolar oxygen pressure), it is less widely used and more expensive.

14.4.4 Respiratory Muscle Strength

The ability to measure respiratory muscle strength can play an important role in the diagnosis and management of patients with neuromuscular disease. Most PFT systems will include maximum inspiratory and expiratory pressure (PImax, PEmax) testing. Other common tests of respiratory muscle strength include sniff nasal inspiratory pressure, cough peak flow, supine VC, and maximum voluntary ventilation.

14.4.5 Forced Oscillation Technique (FOT)

The forced oscillation technique (FOT), of which one approach is impulse oscillometry (IOS), is a noninvasive passive breathing methodology that uses small impulses of flow, which are transmitted toward the respiratory system. The pressure produced by the flow impulses is used to calculate resistance and reactance. FOT can be very useful in children and other patients with cognitive or physical impairments who are unable to perform spirometry testing. FOT has been recognized as a more sensitive test in identifying and quantifying obstructive airways disease and can be used for bronchial challenge testing. FOT has limitations including performance differences between devices and limited reference equations.

14.4.6 Interrupter Technique

The interrupter technique (R_{int}) measures airway resistance by occluding airflow at the mouth for 100 ms. During the cessation of airflow, mouth pressure is sampled (proxy for alveolar pressure) and is compared to flow to generate a resistance value. R_{int} shares many of the advantages and disadvantage of FOT, it is easy for patients to perform, but is less robust than spirometry.

14.4.7 Bronchoprovocation Testing

Bronchoprovocation testing determines the presence or absence of airway hyperresponsiveness, which can aid in the diagnosis of patients with an intermediate pretest probability of asthma. In addition, bronchoprovocation tests can be used to rule out asthma in specific situations (e.g., clearance for military service). Bronchoprovocation tests can act directly or indirectly on airway smooth muscle. Methacholine inhalation can produce bronchoconstriction by acting directly on airway smooth muscle. Mannitol, exercise, cold air, and eucapnic voluntary hyperventilation are examples of indirect challenges. It is probably advantageous for laboratories to offer both a direct and one or more indirect tests since patients have different sensitivity profiles. All bronchoprovocation tests require high-quality spirometry to distinguish true physiologic responses from changes in spirometry technique. Technologists who are still developing spirometry skills should be supervised when performing bronchoprovocation testing. Exercise bronchoprovocation testing requires the technologists to have experience with performing exercise testing and be certified in basic cardiac life support.

14.4.8 Cardiopulmonary Exercise Testing

Cardiopulmonary exercise testing (CPET) involves physically stressing the heart, lungs, and circulatory system, to simultaneously evaluate the cardiovascular, ventilatory, and cellular systems. The test involves the use of an exercise device such as a cycle ergometer, treadmill, or arm ergometer (for those with limb limitations) to achieve maximum exercise capacity. The metabolic system measures flow, volume, and gas analysis. These measurements allow for the integration and calculations of metabolic demand during exercise, as well as the characterization of ventilatory kinetics and flow limitation. CPET requires highly skilled technologists who understand exercise physiology, cardiac function including electrocardiogram interpretation, exercise protocols, and the setup and maintenance of the testing system. The laboratory offering CPET must perform tests frequently to maintain technologist and physician proficiency.

14.4.9 Metabolic Studies

Systems used to measure the metabolic characteristics during exercise also have the ability to determine resting energy expenditure (REE). Indirect calorimetry allows for the estimation of caloric needs by substrate to manage nutritional demands. There are two testing methodologies used, open-circuit and closed-circuit calorimetry. The open circuit is most commonly used in the outpatient clinical practice.

14.4.10 Field Walking Tests

Field walking tests are performed to assess functional capacity in patients with chronic respiratory disease. There are three types of field walking tests: 6-min walk tests (6MWT), incremental shuttle walk test (ISWT), and endurance shuttle walk test (ESWT). The 6MWT is performed in an unfixed track with a minimum length of 30 m. Both the ISWT and ESWT are performed using fixed tracks 10 m in length with two cones inset 0.5 m from each end. The ERS/ATS has outlined the universal equipment required for all field exercise tests. It is important that the laboratory and technologists closely follow the ERS/ATS recommendations (including patient instructions) because inconsistencies in the test procedure can affect the test results. It is also important to make a distinction between a field walking test and an oxygen titration study.

14.4.11 *Arterial Blood-Gas Analysis*

Arterial blood-gas (ABG) analysis is an invasive test performed to evaluate oxygenation, ventilation, and acid-base status. If the blood-gas analyzer contains a hemoximeter, hemoglobin, oxyhemoglobin, carboxyhemoglobin, and methemoglobin can also be measured. Hemoglobin and carboxyhemoglobin can be used to adjust DL_{CO}. ABG analysis is more accurate than pulse oximetry and can be used during exercise testing. ABG data can also be used to calculate intrapulmonary shunt and perform high-altitude simulation tests (HAST). Managing a blood-gas laboratory requires a sophisticated and meticulously executed QMS program.

14.4.12 *Billing and Reimbursement Practices*

Billing and reimbursement practices for pulmonary diagnostic testing are diverse and depend on a country's private or government payer practices. In the United States, current procedural terminology (CPT) codes are used as a standardized methodology to describe the procedures that are billed. Many privately funded organizations have a fee-for-service payment structure, whereas a public healthcare organization might receive payment for the procedures performed from the government-funded health insurance program. Regardless of the billing and payer process, the laboratory should have a methodology of verifying correct billing codes or processes to ensure accurate charges have been entered into the billing system.

14.4.13 *Appointment Scheduling*

The appointment scheduling process should be carefully considered and clearly defined in a workflow document. Efficient scheduling and testing of patients improve laboratory productivity and patient satisfaction. Absenteeism is reduced when patients are given a reminder (e.g., telephone call or paper appointment notification) of their test date and time. Patients should be provided with pretest instructions giving them guidance on how to prepare for their test (e.g. proper attire, fasting, medication use, etc.). The time allotted for patient testing should provide the technologist with enough time to capture acceptable and repeatable data according to ATS/ERS technical standards. Specific policies in accordance with government and health system regulations should be in place to protect patient privacy before, during, and after testing.

14.4.14 *Report Formatting*

The quality and content of test reports can have a substantial impact on test interpretation. Demographic data such as name, numeric identifiers, date of birth, age, sex, race, height, and weight must be included. The calibration date, test indication, ordering physician, technologist, and reference equations should also be included in the report header. PFT indices that do not aid in test interpretation should not be included in the report. Each reported index should include the following: measured value, reference mean (predicted), reference range, percent of mean, and z-score (see Fig. 14.6). Flow-volume loops and time/volume graphs should be included in the report. Longitudinal data should also be available for the interpreter. The laboratory should avoid having multiple reports for the same test to promote uniformity. Laboratories should follow the recommendations for standardizing the reporting of PFTs published by the American Thoracic Society.

14.4.15 *Infection Control*

Infection control and prevention protects patients and staff from infectious microorganisms. Infection control begins with handwashing hygiene and personal protective equipment use. Mouthpieces, nose clips, and filters should be not be reused. Flow sensors should be disinfected according to the manufacturer's recommendations. The use of filters does not eliminate the need for regular cleaning and disinfection of the PFT system. Patients with active tuberculosis or other airborne infectious

Name: **Anonymous Doe** MRN: ****** Sex: **F** DOB:**10/29/1945** Age:**71** Race: **W**
Height: **67 in** Weight: **287 lb** BMI: **45.0** Diagnosis: **Pulmonary fibrosis, unspecified**
Room: **OP** Acct#: **********
Tech: [redacted] Attending: **Pulmonary** Referring: [redacted]

ATS/ERS compliant tests earn a ✔ : Spiro ✔ DLCO ✔ LV/Raw ✔ Predicteds: Spiro GLI 2012, DLCO Cotes, LV Quanjer

Spirometry (BTPS)			**Pre Bronchodilator**					**Post Bronchodilator**			
		Actual	Range		Predicted	% Pred	Z-score	Actual	% Pred	% Change	Z-score
StartTime		13.25	----	----	----	----	----	13.57	----	--	----
FVC	L	1.64	2.24	3.95	3.09	53	-2.87	1.67	54	2	-2.81
FEV_1	L	1.45	1.72	3.03	2.37	61	-2.29	1.52	64	5	-2.12
FEV_1 / FVC	%	88	64	91	78	113	1.48	91	117	3	1.93

Fig. 14.6 Pulmonary function report header and data presentation

diseases should be tested in a negative-pressure room. Isolation precautions and personal protective equipment (e.g. N-95 mask) should be worn by testing personnel.

14.5 Summary

Several key components of a PFL aligned with ATS/ERS standards and quality systems have been reviewed. The personnel and medical direction are key factors in all laboratories. Selection of equipment, installation, and quality control ensure equipment functionality. Answering the clinical question asked of testing occurs through the availability, selection, and interpretation of the appropriate PFTs. Ensuring data integrity and patient safety is at the core of all well-managed PFLs. The goal is data that is accurate and precise for clinical decision-making.

14.5.1 Illustrative Cases

Case #1

An 18-year-old female with chronic asthma undergoes annual spirometry testing. Recently the patient became compliant with inhaled corticosteroid therapy. As a consequence, her asthma control test improved and her FE_{NO} declined from 65 ppb to 35 ppb. However, at the same time, the patient's FEV_1 declined from 80% of predicted last year to 75% of predicted. The interpreting physician verifies that both tests were performed correctly and that the spirometer passed the calibration verification testing prior to both tests. The interpreting physician notices that the decline in the FEV_1 percent of predicted is accompanied by a 300 ml increase in the absolute value.

The discordance between the absolute FEV_1 value and the percent of predicted in this patient was the result of noncontinuous reference equations. The spirometer was programmed to use the Zapletal reference equations for children and adolescents. However, when the patient turned 18 years old, the reference equation changed to Quanjer (1993). This phenomenon has been called the "switching and stitching together of reference equations" which can cause significant shifts in the predicted value. In this patient, the predicted FEV_1 jumped from 2.5 L (Zapletal) at age 17 to 3.07 L (Quanjer 1993) at age 18 resulting in a lower percent of predicted despite an increase in the absolute value. Using all-age reference equations for PFTs eliminates the "switching and stitching" problem. For example, in this patient, using the all-age GLI equations (age 3–95 years) for spirometry would have reported an FEV_1 percent of predicted of 67% based on a predicted value of 2.98 L at age 17 and a percent of predicted of 77% based on a predicted value of 3.00 L at age 18. Using the GLI equations for this patient would have accurately reflected the improvement in lung function and asthma control.

Case #2

Weekly syringe DL_{CO} simulation testing was completed at PFL. Environmental conditions on the day of testing were as follows: temperature 24 degrees C, barometric pressure 759 mmHg, and humidity 50%. Calibration of the device was completed and acceptable. Table 14.2 lists the results obtained while performing a weekly syringe DL_{CO} with a 3-liter syringe.

In this case, the absolute DL_{CO} is acceptable. The inspired volume (V_I) is acceptable on both trials. However the V_A is increased and unacceptable. V_A is equal to the V_I times the change in expired tracer gas. Because the V_I is acceptable, the elevated V_A is due to either increased mechanical dead space or an inaccurate measurement of the tracer gas. The system dead space including filter dead space is entered into the DL_{CO} system software on installation and generally is not changed. The technologist was asked to review the technique used and evaluate any deviation from the written procedure or potential equipment problems. The gas analyzer was found to be linear and within an acceptable range likely ruling out the possibility of an inaccurate measurement of the tracer gas. The technologist disclosed that she added large bore tubing between the mouthpiece and the calibration syringe to perform the procedure. Once the tubing was removed and the DL_{CO} simulation was repeated, the V_A was acceptable. The written procedure was updated to clarify the correct connections for the procedure and the technologist received additional training. This case study emphasizes two different issues. Not all QC failures are related to equipment, and QC procedures must be clearly explained in a standard operating procedure document.

Case #3

A 31-year-old female presented to her physician complaining of a cough, throat tightness, and episodic shortness of breath following an upper respiratory illness. The patient denied wheezing. Physical exam was normal other than obesity (body mass index 38). A chest radiograph, spirometry, and DL_{CO} were ordered. The PFT results are displayed in Table 14.3 and Fig. 14.7.

Table 14.2 Results from a DL_{CO} simulation test

	Trial #1	Trial #2	Expected values
DL_{CO} (ml/min/mmHg) STPD	0.2	0.1	<0.5 ml/min/mmHg or 0.166 SI units
VI (L) BTPS	3.35	3.33	3.08–3.40
VA (L) BTPS	4.42	4.36	3.11–3.70

Table 14.3 Pulmonary function test #1

	Pre	Post	Predicted	% Predicted
FVC	2.10	2.11	3.42	61%
FEV1	0.89	1.36	2.90	31%
FEV1/FVC %	42.4	64.5		
DLCO		8.0	23.6	34%

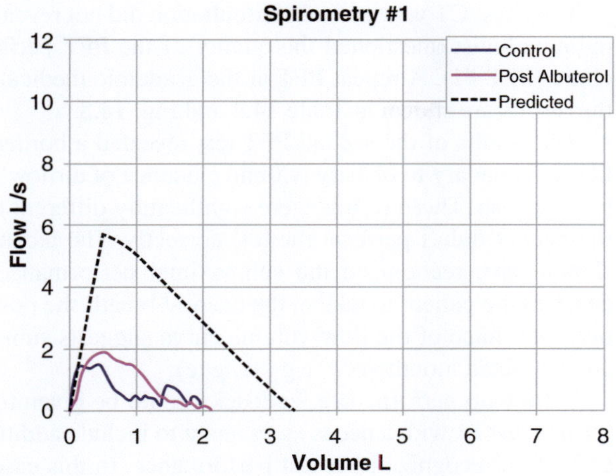

Fig. 14.7 Flow-volume loop recorded in a patient complaining of cough, throat tightness, and shortness of breath

Table 14.4 Pulmonary function test #2

	Pre	Post	Predicted	% Predicted
FVC	2.55	2.48	3.42	75%
FEV1	2.27	2.25	2.90	78%
FEV1/FVC %	89	90.7		
DLCO		24.2	23.6	103%

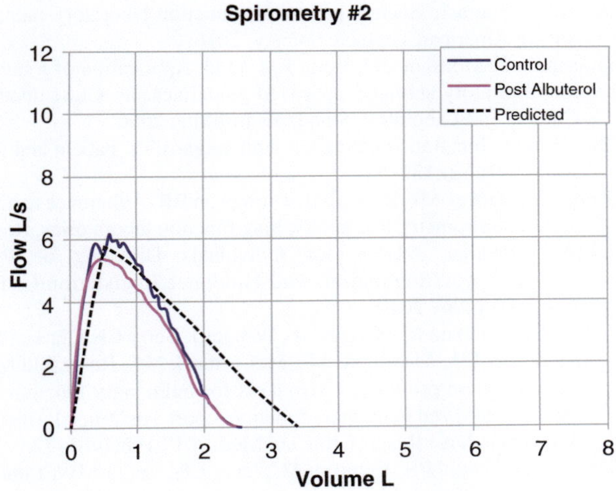

Fig. 14.8 Repeat flow-volume loop recorded in a patient complaining of cough, throat tightness, and shortness of breath

The chest radiograph was normal. The PFT was interpreted as showing severe obstruction with some bronchodilator responsiveness. The DL_{CO} was severely reduced. In response, the physician ordered a computed tomography (CT) scan of the chest and referred the patient to a pulmonologist at an academic medical center for further evaluation.

The chest CT was normal. Auscultation did not reveal wheezing in the chest. The pulmonologist questioned the quality of the PFT performed at the patient's local clinic (PFT #1). A repeat PFT at the academic medical center's PFL was ordered; the results are shown in Table 14.4 and Fig. 14.8.

The results of the second PFT test revealed a borderline restrictive defect most likely secondary to obesity with no evidence of airflow obstruction or bronchodilator response. These results were significantly different than test #1 simply because the patient didn't perform the test correctly. The technologist performing the test should have recognized the submaximal performance with each maneuver and coached the patient to take in the deepest breath she possibly could before exhaling out. The shape of the flow-volume curve suggests submaximal effort and possibly an obstructed mouthpiece (e.g., tongue)

Follow-up performance feedback should be given to the technologist who performed test #1 with a needs assessment to include additional education and training on how to recognize poor test performance. In this case scenario, the technologist and physician failed to recognize poor-quality test performance, which resulted in unnecessary diagnostic testing. Weight is an important measurement to obtain prior to testing. Although weight should not affect the predicted values, it can affect how the test is interpreted.

Selected References

American Thoracic Society pulmonary function laboratory management and procedure manual. 3rd ed: American Thoracic Society; 2016.

Blonshine S, Mottram CD, Berte LM, et al. Application of a quality management system model for respiratory services: approved guidelines. In: CLSI document HS4-A2. 2nd ed. Wayne: Clinical and Laboratory Standards Institute; 2006.

Blonshine S. Integrating education with diagnostics, patient and technologist. Respir Care Clin N Am. 1997;3(2):139–54.

Borg BM, Hartley MF, Bailey MJ, Thompson BR. Adherence to acceptability and repeatability criteria for spirometry in complex lung function laboratories. Respir Care. 2012;57(12):2032–8.

CLIA Personnel Policies for Individuals Directing or Performing Non-waived Tests. www.cms.gov/Regulations-and-Guidance/Legislation/CLIA/Downloads/PSV-FAQs.pdf. Accessed 1 Nov 2017.

Culver BH, Graham BL, Coates AL, Wanger J, Berry CE, Clarke PK, Hallstrand TS, Hankinson JL, Kaminsky DA, MacIntyre NR, McCormack MC, Rosenfeld M, Stanojevic S, Weiner DJ. ATS Committee on proficiency standards for pulmonary function laboratories. Recommendations for a standardized pulmonary function report. An Official American Thoracic Society Technical Statement. Am J Respir Crit Care Med. 2017;196:1463–72.

Dweik RA, Boggs PB, Erzurum SC, Irvin CG, Leigh MW, Lundberg JO, et al. An official ATS clinical practice guideline: interpretation of exhaled nitric oxide levels (FENO) for clinical applications. Am J Respir Crit Care Med. 2011;184(5):602–15.

Graham BL, Brusasco VB, Burgos F, Cooper BG, Jensen R, Kendrick A, et al. ERS/ATS standards for single-breath carbon monoxide uptake in the lung. Eur Respir J. 2017;49(1):2017.

Haynes JM, Sweeney EL. The effect of telephone appointment-reminder calls on outpatient absenteeism in a pulmonary function laboratory. Respir Care. 2006;51(1):36–9.

Haynes JM. Quality assurance of the pulmonary function technologist. Respir Care. 2012;57(1):114–22.

Holland AE, Spruit MA, Troosters T, Puhan MA, Pepin V, Saey D, et al. An official European Respiratory Society/American Thoracic Society technical standard: field walking tests in chronic respiratory disease. Eur Respir J. 2014;44:1428–46.

HS4-A2. Application of a quality system model for respiratory services, approved guideline. Wayne: Clinical Laboratory Standards Institute; 2006.

Jensen R, Leyk M, Crapo R, Muchmore D, Berclaz PY. Quality control of DLCO instruments in global clinical trials. Eur Respir J. 2009;33(4):828–34.

Kirkby J, Aurora P, Spencer H, Rees S, Sonnappa S, Stocks J. Stitching and switching: the impact of discontinuous lung function reference equations. Eur Respir J. 2012;39(5):1256–57.

Miller MR, Crapo R, Hankinson J, Brusasco V, Burgos F, Casaburi R, et al. General considerations for lung function testing. Eur Respir J. 2005a;26(1):153–61.

Miller MR, Crapo R, Hankinson J, Brusasco V, Burgos F, Casaburi R, et al. General considerations for lung function testing. Eur Respir J. 2005b;26(1):153–61.

Miller MR, Hankinson J, Brusasco V, Burgos F, Cassaburi R, Coates A, et al. Standardisation of spirometry. Eur Respir J. 2005c;26(2):319–38.

Mottram CD. Pulmonary function testing equipment. In: Mottram CD, editor. Ruppel's manual of pulmonary function testing. 11th ed. St. Louis: Elsevier; 2018. p. 363–414.

Oostveen E, MacLeod D, Lorino H, Farré R, Hantos Z, Desager K, Marchal F. ERS task force on respiratory impedance measurements. The forced oscillation technique in clinical practice: methodology, recommendations and future developments. Eur Respir J. 2003;22(6):1026–41.

Patout M, Sesé L, Gille T, Coiffard B, Korzeniewski S, Lhuillier E, et al. Does training respiratory physicians in clinical respiratory physiology and interpretation of pulmonary function testing improve core knowledge? Thorax. 2018;73:78–81.

Porszasz J, Blonshine S, Cao R, Paden HA, Casaburi R, Rossiter HB. Biological quality control for cardiopulmonary exercise testing in multicenter clinical trials. BMC Pulm Med. 2016;16:13.

Quanjer PH, Tammeling GJ, Cotes JE, Pedersen OF, Peslin R, Yernault JC. Lung volumes and forced ventilatory flows. Eur Respir J. 1993;6 Suppl 16:5–40.

Quality management system: a model for laboratory services, Approved guideline. CLSI document 4. Wayne: Clinical Laboratory Standards Institute; 2011.

Quanjer PH, Stanojevic S, Cole TJ, Baur X, Hall GL, Culver BH, et al. Multi-ethnic reference values for spirometry for the 3-95-yr age range: the global lung function 2012 equations. Eur Respir J. 2012;40(6):1324–43.

Wanger J, Clausen JL, Coates A, Pedersen OF, Brusasco V, Burgos F, et al. Standardisation of the measurement of lung volumes. Eur Respir J. 2005;26(3):511–22.

Zavorsky GS, Hsia CC, Hughes JM, Borland CD, Guénard H, van der Lee I, et al. Standardisation and application of the single-breath determination of nitric oxide uptake in the lung. Eur Respir J. 2017;49(2):1600962.

Index

D. A. Kaminsky, C. G. Irvin (eds.), *Pulmonary Function Testing*, Respiratory Medicine, https://doi.org/10.1007/978-3-319-94159-2

MIX
Papier aus verantwortungsvollen Quellen
Paper from responsible sources
FSC® C105338

If you have any concerns about our products,
you can contact us on
ProductSafety@springernature.com

In case Publisher is established outside the EU,
the EU authorized representative is:
Springer Nature Customer Service Center GmbH
Europaplatz 3, 69115 Heidelberg, Germany

Printed by Libri Plureos GmbH
in Hamburg, Germany